Musculoskeletal Ultrasound in Orthopedic and Rheumatic disease in Adults

Fabio Martino • Enzo Silvestri
Davide Orlandi
Editors

Musculoskeletal Ultrasound in Orthopedic and Rheumatic disease in Adults

Springer

Editors
Fabio Martino
Radiology
Sant'Agata Diagnostic Center
Bari, Italy

Enzo Silvestri
Radiology
Alliance Medical
Genova, Genova, Italy

Davide Orlandi
Department of Radiology
Ospedale Evangelico Internazionale
Genova, Genova, Italy

ISBN 978-3-030-91201-7 ISBN 978-3-030-91202-4 (eBook)
https://doi.org/10.1007/978-3-030-91202-4

This Springer imprint is published by the registered company Springer Nature Switzerland AG
The registered company address is: Gewerbestrasse 11, 6330 Cham, Switzerland

Foreword

It is my great honor to write a preface for the book of my dear friends Martino, Silvestri, and Orlandi.

Some may think that in 2021, a text on ultrasonography might be no longer necessary. Having read the book, I must say that I am, on the contrary, deeply convinced that it is extremely relevant and useful.

The combination of images and diagrams, both anatomical and pathological, allows for a clear understanding of even the most complicated anatomy and the most sophisticated semiotics and eases the comprehension of the elements, which lead to a clear differential diagnosis among different pathologies.

This text addresses with great didactic ability the various diagnostic challenges and most importantly has a very contemporary conception and efficient chapter organization; moreover, the presence of illustrative didactic diagrams is highly effective.

The goal, in my opinion, has been fully achieved.

On top of everything already said, I must add that the three editors possess great experience and unquestionable knowledge and come from an Italian school, which across the years has engaged with the orthopedic, rheumatologic, and surgical worlds in extremely high-level international settings.

The confrontation and exchange with other specialists emerge clearly in the way the diagnostic challenges are approached from a clinical point of view, keeping a watchful eye on the subsequent therapeutical options.

In this text, ultrasonography is not only dignified but also raised to an exceptionally high level, comparable in its specificity to that of other diagnostic methods.

In conclusion, I would like to thank my friends for the effort they have made, whose outcome is a book of absolute value that will remain among the "important" ones.

Carlo Masciocchi
Direttore della U.O.C. di Radiologia universitaria
del P.O. San Salvatore della suddetta ASL e della
U.O. di Radioterapia dell'Ospedale San Salvatore dell'Aquila,
L'Aquila, Italy

Contents

Contributors

Alberto Aliprandi Responsabile Servizio di Radiologia, Istituti Clinici Zucchi, Monza (MB), Italy

Gian Nicola Bisciotti Kinemove Rehabilitation Centers, Pontremoli (SP), Italy

Davide Bizzoca Orthopedic & Trauma Unit, Department of Basic Medical Sciences, Neuroscience and Sense Organs, University of Bari "Aldo Moro", AOU Consorziale "Policlinico", Bari, Italy

Marco Di Carlo Clinica Reumatologica, Dipartimento di Scienze Cliniche e Molecolari, Università Politecnica delle Marche, Jesi (Ancona), Italy

Marina Carotti Clinica di Radiologia, Dipartimento di Scienze Radiologiche – Azienda Ospedali Riuniti di Ancona Universita' Politecnica delle Marche, Ancona, Italy

Luca Cavagnaro Ortopedia e Traumatologia 2- Joint Replacement, Unit/ Bone Infection Unit, Ospedale Santa Corona, Pietra Ligure (SV), Italy

Matteo De Cesari Department of Radiology, Ospedali del Tigullio, Lavagna, Italy

Edoardo Cipolletta Clinica Reumatologica, Dipartimento di Scienze Cliniche e Molecolari, Università Politecnica delle Marche, Jesi (Ancona), Italy

Carlo Faletti Direttore tecnico Radiodiagnostica Centro Diagnostico Cernaia, Asti Direttore scientifico Master MSK di II livello, Università degli studi di Torino, Turin, Italy

Massimo De Filippo Director of Diagnostic an Interventional Unit, Azienda Ospedaliero-Universitaria di Parma, Parma, Italy

Professor of Radiology, Department of Medicine and Surgery, University of Parma, Parma, Italy

Emilio Filippucci Clinica Reumatologica, Dipartimento di Scienze Cliniche e Molecolari, Università Politecnica delle Marche, Jesi (Ancona), Italy

Salvatore Guarino Department of Radiology, Monaldi Hospital, AORN Ospedali dei Colli, Naples, Italy

Armanda De Marchi Radiologia CIDIMU: Centro Italiano di Diagnostica Medica Ultrasonica, Torino, Italy

Department of Imaging, Azienda Ospedaliera Città della Salute e della Scienza, CTO Hospital, Torino, Italy

Fabio Martino Radiology, Sant'Agata Diagnostic Center, Bari, Italy

Radiologist Diagnostic an Interventional Unit, Azienda Ospedaliero-Universitaria di Parma, Parma, Italy

Gianluigi Martino Institute of Radiology, University of Bari, Bari, Italy

Elena Massone Postgraduate School of Radiology, Genoa University, Genova, Italy

Department of Radiology, Ospedale Santa Corona, Pietra Ligure (SV), Italy

Biagio Moretti Orthopedic & Trauma Unit, Department of Basic Medical Sciences, Neuroscience and Sense Organs, University of Bari "Aldo Moro", AOU Consorziale "Policlinico", Bari, Italy

Lorenzo Moretti Orthopedic & Trauma Unit, Department of Basic Medical Sciences, Neuroscience and Sense Organs, University of Bari "Aldo Moro", AOU Consorziale "Policlinico", Bari, Italy

Alessandro Muda Department of Radiology, IRCCS Policlinico San Martino-IST, Genova, Italy

Davide Orlandi Radiology, Alliance Medical, Genova, Italy

Department of Radiology, Ospedale Evangelico Internazionale, Genova, Italy

Radiology Unit, Ospedale Evangelico Internazionale, Genova, Italy

Department of Diagnostic Imaging, Ospedale Evangelico Internazionale, Genova, Italy

Ernesto La Paglia Department of Radiology, Humanitas Cellini, Torino, Italy

Francesco Pagnini Radiologist, Diagnostic an Interventional Unit, Azienda Ospedaliero-Universitaria di Parma, Parma, Italy

Giulio Pasta Specialista in Radiologia e Diagnostica per Immagini, Studio Associato di Radiologia Dr. Pasta, Emilia-Romagna, Italy

Francesco Di Pietto Dipartimento di Diagnostica per Immagini "Pineta Grande Hospital", Castel Volturno, Italy

Giovanni Rusconi Dipartimento di Diagnostica per Immagini "Pineta Grande Hospital", Castel Volturno (CE), Italy

Fausto Salaffi Clinica Reumatologica, Dipartimento di Scienze Cliniche e Molecolari, Università Politecnica delle Marche, Jesi (Ancona), Italy

Giuseppe Sepolvere Department of Anesthesia and Cardiac Surgery Intensive Care Unit, San Michele Hospital, Maddaloni, Italy

Enzo Silvestri Radiology, Alliance Medical, Genova, Italy

Mario Tedesco Department of Anesthesia and Intensive Care Unit and Pain Therapy, Mater Dei Hospital, Bari, Italy

Umberto Viglino Postgraduate School of Radiology, Genoa University, Genova, Italy

Piero Volpi IRCCS Humanitas Research Hospital, Milano, Italy

Marcello Zappia Musculoskeletal Radiology Unit, Istituto Diagnostico Varelli, Napoli, Italy

Dipartimento di Medicina e Scienze della Salute, Università degli Studi del Molise (CB), Campobasso, Italy

Part I

Sonographic Semiology in Musculoskeletal Pathologic Involvement

Osseous and Cartilaginous Surface

1

Enzo Silvestri, Davide Orlandi,
and Elena Massone

Contents

1.1 Sonographic and Doppler Normal Anatomy

1.1.1 Cartilage

Cartilage is a greatly specialized type of flexible, semitransparent, and elastic, connective tissue, mainly composed of water (70–80% by wet weight). It is avascular and aneural.

This tissue is formed by cartilage cells scattered through a glycoprotein material that is strengthened by collagen fibers.

In the musculoskeletal system there are two types of cartilage: *hyaline* and *fibrocartilage*.

Fibrocartilage (also called *white cartilage*) is a specialized type of cartilage that contains more collagen and is more resistant at tensile strength. It is found in areas requiring tough support or great tensile strength, such as between intervertebral disk, at the pubic and other symphyses, and at sites connecting tendons or ligaments to bones.

Hyaline cartilage is the most common variety of cartilage. It is found in costal cartilage, epiphyseal plates, and covering bones in joints (articular cartilage). The free surfaces of most hyaline cartilage (but not articular cartilage) are covered by a layer of fibrous connective tissue (perichondrium). It is stratified and divided into four zones (Fig. 1.1): superficial (called also tangential zone), middle, deep, and calcified.

The orientation of collagen fibers varies through the four zones of articular cartilage in order to give better tensile strength.

E. Silvestri
Radiology, Alliance Medical, Genova, Italy

D. Orlandi (✉)
Department of Radiology, Ospedale Evangelico Internazionale, Genova, Italy

E. Massone
Department of Radiology, Ospedale Santa Corona, Pietra Ligure (SV), Italy

F. Martino et al. (eds.), *Musculoskeletal Ultrasound in Orthopedic and Rheumatic disease in Adults*,
https://doi.org/10.1007/978-3-030-91202-4_1

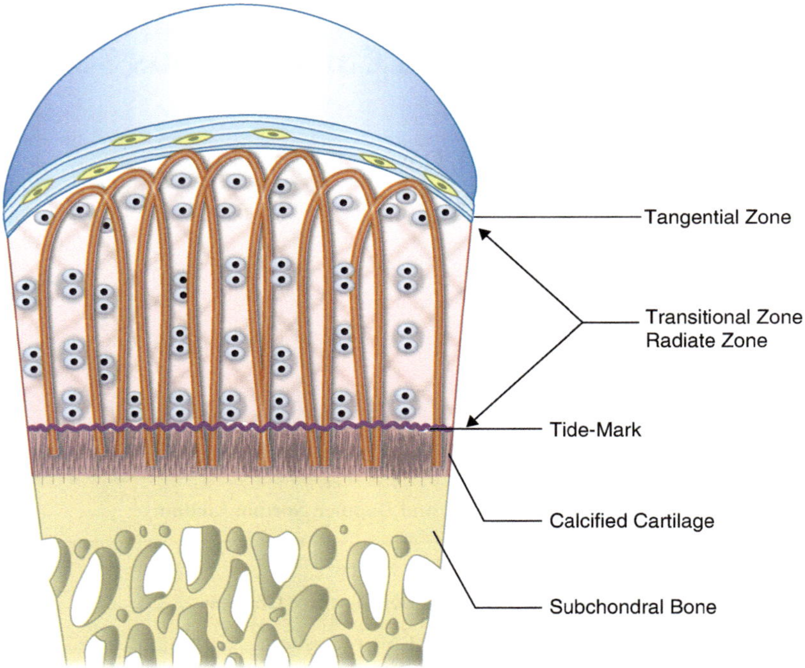

Fig. 1.1 Anatomical diagram of hyaline cartilage structure

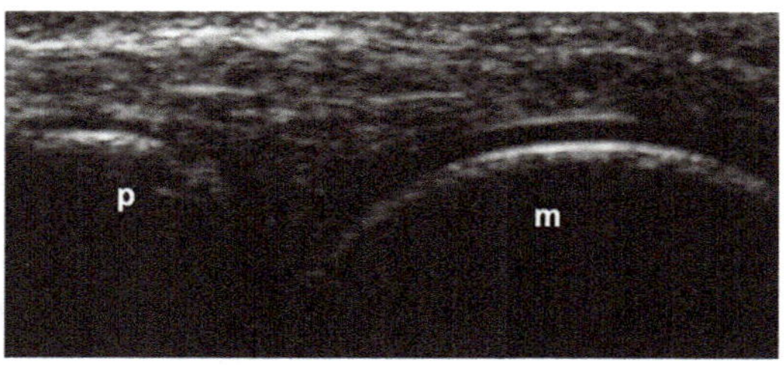

Fig. 1.2 Healthy subject. Longitudinal dorsal US scan of the second metacarpophalangeal joint obtained with a 5–13 MHz broadband linear transducer. The articular cartilage of the metacarpal head appears as a homogeneous anechoic layer with clearly defined hyperechoic contours. *m* metacarpal head; *p* proximal phalanx

Hyaline cartilage is detectable by ultrasonography as a homogeneously hypo-anechoic layer (high water content) delimited by thin, sharp, and hyperechoic margins (superficial margin: synovial space-cartilage interface; deep margin: bone-cartilage interface) (Fig. 1.2). *Sharp margins* and *homogeneity of the echotexture* are hallmarks of normal cartilage (Fig. 1.3).

The synovial space-cartilage interface is slightly thinner than the bone-cartilage interface. Both margins are best visualized when the direction of the ultrasound (US) beam is perpendicular to the cartilage surface.

The pronounced difference in chemical structure between articular cartilage and subchondral bone allows easy detection of the deep margin, while the superficial margin requires careful examination techniques for clear identification.

Optimization of the visualization of the cartilage margins is essential for measuring the cartilage thickness.

Cartilage thickness ranges from 0.1 mm on the articular surface of the head of the proximal phalanx to 2.6 mm on the lateral femoral condyle of the knee joint. The inter-observer reproducibility of measurements of cartilage thickness seems to be relatively good.

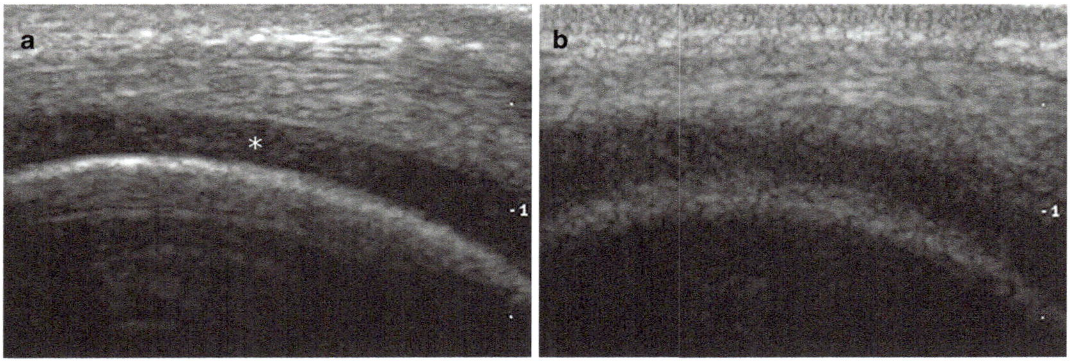

Fig. 1.3 (**a** and **b**) Healthy subject. Knee. Suprapatellar longitudinal scan of the articular cartilage of the lateral femoral condyle obtained with a 5–10 MHz broadband linear transducer. (**a**) Normal features of the articular cartilage (*) obtained with the ultrasound beam directly perpendicular to the cartilage surface. (**b**) Apparent loss of sharpness of the cartilage margins due to imperfect insonation angle

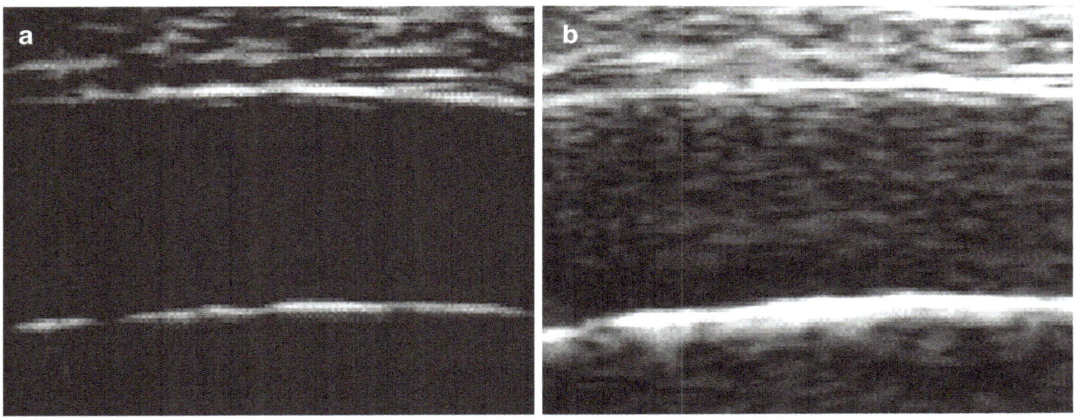

Fig. 1.4 (**a** and **b**) Healthy subject. Knee. Suprapatellar longitudinal scan of the articular cartilage of the lateral femoral condyle obtained with an 8–16 MHz broadband linear transducer. Both images show the characteristic homogeneous echotexture of the cartilage layer. (**a**) Anechoic, obtained with low levels of gain. (**b**) Hypoechoic, obtained with relatively higher levels of gain

These sonographic features are remarkably similar at different anatomic sites and largely dependent upon the equipment settings.

The typical anechoic pattern is obtained at lower levels of gain (Fig.1.4a and b).

The relative lack of echoes and the sharpness of the synovial space-cartilage interface and of the cartilage-bone interface are the main features of a healthy tissue.

Many different factors contribute to the final sonographic visualization of the hyaline cartilage:

- Size of the acoustic window
- Operator experience
- Transducer frequency
- Patient position

US examination may show a wide range of possible changes such as loss of sharpness, loss of clarity of the cartilaginous layer, joint space narrowing, or increased intensity of posterior bone-cartilage interface.

In order to reduce misinterpretation, multiplanar examination and comparison with the contralateral side must be carried out.

Hyaline cartilage can be examined at different anatomical sites, including hip, knee, shoulder, elbow, and metacarpophalangeal joints.

The complex anatomical structure of the knee joint poses particular acoustic barriers to accurate evaluation of the cartilage, meaning that only femoral condylar cartilage can be assessed.

The weight-bearing surfaces of the femoral condyles can be assessed by transverse suprapatellar scanning with the knee in maximal flexion or with an infrapatellar transverse scan with the leg fully extended.

Suprapatellar scanning of weight-bearing area can be difficult in patients with limited degrees of flexion due to pain.

Further assessment of the weight-bearing cartilage of the medial femoral condyle can also be obtained by the medial parapatellar view with the knee in maximal flexion. The transverse suprapatellar scan of the knee demonstrates that, in healthy subjects, the femoral cartilage typically appears as a clear-cut, wavy hypo-anechoic layer, with upper concavity, which is thicker at the level of the intercondyloid fossa (Fig. 1.5). This particular scan should be carried out with the knee flexed to an angle of at least 90°. A panoramic view of the entire cartilaginous profile can best be obtained with wide footprint and medium-frequency probes (not higher than 10 MHz). Linear probes do not allow the ultrasound beam to reach the cartilaginous layer with the same angle of incidence, leading to apparent inhomogeneity in the cartilaginous echotexture and profile of the margins.

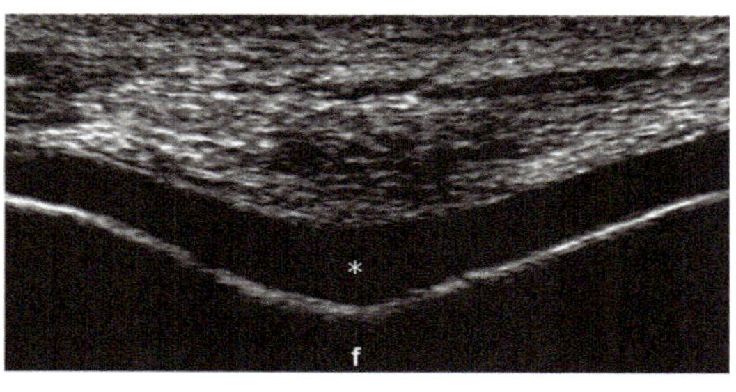

Fig. 1.5 Transverse view of the knee. Articular cartilage (*) appears as a curved anechoic band. The image was obtained with a 7–14 MHz broadband linear transducer. *f* femur

In addition, the transverse scan demonstrates the femoral cartilage most clearly at the level of peripheral portions of femoral condyles. Conversely, longitudinal scans carried out on contiguous planes allow for accurate evaluation of the profile of the condylar cartilage, from its most proximal portions that articulate with the patella to the more distal portions that relate to the tibial plateau (Fig. 1.3).

Recent data showed that US scanning approach allows similar diagnostic performance compared to routine MRI for knee cartilage defects at the femoral trochlea. Diagnostic performance of US has been tested even using arthroscopic findings as a gold standard with a notably high correlation. Moreover, US is more accessible, easier to perform, and less expensive than MRI, with potential advantages of easier initial screening and assessment of cartilage defects. However, because weight-bearing sites at the femoral condyles and tibial plateau cannot be assessed with US, this represents a significant limitation of such method.

Articular cartilage of the metacarpal head can be evaluated by longitudinal and transverse dorsal scans with the metacarpophalangeal joint held in maximal flexion. Standard longitudinal dorsal and volar scans may also be useful.

Higher frequency probes (>10 MHz) must be used in order to study the articular cartilage of the metacarpal head. Particular attention must be paid to the identification of the superficial margin that, in healthy subjects, appears as a thin hyperechoic line (of about a tenth of a millimeter thick), visible in tracts perpendicular to the direction of the ultrasound beam. This must be identified in order to obtain a correct measurement of the cartilaginous thickness. In a healthy subject, the thickness of the cartilage of the metacarpal head can vary between 0.2 and 0.5 mm.

Ultrasound can also provide a good insight even in some fibrocartilaginous structures such as knee menisci and triangular fibrocartilage complex (TFCC), which will be extensively treated in Chap. 2.

1.1.2 Osseous Tissue

Bone tissue is a biological tissue characterized by a remarkable hardness and resistance. It has a honeycomb-like structure internally, which helps to give the bone rigidity. Bone tissue is made up of different types of bone cells; osteoblasts and osteocytes are involved in the formation and mineralization of bone; osteoclasts are involved in the resorption of bone tissue. All these cells are entrenched in a matrix of collagen fibers that provide a surface for inorganic salt crystals to adhere.

Bones protect the various organs of the body, produce red and white blood cells, store minerals, provide structure and support for the body, and enable mobility.

Bones come in a variety of shapes and sizes and have a complex internal and external structure.

Based on shape, bones can be classified into three types:

- *Long bones* (e.g., femur, humerus, phalanges): characterized by a more developed dimension than the other two (precisely, the length compared to the thickness). A long bone has two parts: the **diaphysis** and the **epiphysis**. The diaphysis is the tubular shaft that runs between the proximal and distal ends of the bone. The hollow region in the diaphysis is called the **medullary cavity** (**endosteum**), which is filled with yellow marrow. The walls of the diaphysis are composed of dense and hard **compact bone**. The epiphysis is the rounded end of a long bone which is filled with spongy bone. Red marrow fills the spaces in the spongy bone. Each epiphysis meets the diaphysis at the metaphysis, the narrow area that contains the **epiphyseal plate** (growth plate), a layer of hyaline (transparent) cartilage in a growing bone. When the bone stops growing in early adulthood (approximately 18–21 years), the cartilage is replaced by osseous tissue and the epiphyseal plate becomes an epiphyseal line. A fibrous membrane called the **periosteum** (peri- = "around" or "surrounding") covers the outer surface of the bone. It contains blood vessels, nerves, and lymphatic vessels that nourish compact bone. Tendons and ligaments also attach to bones at the periosteum. The periosteum covers the entire outer surface except where the epiphyses meet other bones to form joints. In this region, the epiphyses are covered with **articular cartilage**, a thin layer of cartilage that reduces friction and acts as a shock absorber.
- *Flat bones* (scapula, skull, and sternum): two dimensions more developed than the third (in fact they are bones with a very small thickness, if compared to the total area of the bone).
- *Short bones* (vertebrae and the carpal bones): small, stocky bones, with all three dimensions of the same order of magnitude. It consists of a central part called the diaphysis and two vaguely rounded ends, called the epiphysis. During the development of the skeleton, between the diaphysis and the epiphysis there is a layer of cartilage, called conjugation cartilage or epiphyseal disk. As long as this cartilage is not mineralized and ossified, bone lengthening is possible. The bone is totally covered by a dense elastic connective membrane, called the periosteum; the exceptions are the epiphyseal articular surfaces which are instead covered by a hyaline cartilage incrustation. The interior of the diaphyseal cavity as well as that of the epiphyses is instead covered by a layer of paving cells called the endosteum.

The high-impedance difference between bone and soft tissue such as muscle, fat, or water causes an almost complete reflection of the acoustic waves at the bone's surface. As a result, the bone surface is seen, and the underlying structures are not seen ("shadow region").

So the interior bone surfaces cannot be imaged with US imaging. The high-intensity feature depicting bone boundary response looks like a line with a shape closely resembling the surface (Fig. 1.6). The bone surface appearance in US has a thickness which can reach a value of 4 mm in certain cases. The response thickness is affected by the inclination of the image surface with respect to the US transducer.

The greater the inclination of the imaged surface, the greater the response thickness.

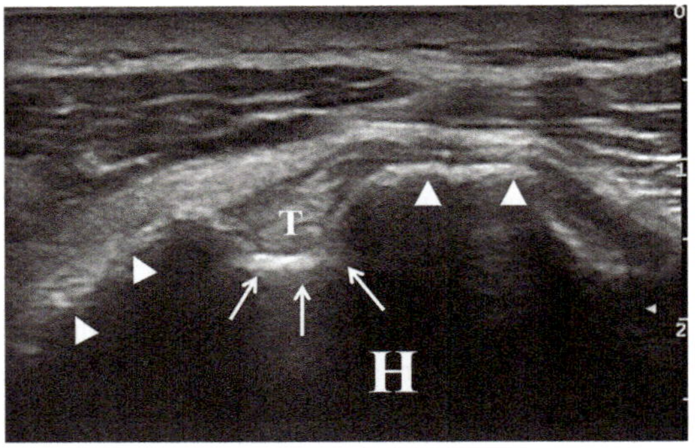

Fig. 1.6 Bone surface appearance; anterior transversal view of humeral head: (H) bone surface (arrowheads), bicipital groove (arrows), long head of biceps tendon (T)

1.2 Osteochondral Degenerative Changes

These include:

- Loss of sharpness of the synovial space-cartilage
- Loss of transparency of the cartilaginous layer (it reflects pathological changes such as fibrillation of cartilage and cleft formation)
- Cartilage thinning and subchondral bone profile irregularities (most common US findings in advanced osteoarthritis) (Fig. 1.7a and b)

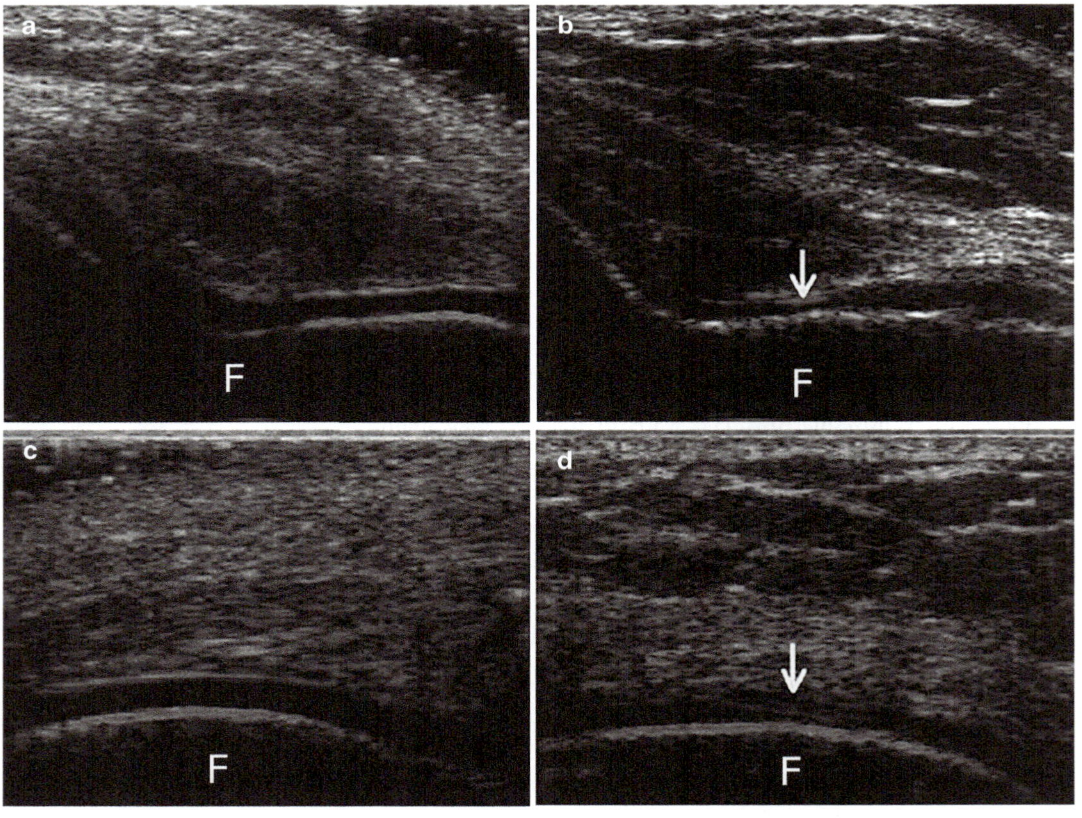

Fig. 1.7 (**a** and **b**) Osteoarthritis. Transverse (**a** and **b**) and longitudinal (**c** and **d**) suprapatellar US scans of the knee. (**a** and **c**) Normal cartilage features. (**b** and **d**) Loss of sharpness of the superficial margin and circumscribed thinning (arrows) of the cartilage layer of the medial femoral condyle (**F**)

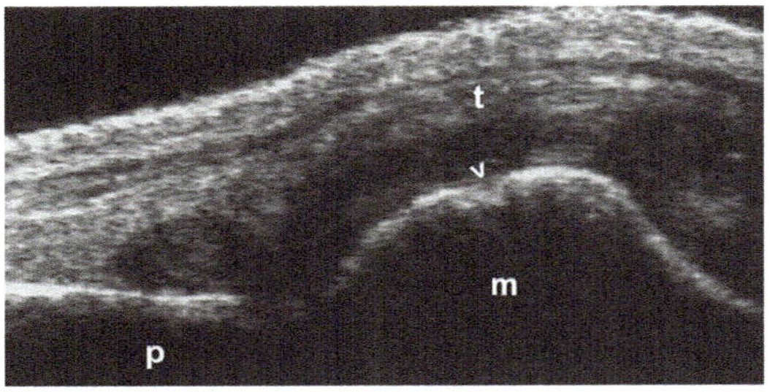

Fig. 1.8 Rheumatoid arthritis. Longitudinal dorsal scan of a metacarpophalangeal joint shows proliferative synovitis with early erosive changes. Complete loss of the cartilage layer of the metacarpal head with initial subchondral involvement (arrowhead). *m* metacarpal head; *p* proximal; *t* tendon

1.3 Osteochondral Erosive Lesion

US can visualize pre-erosive changes (such as in rheumatoid arthritis), particularly at the level of the metacarpophalangeal joint, together with loss of the cartilage layer and irregularities of the subchondral bone (Fig. 1.8).

Several studies in rheumatoid arthritis have confirmed that ultrasonography permits accurate and detailed analysis of the anatomical changes induced by the inflammatory process and is more sensitive than conventional X-rays for the detection of bone erosions.

Bone erosions' US appearance looks like oval well-defined cortical breaks with an irregular floor visible in transverse and longitudinal planes, in most cases filled by hyperperfused synovial pannus (Fig. 1.9).

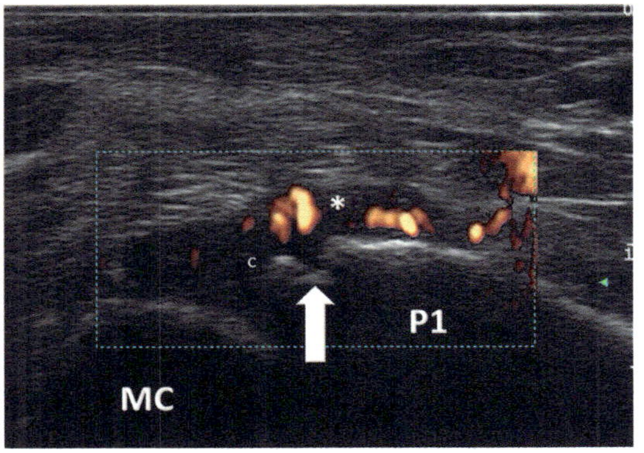

Fig. 1.9 Second metacarpophalangeal joint, US color power Doppler longitudinal scan: metacarpal head (MC) and cartilage (c), first phalanx (P1), bone erosion (arrow), hypertrophic and hyperemic synovia (asterisk)

1.4 Bone Fracture

Fractures can be visualized as a break in the hyperechoic cortical surface and the developing hematoma, and subsequent callus formation can be visualized from an early stage starting as an anechoic (dark) shadow, with a similar appearance to articular cartilage, becoming increasingly hyperechoic with calcification such that the normal appearance of cortical bone is restored (Fig. 1.10).

Ultrasound can be used:

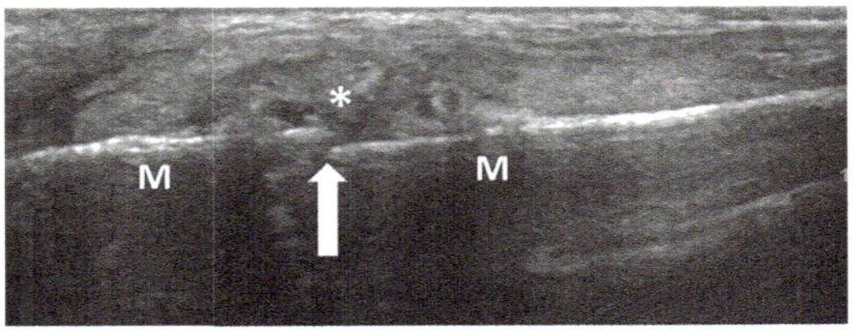

Fig. 1.10 Third metatarsal bone, US longitudinal scan: bone (M), fracture (arrow), reactive tissue thickening (asterisk)

- To diagnose common pediatric fractures
- To detect occult injuries and stress fractures in adults
- To judge reduction of distal radius fractures in real in the emergency department
- To detect long bone fractures in the resuscitation setting
- To monitor callus progression and fracture union
- With the advent of 3D image processing, to study a fracture site from multiple angles and compile them into a 3D reconstruction

Further Readings

Aisen AM, McCune WJ, MacGuire A, et al. Sonographic evaluation of the cartilage of the knee. Radiology. 1984;153:781–4.

Backhaus M, Burmester GR, Gerber T, et al. Guidelines for musculoskeletal ultrasound in rheumatology. Ann Rheum Dis. 2001;60:641–9.

Cao J, Zheng B, Meng X, Lv Y, Lu H, Wang K, Huang D, Ren J. A novel ultrasound scanning approach for evaluating femoral cartilage defects of the knee: comparison with routine magnetic resonance imaging. J Orthop Surg Res. 2018;13(1):178.

Castriota-Scanderbeg A, De Micheli V, Scarale MG, et al. Precision of sonographic measurement of articular cartilage: inter- and intraobserver analysis. Skeletal Radiol. 1996;25:545–9.

Disler DG, Raymond E, May DA, et al. Articular cartilage defects: in vitro evaluation of accuracy and interobserver reliability for detection and grading with US. Radiology. 2000;215:846–51.

Grassi W, Tittarelli E, Pirani O, et al. Ultrasound examination of metacarpophalangeal joints in rheumatoid arthritis. Scand J Rheumatol. 1993;22:243–7.

Grassi W, Cervini C. Ultrasonography in rheumatology: an evolving technique. Ann Rheum Dis. 1998;57:268–71.

Grassi W, Lamanna G, Farina A, Cervini C. Sonographic imaging of normal and osteoarthritic cartilage. Semin Arthritis Rheum. 1999;28:398–403.

McCune WJ, Dedrick DK, Aisen AM, MacGuire A. Sonographic evaluation of osteoarthritic femoral condylar cartilage. Correlation with operative findings. Clin Orthop. 1990;254:230–5.

Razek A, Fouda N, Elmetwaley N, et al. Sonography of the knee joint. J Ultrasound. 2009;12(2):53e60.

Saarakkala S, Waris P, Wasris V, Tarkiainen I, Karvanen E, Aarnio J, Koski JM. Diagnostic performance of knee ultrasonography for detecting degenerative changes of articular cartilage. Osteoarthritis Cartilage. 2012 May;20(5):376–81.

Schmitz RJ, Wang HM, Polprasert DR, Kraft RA, Pietrosimone BG. Evaluation of knee cartilage thickness: A comparison between ultrasound and magnetic resonance imaging methods. Knee. 2017;24(2):217–23.

Sheperd DET, Seedhom BB. Thickness of human articular cartilage in joints of the lower limb. Ann Rheum Dis. 1999;58:27–34.

Synovial Spaces

2

Davide Orlandi, Enzo Silvestri,
and Alessandro Muda

Contents

2.1 Sonographic and Doppler Normal Anatomy

The synovial cavity (Fig. 2.1) is the space found between bone segments and articular capsule; it is delimited by a fibrous wrap internally covered by a synovial membrane and contains a slight film of synovial fluid. The synovial cavity consists, depending on where it is found, of the joint cavity, the bursae, and the tendon sheaths.

The synovial fluid has a variable volume according to the dimension of the articular cavity and it represents, physiologically, a thin veil to protect the cartilage surface; it acts as a lubricant and it has nourishing functions for the cartilage itself. The synovial fluid is filtered from the blood plasma and it contains a maximum of 200 cell/cc. It also contains electrolytes, glucose, enzymes, immunoglobulins, and proteins mainly originating from blood, with the addition of mucin, mostly hyaluronic acid, which is well represented. The mucin makes the synovial fluid viscous, elastic, and plastic.

D. Orlandi (✉)
Department of Radiology, Ospedale Evangelico Internazionale, Genova, Italy

E. Silvestri
Radiology, Alliance Medical, Genova, Italy

A. Muda
Department of Radiology, IRCCS Policlinico San Martino-IST, Genova, Italy

F. Martino et al. (eds.), *Musculoskeletal Ultrasound in Orthopedic and Rheumatic disease in Adults*,
https://doi.org/10.1007/978-3-030-91202-4_2

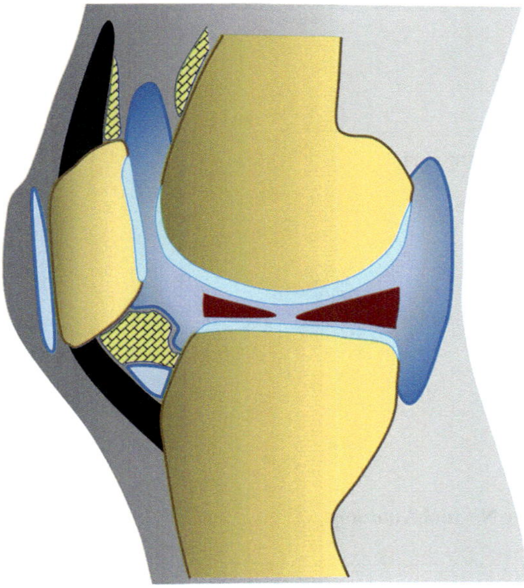

Fig. 2.1 Anatomical diagram of a synovial joint. Insertion and development of the articular capsule with the synovial membrane (in blue), articular cartilage (in turquoise), bursae (in blue), fat pads (honeycomb), and menisci (in red) are clearly shown

The articular capsule consists of intertwisted bundles of connective fibrous tissue, whose insertion onto bone occurs as a continuous line. At some points the capsule is strengthened by the intrinsic capsular ligaments, represented by local thickenings (made of fibrous or fibroelastic tissue) of the capsule itself, where the fiber bundles become parallel. The articular capsule is internally covered by the synovial membrane. The synovial membrane is a connective tissue of mesenchymal origin, covering any exposed osseous surface, the synovial bursae in communication with the joint cavity, and the intracapsular ligament and tendons; it is not present on meniscal and discal surfaces and it stops right before the edge of joint cartilage, the peripheral area of which, only a few millimeters thick, constitutes a zone of transition from synovial membrane to cartilage.

In the synovial cavities of some joints, adipose tissue is stored in specific regions, forming mobile and elastic pads that fill in the spaces of the articular cavity. Such fat pads, when the joint moves, adapt to the changes of shape and volume of the synovial cavity, supporting the lubrication of the joint surfaces.

The synovial membrane is made of a cellular intima lying on a fibrovascular subintimal lamina consisting of abundant loose areolar tissue, collagen, and elastic fibers. When the synovial membrane covers the intracapsular tendons or ligaments, the subintima is hardly identifiable as a separate layer, being fused together with the capsule, the ligament, or the adjacent tendon.

The synovial intima is made of cells, called synoviocytes A and B, whose function is to remove the debris found in the joint cavity and to synthesize some molecules for the synovial fluid. The synoviocytes do not actively proliferate under basal conditions, while the speed of cellular division is considerably increased after trauma and acute hemarthrosis.

The bursae are virtual spaces localized in specific regions of the joint where high friction between closely opposing structures occurs. The bursae can be visualized almost solely in pathologic conditions, because they physiologically contain a slight film of synovial fluid. As above, the bursae are covered by the synovial membrane that continues from the synovial membrane of the articular cavity, so that it constitutes communicating bursae where the synovial fluid is freely circulating.

The communicating bursae have a further biomechanical function: they decrease the endoarticular pressure when there is a fluid collection in the joint cavity.

Normally, the synovial cavities are barely visible or invisible with US, whereas they can be easily evaluated when a thickening of the synovial membrane or a joint fluid collection occurs. The size of the synovial cavity of the hip can be depicted and measured by US using a sagittal view passing through the femoral head—the lower limb externally rotated 10–15°; in healthy subjects the interposed distance between the femoral neck outline and the articular capsule has a mean value of 5.1 mm (range 3–7 mm). There is no evident relationship between the sonographic size of the synovial cavity and age, gender, height, or body weight; the maximum difference between one side and the contralateral side is about 1 mm. In the knee, the only synovial cavity accessible to US is the suprapatellar recess. The examination can be performed through suprapatellar longitudinal and axial views, with the patient lying supine with the knee in the extended position. The suprapatellar recess appears as a hypoechoic flat structure, with a regular and clear contour, whose anteroposterior diameter does not measure more than 3–4 mm. Dynamic assessment, performed during the contraction of the quadriceps femoris muscle, shows a slight increase both in the anteroposterior diameter and in the recess length.

The increase in fluid collection during this phase, related to the mean sagittal diameter increase of the bursa (1 mm), can be related to the simultaneous contraction of the suprapatellar recess tensor muscle. This small muscle drags the bursa, causing a vacuum effect that causes the bursa to be filled with fluid coming from the joint cavity. In people who are fit, compared to those who lead a sedentary life, the suprapatellar recess diameter does not change, but it is well visualized in 25% and 66% of patients, respectively, according to the relaxation and the contraction of the quadriceps femoris. The synovial membrane contour can be indirectly assessed when the suprapatellar recess is distended by synovial fluid. It appears as a thin echoic band of 1.7 mm (mean value). The anterior synovial layer of the suprapatellar recess is usually more easily identified than the deep layer. The first can be easily assessed thanks to the different echogenicity of the overlying quadriceps tendon, which appears moderately echoic, while the latter is strictly contiguous with the pre-femoral fat pad, which is echoic and has a maximum thickness of about 1 cm. Normally the synovial fluid in the sub-quadricipital recess is homogeneously hypoanechoic and any change is related to pathology (Fig. 2.2).

The articular capsule is extremely thin and can be barely identified by ultrasound in physiological situations, whereas acute, inflammatory, or post-traumatic pathology makes it easily visible because of the natural acoustic window provided by the joint fluid collection.

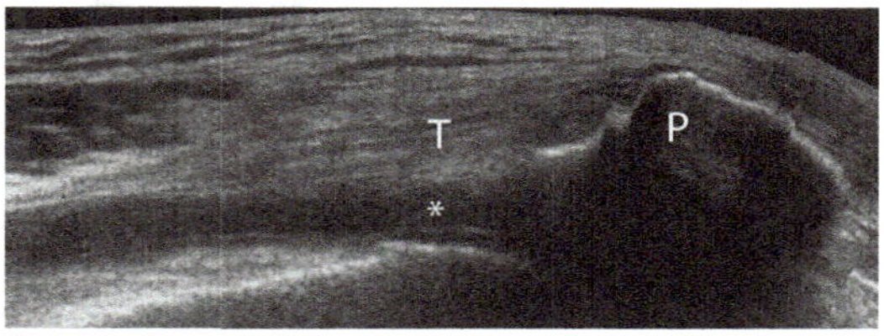

Fig. 2.2 Longitudinal extended field-of-view (EFOV) US scan of anterior compartment of the knee. Small amount of fluid in the joint (*) and distension of suprapatellar capsular recess. *T* quadriceps tendon; *P* patella

In order to identify the capsule, it is necessary to have precise anatomical reference points, joint by joint.

The articular capsule appears as a thin hyperechoic layer, hard to differentiate from the adjacent tendons and ligaments that have very similar echogenicity.

In the shoulder, the superior edge of the capsule corresponds to the inferior echoic edge of the tendons of the rotator cuff muscles (supraspinatus, infraspinatus, and teres minor); it is only when pathology occurs, such as an adhesive capsulitis—causing thickening and retraction—that the capsule can be identified as a marked irregularity of the inferior profile of the rotator cuff tendons. The axillary recess of the inferior edge of the capsule is more easily explored. The articular capsule of the knee can be easily assessed in the internal and external compartments, where the collateral ligaments delineate the capsule borders. The same procedure can be applied to assess any other joint of the hand and foot.

Ultrasound is a highly sensitive technique for the detection of even minimal fluid collections and it still represents a particularly useful diagnostic tool to quantify fluid and to monitor its evolution.

The considerable sensitivity of the identification of synovial fluid collection, the highly detailed anatomical depiction, and the real-time visualization of tissues make US the ideal imaging technique for interventional guided procedures, such as arthrocentesis.

Thanks to US, the aspiration of synovial fluid is possible even when the joint collection is minimal.

Pathologic conditions that can be assessed within the synovial cavity with US include hydrarthrosis, pneumohydrarthrosis, pyarthrosis, hemarthrosis, lipohemarthrosis, bursitis, tenosynovitis, and synovial thickening.

The **menisci** are fibrocartilaginous structures that partially divide an articular cavity. They are present in the knee, wrist, acromioclavicular, sternoclavicular, and temporomandibular joints. The menisci are derived from a condensation of the intermediate layer of the mesenchymal tissue to form attachments to the surrounding joint capsule. Their shape is characteristic for each joint and is vital for normal biomechanics and joint stability. Particularly at knee and wrist levels, ultrasound can visualize and evaluate the meniscal structure, as a possible alternative to MRI, rapidly and less costly performed. Menisci appear as a wedge-shaped echogenic formation. The usefulness of ultrasound in the diagnosis of lesions of the menisci of the knee remains controversial. According to some authors, ultrasonography has high accuracy in detecting the presence of tears in menisci, and can be used as a point-of-injury diagnostic modality for meniscal injuries. According to others, it is considered as a useful tool to image the meniscus, but there are no reliable data on its accuracy. Therefore, it appears to be useful for the screening of meniscal tears but detection of the morphology of meniscal tears seems insufficient compared to MRI. Both in coronal (for the body) and sagittal (for the anterior or posterior horn) section planes, the normal meniscus appears with the characteristic triangular shape, homogeneously hyperechoic (Fig. 2.3 a and b). The prevalent limit of the method is represented by the poor evidence of meniscus internal margin. Usually, there is a better evidence of the medial meniscus with respect to the lateral one, and of the posterior horn with respect to the body and the anterior one.

The TFCC consists of the triangular fibrocartilage proper (TFC), the dorsal and volar radioulnar ligaments, the ulnar collateral ligament, the meniscal homologue, the sheath of the extensor carpi ulnaris, and the ulnolunate and ulnotriquetral ligament.

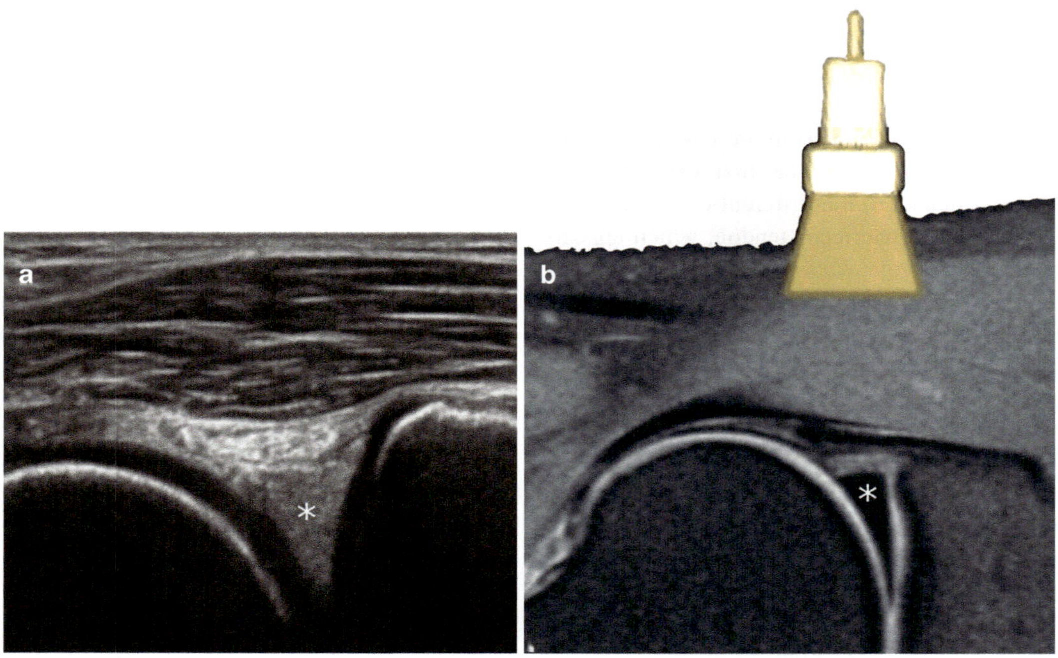

Fig. 2.3 Ultrasound (**a**) and MRI (**b**) appearance of normal meniscus (*)

According to Taljanovic et al. the TFC disk was considered normal if it was seen as homogeneously echogenic triangular tissue in the proper anatomic location at the articular aspect of the ulnar head. It was considered torn if hypoechoic clefts or defects were seen in the substance of the TFC disk. If some irregularity of the TFC disk was observed without a frank cleft on sonography it was considered partially torn.

Usually, a linear transducer of 7–11 MHz is used for TFCC examination. The patient is examined while sitting upright, with the hand placed on a cushion and fully pronated and then supinated.

2.2 Joint Effusion

A collection of fluid within the synovial cavity causes the swelling of the involved joint. In *hydrarthrosis*, US shows fluid collection within the cavity, which has an anechoic appearance with dorsal acoustic enhancement (Fig. 2.4a and b).

The amount of fluid within the joint is directly proportional to the severity of the synovial inflammation and to the capability of the capsular wall to expand. In some cases the anechoic appearance of the fluid collection can be inhomogeneous because of the presence of dot-like echoes scattered within the collection itself. This more complicated appearance of the collection may depend on the presence of a fibrinous component within the inflammatory exudate, which can be particularly abundant in relapsing collections and can be visualized as arranged echogenic and inhomogeneous clusters, with a scirrhous conformation.

Pyarthrosis occurs in bacterial arthritis, which is usually rare in patients with normal immune systems, while it is common in children, in immunosuppressed patients, in diabetics, and in patients on dialysis. In acute infections with joint fluid collection, it is necessary to sample the fluid in order to prescribe the most appropriate antibiotic therapy.

In chronic infections the fluid collection is usually poor and it is often associated with considerable synovial thickening. In infections the fluid is usually hypoechoic, but it may appear hyperechoic in more superficial joints. In such cases, the synovial hyperemia can be well depicted with the use of Doppler techniques as a complement to grayscale US. However, it should be kept in mind that synovial hyperemia in bacterial arthritis is not a mandatory finding, because it depends on the patient's age, duration of the infection, and immune status. Therefore, since there is no certainty in differentiating septic from aseptic inflammation, it is more suitable to perform a biopsy when clinical suspicion is high.

Hemarthrosis exhibits a peculiar US pattern that changes with time similar to hematoma. Hemorrhagic fluid collections are in fact homogeneously echogenic within the first 2–3 days from onset, due to the presence of a corpuscular content. After the third day, the hemarthrosis shows a progressive reduction in echogenicity due to lytic enzyme release. Eventually, US shows echogenic branches, corresponding to fibrinous clots, crossing the anechoic appearing

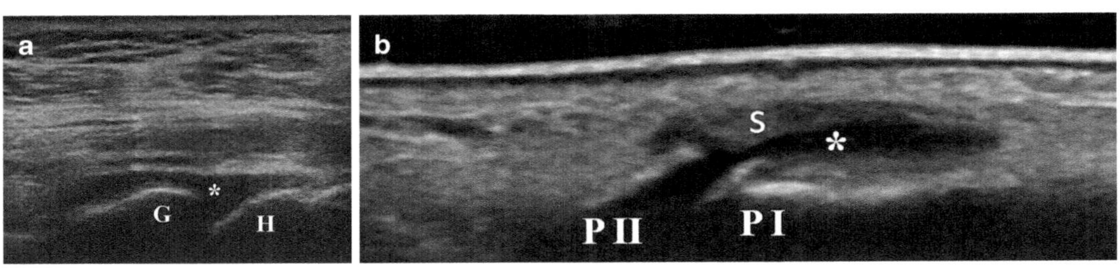

Fig. 2.4 (**a**) Posterior transverse US scan at the level of glenohumeral joint: glenoid (G), humeral head (H), joint. (**b**) Proximal interphalangeal joint (second finger), longitudinal US scan; first phalanx (P I), second phalanx (P II), joint effusion (asterisk), synovial thickening (s)

zone. Occasionally, the post-arthrocentesis follow-up examination demonstrates the presence of *pneumohydrarthrosis*. The presence of gas in the joint cavity produces a highly reflective mist within the anechoic fluid collection, forming an air-fluid level that changes together with the patient's position. When assessing hydrarthrosis and pneumohydrarthrosis, color and power Doppler techniques do not demonstrate significant vascular changes.

Lipohemarthrosis is easily identified by means of US and it appears as a dual-phase collection, showing a fluid-fluid level. The overlying echogenic fraction corresponds to the lipid content, while the underlying fraction is hemorrhagic. When lipohemarthrosis is found in a post-traumatic limb, the presence of a joint fracture can be suspected.

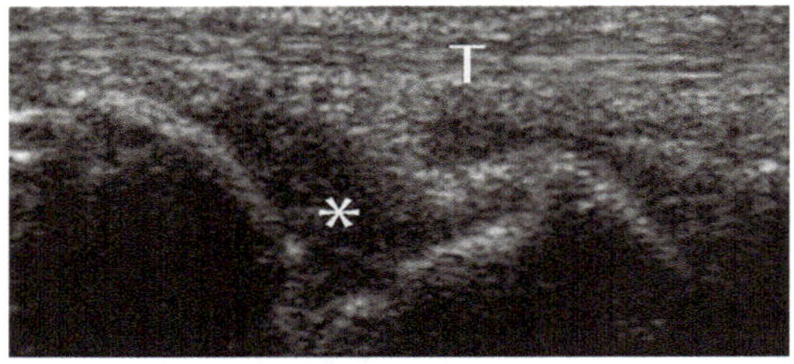

Fig. 2.5 Longitudinal sonogram of wrist, dorsal side in a patient affected by rheumatoid arthritis. Synovial proliferation appears hypoechoic (*). *T* extensor tendons

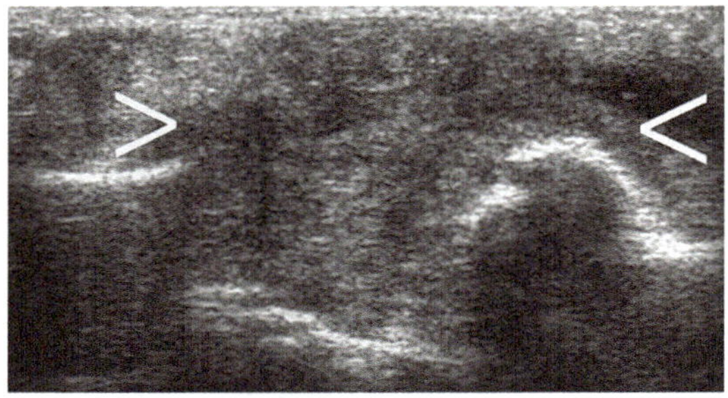

Fig. 2.6 Longitudinal sonogram of wrist, dorsal side. Patient affected by rheumatoid arthritis. In this case, synovial proliferation (arrowheads) has a hyperechoic appearance

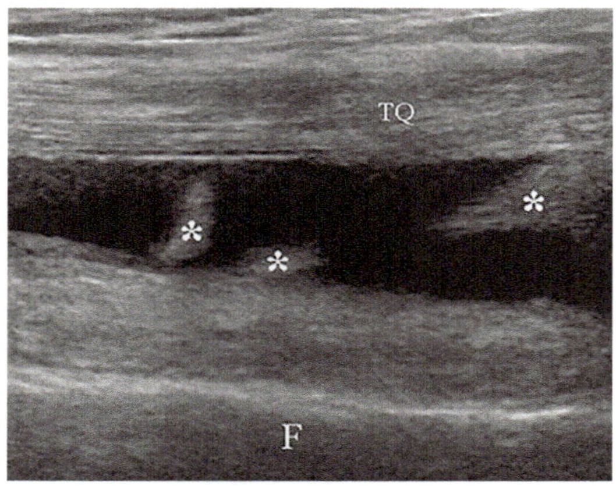

Fig. 2.7 Longitudinal US scan of suprapatellar recess showing a large amount of anechoic fluid collection with hyperechoic synovial proliferation (*). *TQ* quadricipital tendon; *F* femur

2.3 Synovial Inflammation and Proliferation

Hypertrophic or hyperplasic synovial thickening is a condition found in several long-standing inflammatory arthropathies and it can be the cause of bone and cartilage erosion in the joint. US nowadays can identify inflammatory synovial thickening more accurately than clinical examination, especially when small joints such as the metacarpophalangeal and interphalangeal joints are affected, commonly observed in chronic polyarthropathies. Synovial thickening is characterized by heterogeneous echotexture varying from hypoechoic to hyperechoic, depending on the amount of water contained in the synovial tissue (Figs. 2.5 and 2.6).

In larger joints, such as the knee, synovial thickening appears as a succession of irregularly proliferating branches, mildly echoic, jutting out from the synovia into the articular cavity; the assessment of synovial pannus is considerably easier when associated with a fluid collection because it works as a contrast agent (Fig. 2.7).

In pigmented villonodular synovitis, the synovial hypertrophy is usually overabundant, made of thick fusiform villi and gross nodules, with a winding outline surrounded by abundant fluid collection. A similar appearance can be observed in joints affected by relapsing hemarthrosis in hemophilic arthropathies. The continual presence of hemorrhagic effusion irritates the synovial membrane and determines the formation of pannus that starts as a simple thickening and then turns into villous hypertrophy. The sonographer should always keep in mind that synovial hypertrophy is a nonspecific finding and that the differentiation between a nonspecific synovitis and a synovial tumor can be very tricky (hemangioma, synovial sarcoma). A fibrinous exudate can make it difficult to detect the thickened synovial membrane contour, especially when it is abundant, because it may simulate the US pattern of synovial hyperplasia. In these cases, when fluid and hypertrophic synovial cannot be differentiated it is possible to use dynamic and compressive maneuvers. Such a technique allows the fluid to be "squeezed out" from the hypertrophic synovial wall and the differentiation of the two articular contents.

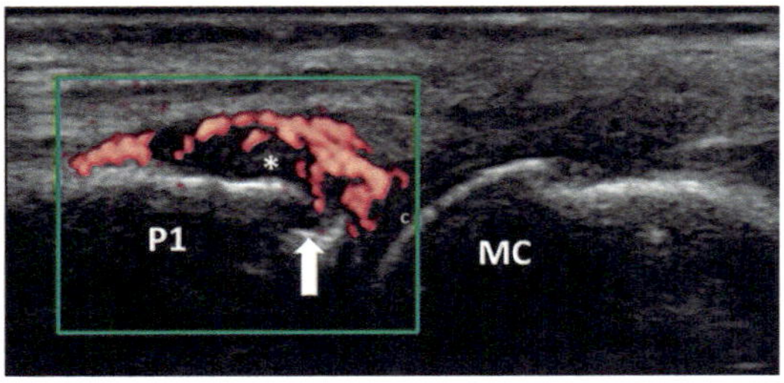

Fig. 2.8 Second metacarpophalangeal joint, US color power Doppler longitudinal scan: metacarpal head (MC) and cartilage (c), first phalanx (P1), bone erosion (arrow), synovial hyperemic proliferation (asterisk)

When doubt persists with grayscale US, power and color Doppler techniques can be applied to differentiate the fluid from the proliferating tissue, with the presence or absence of vascular signals (Fig. 2.8).

The role of Doppler techniques for the assessment of synovial vascularization in rheumatoid arthritis is very important. In rheumatoid arthritis, the formation of pannus is a crucial event in the pathogenesis of articular degeneration. Neoangiogenesis is an important pathological element in rheumatoid synovitis. Since hypervascularization is proportional to the degree of inflammation of the synovial pannus, it is fundamental to study and quantify the vascular signals in order to evaluate the aggressiveness of the pannus itself. Power Doppler is able to assess the increased vascularization involving synovial hyperplasic tissue and consequently to give information regarding the activity of the synovial pannus (Fig. 2.9a and b).

Despite attempts at semiquantitative or quantitative evaluation of the vascularization by means of dedicated software, the technique is limited by poor reproducibility. Nevertheless, the recent availability of power Doppler techniques in association with the use of contrast agents (contrast-enhanced power Doppler—CePD) has allowed a more detailed analysis of the synovial

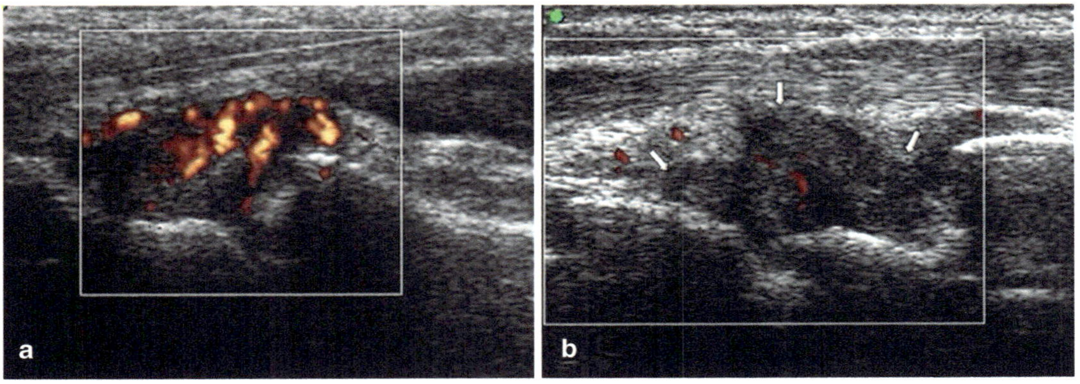

Fig. 2.9 Patient with rheumatoid arthritis. (**a**) The power Doppler scan shows a high degree of hyperperfusion, an expression of hyperactive pannus. (**b**) Follow-up during therapy. A significant reduction in flow signal is shown within the pannus (arrows)

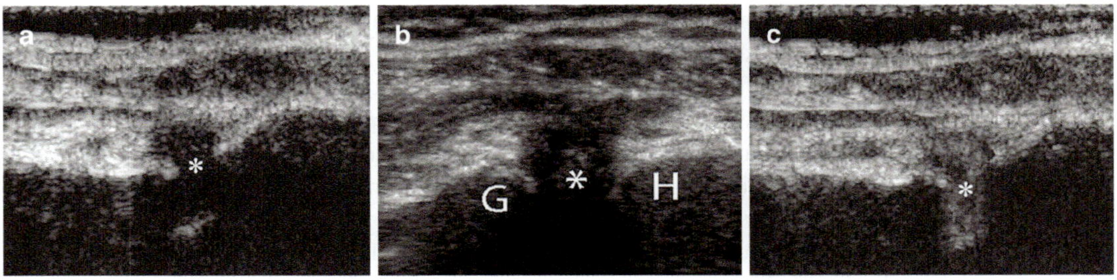

Fig. 2.10 Patient with rheumatoid arthritis. (**a**) Shoulder, posterior scan. Expansion of posterior capsular recess with inhomogeneous hypoechoic synovial proliferation (*). (**b** and **c**) Images taken before (**b**), and after (**c**), injection of contrast agent (CeUS). These scans show a significant hyperemia of synovial proliferation. The hyperechoic appearance is due to the contrasting microbubbles. *G* posterior margin of humeral glenoid process; *H* posterior aspect of humeral head

vascularization. It should be considered that the information derived from power Doppler and CePD refers exclusively to the macrovascularization of synovial pannus. Such limits have now been overcome by the introduction of new-generation contrast agents that allow quantitative analysis of the synovial microvascularization to be performed by means of grayscale US (contrast-enhanced US—CeUS) (Fig. 2.10a–c).

2.4 Bursitis

Bursae are anatomical entities located near joints (non-communicating bursae) or in direct communication with the joint cavity (communicating bursae). The main function of non-communicating bursae, located at the insertional areas of the anchor tendons of several joints, is to reduce the friction between tendon and bone. Communicating bursae, on the other hand, when an abundant intra-articular fluid collection occurs, function by reducing the joint cavity pressure, by expanding and being filled with the fluid coming from the cavity. Bursitis represents the most common bursal pathology and US is the first-choice diagnostic technique.

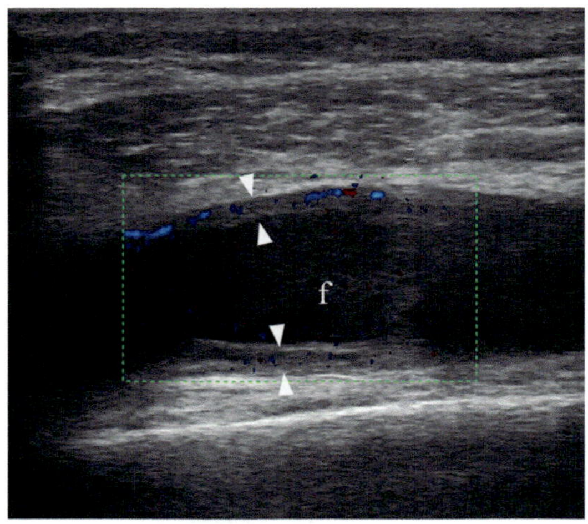

Fig. 2.11 US power color Doppler scan; acute thickening of the bursal wall (arrowheads) with some color spot of hyperemia; fluid effusion (f)

2.4.1 Non-communicating Bursitis

1. Acute traumatic bursitis: affecting several synovial bursae, the bursal expansion follows direct impact or chronic frictional microtrauma. The most commonly involved bursae are the subacromial-deltoid bursa, the prepatellar and deep infrapatellar bursa, the retrocalcaneal and superficialis bursa of the Achilles tendon, and the trochanteric bursa. In acute forms, an increase in anechoic fluid within the bursa is observed (a comparison with the contralateral limb may be useful), while the synovial wall keeps its original thickness (Fig. 2.11a).
2. In chronic forms, the fluid often appears hypoechoic and contains hyperechoic spots consistent with microcalcification, and the bursal walls are thickened (Fig. 2.12a and b).

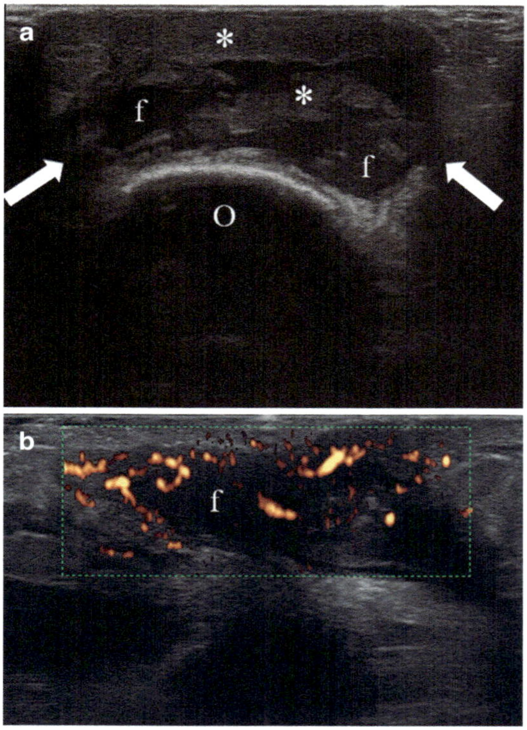

Fig. 2.12 Posterior aspect of elbow, transverse scan: olecranic chronic bursitis (white arrows), fluid distension (f), and synovial thickening and septa (asterisks) (**a**); US color power Doppler longitudinal scan: synovial hyperemia (**b**)

3. Hemorrhagic bursitis: usually following a violent sporting trauma on artificial surfaces and mainly affects the hands and knees. The hemorrhagic effusion may organize and form adhesions or calcifications. Clots and fibrin, appearing as irregular hyperechoic masses, are easily distinguished from synovial hypertrophy because of their mobility and the absence of vascular signal on power or color Doppler analysis.
4. Chemical bursitis: often associated with metabolic disease, and inflammatory and degenerative processes. The most common cause is the monosodium urate crystal deposition in gout.
5. Septic bursitis: difficult to differentiate from chronic inflammatory bursitis, but it is characterized by intrabursal hyperechoic diffuse areas, corresponding to thickened synovial membrane (Fig. 2.13). The presence of gas within the bursa may be consistent with septic bursitis, but the final diagnosis can be obtained by performing a color or power Doppler examination that allows the detection of vascular signals within the soft tissues, indicating an inflammatory hyperemia, or, even better, by sampling the bursal fluid.

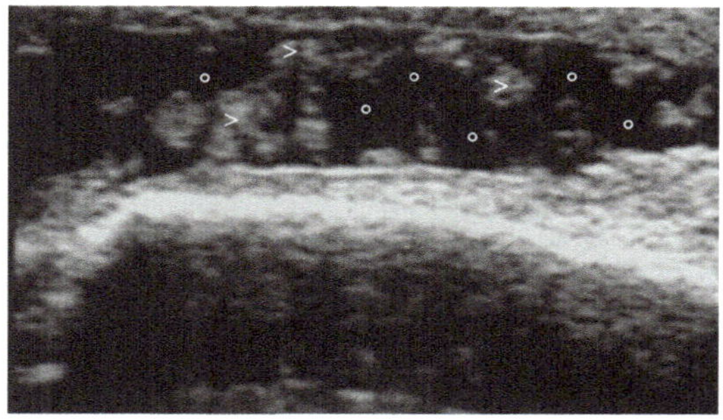

Fig. 2.13 Patient with gout, olecranon bursitis. The bursa is expanded by a small amount of synovial fluid (circles) with some hyperechoic synovial proliferation (arrowheads)

2.4.2 Communicating Bursitis

Communicating synovial bursae develop during adolescence and are characterized by the presence of a tract that connects them to the nearby joint. Their function is to reduce intra-articular pressure in order to avoid the onset of joint complications. The most common communicating bursitis is the medial gastrocnemius and semimembranosus tendon bursitis, with a particularly high incidence in rheumatoid arthritis compared with other rheumatic disorders such as Reiter's syndrome, villonodular arthrosynovitis, Sjogren's syndrome, ankylosing spondylitis, psoriatic arthritis, gonococcal arthritis, and gout (Fig. 2.14a and b).

In long-standing fluid collections, the progressive filling of the bursa leads to the formation of a cyst (Baker's cyst), which can be easily palpated on clinical examination when it reaches considerable dimensions (gigantic cysts) and can be completely visible thanks to panoramic imaging (extended field of view (EFOV)) (Fig. 2.15).

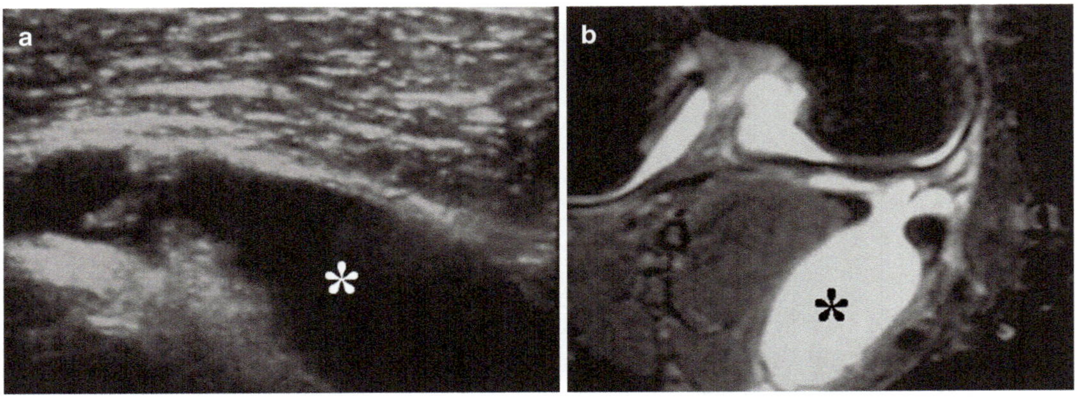

Fig. 2.14 Transverse US scan of popliteal fossa in a patient affected by knee OA. Baker's cyst is shown. (**a**) MR scan of the same patient (axial view, fat suppression technique); cyst (asterisk) (**b**)

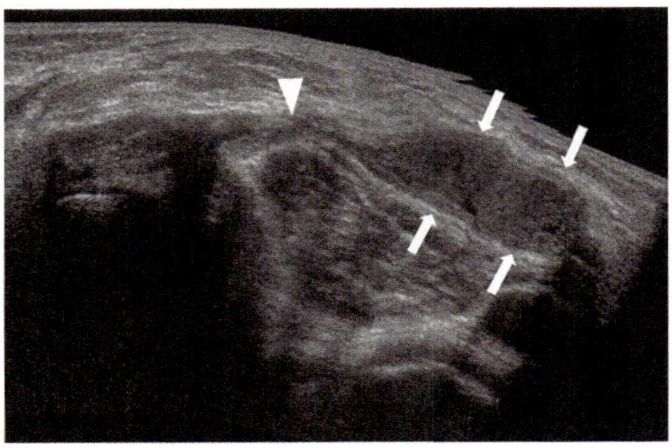

Fig. 2.15 Rheumatoid arthritis; EFOV scan shows the whole extent of a popliteal cyst (arrows) that courses toward the proximal third of the leg; connecting peduncle with the joint (arrowhead)

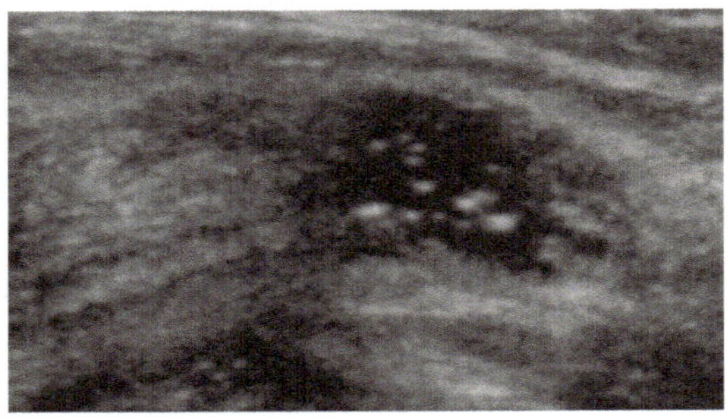

Fig. 2.16 Small popliteal cyst with fluid content and hyperechoic spots, caused by small clots and debris

The US appearance of a Baker's cyst is that of a hypoanechoic pear-shaped cavity, with a well-defined outline, presenting with posterior acoustic enhancement. Communication with the superior aspect of the posteromedial edge of the articular cavity can often be detected at the medial femoral condyle. Echoes within the cyst confirm the presence of debris and clots that, especially when abundant, make the US detection of small popliteal cysts difficult (Fig. 2.16).

The dimension of a Baker's cyst at follow-up can correlate with the clinical progression of arthritis and the efficacy of medical therapy and, in selected cases, US may be used as a guide for the aspiration and injection of the cyst (Fig. 2.17a and b).

When swelling is appreciated in the popliteal fossa, it is necessary to perform an US to differentiate a Baker's cyst from vascular (popliteal artery aneurysms, venous thrombosis) or muscular (different degrees of injuries involving the popliteal fossa muscles) pathologies. In chronic inflammatory arthropathies, hypertrophic synovial tissue is observed, with a particularly abundant and irregular appearance in rheumatoid arthritis. In this case the bursa may grow considerably, surrounding the tendon of the medial gastrocnemius muscle (Fig. 2.18).

Sometimes a gigantic cyst may end up rupturing leading to inflammation of the surrounding adipose tissue and of the myofascial components, so that it clinically simulates a thrombophlebitis (pseudo-thrombophlebitic syndrome). A fresh rupture of a gigantic cyst can be detected by US by hazy appearance of the cyst's fundus, with an

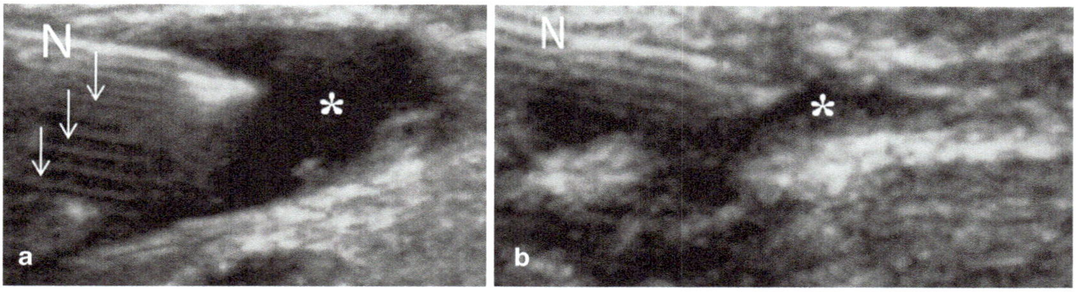

Fig. 2.17 Popliteal cyst before (**a**) and after (**b**) US-guided aspiration. *N* needle, asterisk=cyst. The reverberation artifact is clearly shown (arrows)

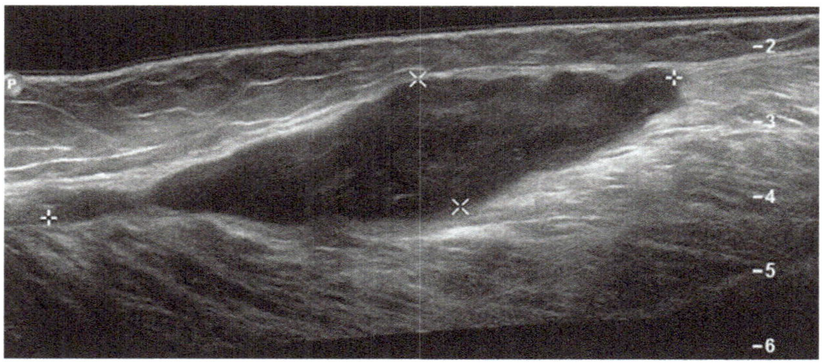

Fig. 2.18 Patient affected with rheumatoid arthritis. The EFoV scan shows the whole extent of a giant popliteal cyst (calipers) that courses toward the proximal third of the leg and has hemorrhagic content

associated free fluid collection located superficially and distally from the cyst itself. When doubt persists, grayscale US and color or power Doppler techniques play a fundamental role in the differential diagnosis. In normal circumstances the subacromial-deltoid bursa of the shoulder does not communicate with the joint cavity, while in cases of complete rupture of the rotator cuff, direct connection between the two cavities is observed (Fig. 2.19a and b).

2.5 Synovial Ganglia

Synovial ganglia are mostly found in the upper limb, particularly at the wrist and hand. The most common location is the carpal dorsum. In this case the cyst usually arises from the scapho-lunate joint because of mucoid degeneration phenomena of the tissues due to repeated microtrauma. US allows the ganglion to be visualized as a typical hypoanechoic nodule, with irregular margins, presenting internal thin hyperechoic septa and a slender peduncle that connects it to the scapho-lunate joint (Fig. 2.20). The application of dynamic maneuvers to the standard ultrasound examination can be particularly useful for the detection of the connecting peduncle and for better assessment of the cyst's relationships with the surrounding tissues.

2.6 Synovial Calcifications

Synovial calcification appears on US as a hyperechoic "platelike" area with posterior acoustic shadowing. The calcified plates, following the synovial membrane outline, have a linear or coarsely wavy appearance and do not move, even when compression is applied with the transducer. This sonographic pattern is typical of synovial osteochondromatosis, but can also be found, less frequently, in chondrocalcinosis and in scleroderma; the calcification process may involve both

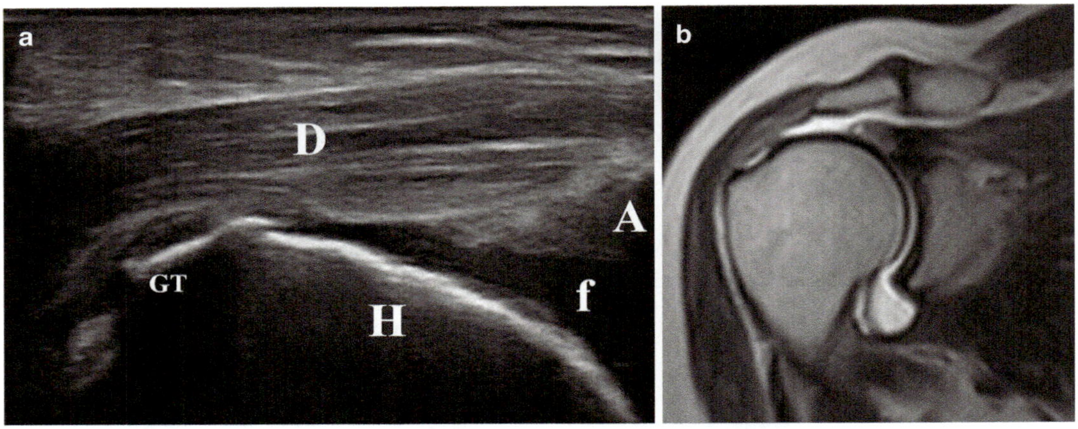

Fig. 2.19 Complete rupture of rotator cuff. (**a**) US coronal scan shows a complete tear of supraspinatus tendon; deltoid muscle (D), humerus (H), great tuberosity (GT), glenohumeral joint and subacromial-deltoid bursa effusion (f), acromion acoustic shadow (A). (**b**) In this case, MR shows the expansion of the articular capsule and subacromial-deltoid bursa (SE T1)

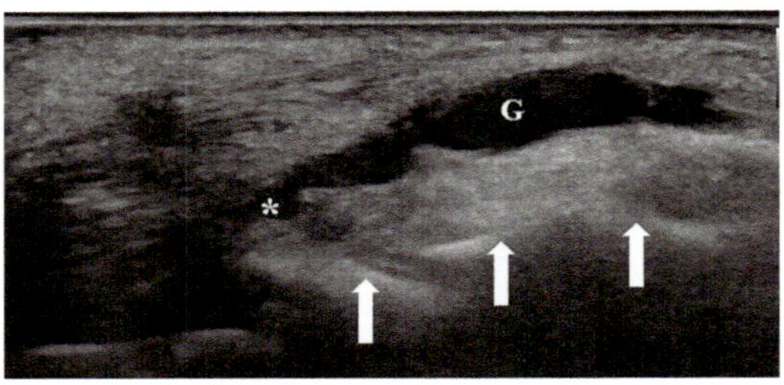

Fig. 2.20 Ganglion cyst of radiocarpal joint (G); peduncle (asterisk), bone surfaces (white arrows)

the synovial membrane of joints and that of mucosal bursae and of tenosynovial sheaths.

2.7 Meniscal Lesions

Currently, meniscal pathology is most often diagnosed based on history, clinical examination, magnetic resonance imaging, and/or arthroscopic visualization. As possible alternative to MRI, high-frequency ultrasound imaging has been reported to be a sensitive method for the evaluation of meniscal injuries and degenerative changes.

Usually MRI fails to identify the crystal deposits in or on the femoral hyaline cartilage, as can crystal depositions in the meniscus fibrocartilage, which conversely can be easily assessed by ultrasound (Fig. 2.21a and b). CPPD crystal deposits in the peripheral portion of the fibrocartilaginous menisci of the knee appear as centrally embedded hyperechoic deposits.

Meniscal pathologic findings are common among persons with knee osteoarthritis. In the knee joint, the menisci play a vital role in joint stability. Thus, mechanical impairment of the meniscus alters the weight-bearing capacities of the tibiofemoral compartments, contributing to the further progression of knee osteoarthritis. Degenerative changes and extrusion of meniscus are being frequently reported in patients with clinically symptomatic osteoarthritis of the knee. Degenerative changes of meniscus appear as loss of homogeneous echostructure, and linear or nodular hypoechoic or echogenic areas, which do not involve an articular surface.

Meniscal extrusion is referred to as meniscal bulging or external displacement with regard to the external aspect of the tibiofemoral compartment. It is thought to be a predictor of meniscal degeneration and tibiofemoral osteoarthritis. Ultrasound exhibits excellent diagnostic performance for the detection of meniscal extrusion compared with MRI. The medial meniscal extrusion assessment is performed using sonographic coronal section at the medial aspect of the knee,

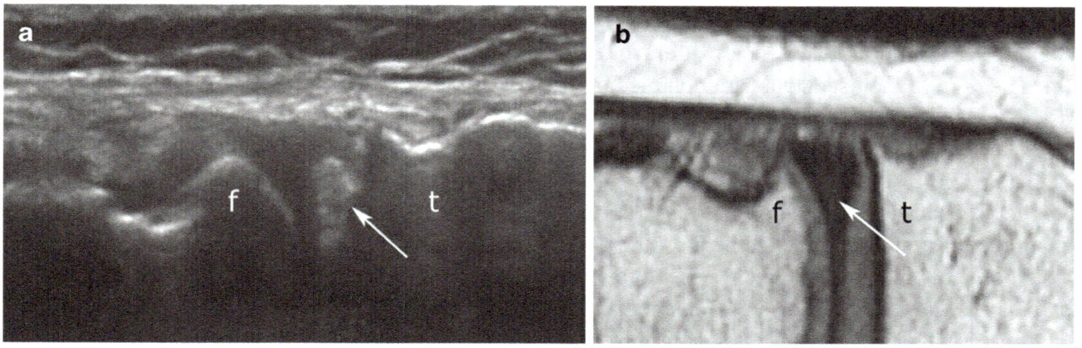

Fig. 2.21 (**a**) Knee ultrasound. Hyperechoic, oval shaped structure of CPPD deposition (arrow) is seen between lateral bony outlines of femur and tibia. (**b**) Knee MRI in same patient. CPPD deposition cannot be visualized by this MRI

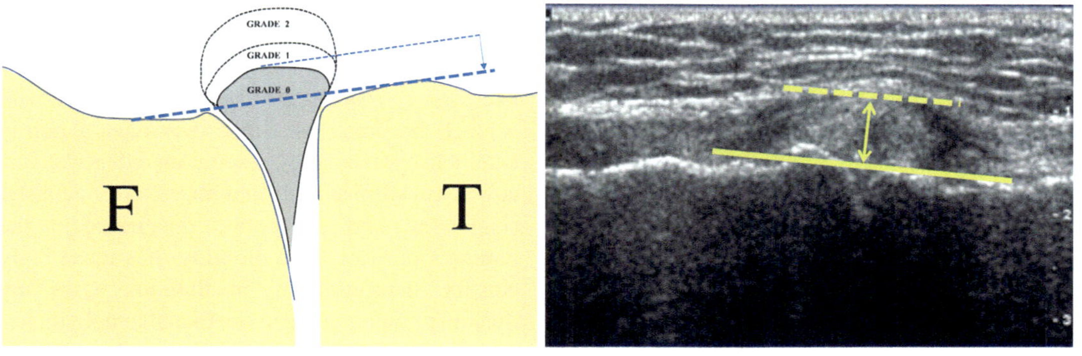

Fig. 2.22 Ultrasound evaluation of meniscal extrusion. A distance less than 2 mm is normal (grade 0), while the extrusion is moderate (grade 1) when the distance is between 2 and 4 mm, and is severe (grade 2) if it exceeds 4 mm

along the medial collateral ligament, with patient in supine position, and fully extended knee. A reference line is drawn tangent to the bone profile of medial aspect of femur and tibia at joint level (excluding osteophytes). The extent of meniscal extrusion can be assessed by semiquantitative grading system, based on the measurement of distance between the reference line and the most prominent point on external profile of meniscus. A distance less than 2 mm is normal (grade 0), while the extrusion is moderate (grade 1) when the distance is between 2 and 4 mm, and is severe (grade 2) if it exceeds 4 mm (Fig. 2.22a and b).

The meniscal cyst can represent a degenerative process of the meniscus, as a consequence of local mucoid degeneration. A fluid collection is formed in the meniscus which, through a horizontal cleavage, flows into the parameniscal soft tissues, forming a parameniscal cyst. Ultrasound has proven to be a sensitive modality for detecting parameniscal cysts and also a useful tool for guiding the needle in its transcutaneous evacuation. It typically appears as an anechoic thin-walled cyst located in the parameniscal soft tissue. A meniscal horizontal tear, which probably communicates with the cyst, coexists not infrequently (Fig. 2.23). It is more common in the lateral compartment of the knee than in the medial one.

A meniscal tear is a disruption of the structure of the meniscus affecting its integrity and stability, and thus its ability to absorb shock. Clinical examination still plays an important role in diagnosing meniscal tears, but accurate diagnosis depends upon imaging, which is largely represented by MR imaging as "gold standard" for confirming and assessing meniscal tears. Ultrasound is another, less used, useful diagnostic test for assessing meniscal tears (Fig. 2.24). The highest sensitivity and accuracy of ultrasound in the detection of meniscal tears are obtained in the assessment of the horizontal tear and complex one; instead, the radial tear is almost never detected.

Meniscocapsular separation results from disruption of the meniscotibial ligaments of the posterior horn of the medial meniscus, frequently associated with anterior cruciate ligament damage. This meniscal injury, also called ramp lesion, when mild, can be responsible for persistent gonalgia; it may escape the MRI assessment and be difficult to detect in arthroscopy. Instead, ultrasonography can be not only diagnostically useful, but also useful in assisting arthroscopic surgery. In summary, the ultrasound does not represent the first-level imaging for detecting meniscal diseases, surely surpassed by the MRI in this role, but it can certainly participate usefully in their diagnosis, particularly in meniscocapsular separation.

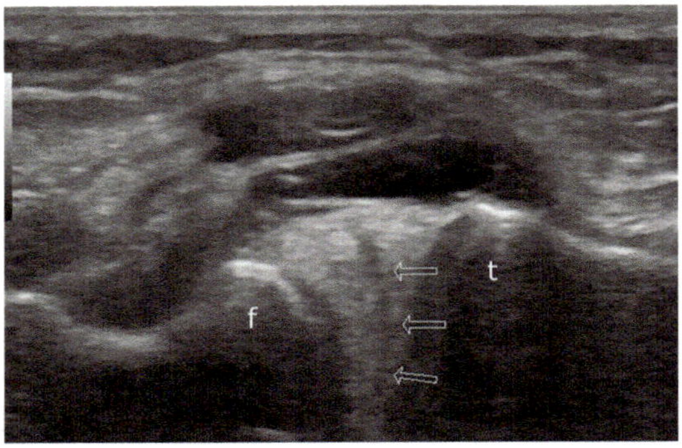

Fig. 2.23 Ultrasound appearance of a horizontal meniscal tear (arrows) seen between the bony outlines of femur (f) and tibia (t)

2.8 Endoarticular Loose Bodies

These can be found in all joints but mostly the knee, where they can be easily detected when located in the suprapatellar recess. Loose bodies occur in several pathologies such as osteochondritis dissecans, osteochondral fractures, osteonecrosis, osteoarthritis, and synovial osteochondromatosis. Since they have a highly calcified content, they appear on US as hyperechoic curvilinear bodies, with posterior acoustic shadowing, and are mobile, depending on the patient's position. The mobility of a loose body can be demonstrated, in dubious cases, by dynamic passive maneuvers that also help differentiate it from gross osteophytes. When a loose body contains osteochondral tissue, the cartilaginous covering (hypoechoic) can be differentiated from the bony component (Fig. 2.25a–c).

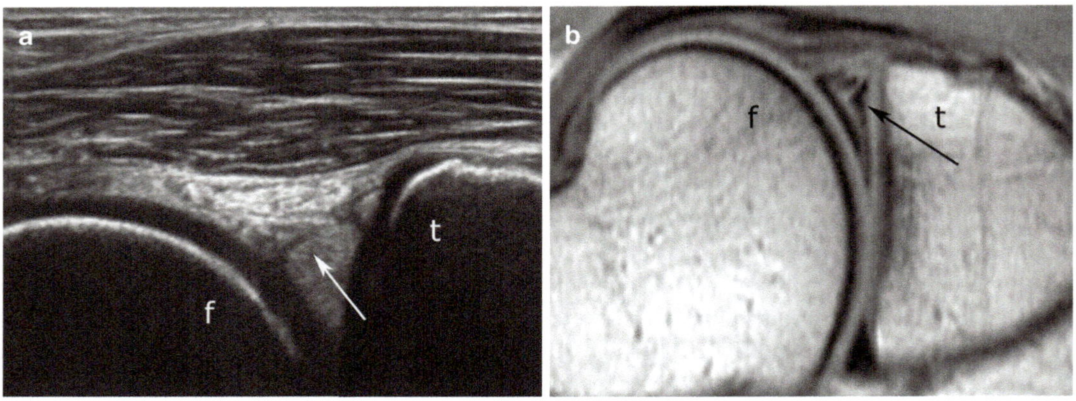

Fig. 2.24 Ultrasound (**a**) and MRI (**b**) appearance of an oblique meniscal tear (arrow). Note that ultrasound is able to clearly visualize the superficial aspect of the tear but offers a really poor detection of its deeper aspect. *f* femur; *t* tibia

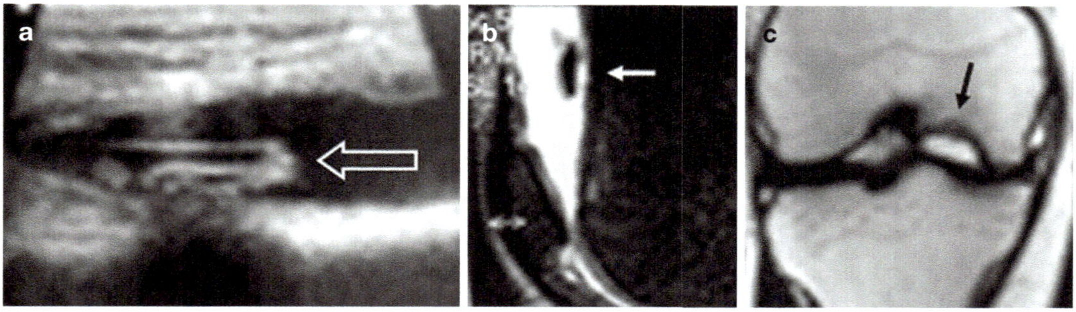

Fig. 2.25 Loose endoarticular osteochondral body in the suprapatellar recess. (**a**) The US scan shows a double-layered loose body (empty white arrow) due to its dual composition (cartilage and bone). The MR scan (fat suppression technique) (**b**) confirms the presence of the loose body in the suprapatellar recess (white arrow) and (**c**) shows the osteochondral detachment location (black arrow) on the femoral condyle (TSE T2)

Further Readings

Bianchi S, Martinoli C. Detection of loose bodies in joints. Radiol Clin North Am. 1999;37:679–90.

Bianchi S, Martinoli C, Bianchi-Zamorani M, Valle M. Ultrasound of the joints. Eur Radiol. 2002;12:56–61.

Cardinal E, Buckwalter KA, Braunstein EM, Mih AD. Occult dorsal carpal ganglion: comparison of US and MR imaging. Radiology. 1994;193:259–62.

Carotti M, Salaffi F, Manganelli P, et al. Power Doppler sonography in the assessment of synovial tissue of the knee joint in rheumatoid arthritis: a preliminary experience. Ann Rheum Dis. 2002;61:877–88.

De Flaviis L, Musso MG. Hand and wrist. Clin Diagn Ultrasound. 1995;30:151–78.

Fitzgerald O, Bresnihan B. Synovial vascularity is increased in rheumatoid arthritis: comment on the article by Stivens et al. (letter). Arthritis Rheum. 1992;35:1540–1.

Gibbon WW. Applications of ultrasound in arthritis. Semin Musculoskelet Radiol. 2004;8:313–28.

Gibbon WW, Wakefield RJ. Ultrasound in inflammatory disease. Radiol Clin North Am. 1999;37:633–51.

Grobbelaar N, Bouffard JA. Sonography of the Knee, a pictorial review. Semin Ultrasound CT MR. 2000;21:231–74.

Hlavacek M. The role of synovial fluid filtration by cartilage in lubrification synovial joints. Squeeze film lubrification: homogeneous filtration. J Biomech. 1993;26:1151–60.

Klauser A, Frauscher F, Schirmer M, et al. The value of contrast enhanced color Doppler ultrasound in the detection of vascularization of finger joint in patients with rheumatoid arthritis. Arthritis Rheum. 2002;46:647–53.

Klauser A, Demharten J, De Marchi A, et al. Contrast enhanced gray-scale sonography in assessment of joint vascularity in rheumatoid arthritis: result from the IACUS study group. Eur Radiol. 2005;15:2404–10.

Mahdy NS, Sakr HM, Allam AE. The role of ultrasound in evaluation of meniscal injury. Egypt J Hosp Med. 2018;72(10):5490–4.

Martino F, Angelelli G, Ettorre GC, et al. Aspetto normale della borsa sovrarotulea nell'ecografia del ginocchio. Radiol Med. 1992;83:43–8.

Newman JS, Adler R, Bude RO, Rubin J. Detection of soft-tissue hyperemia: value of power Doppler sonography. AJR Am J Roentgenol. 1994;163:385–9.

Nogueira-Barbosa MH, Gregio-Junior E, Lorenzato MM, Guermazi A, Roemer FW, Chagas-Neto FA, Crema MD. Ultrasound assessment of medial meniscal extrusion: a validation study using MRI as reference standard. AJR Am J Roentgenol. 2015;204(3):584–8.

Roberts D, Miller TT, Erlanger SM. Sonographic appearance of primary synovial chondromatosis of the knee. J Ultrasound Med. 2004;23:707–9.

Schmidt WA, Volker L, Zacher J, et al. Colour Doppler ultrasonography to detect pannus in knee joint synovitis. Clin Exp Rheumatol. 2000;18:439–44.

Shetty AA, Tindall AJ, James KD, Relwani J, Fernando KW. Accuracy of hand-held ultrasound scanning in detecting meniscal tears. J Bone Joint Surg Br. 2008 Aug;90(8):1045–8.

Silvestri E, Martinoli C, Onetto F, et al. Valutazione dell'artrite reumatoide del ginocchio con color Doppler. Radiol Med. 1994;88:364–7.

Steiner E, Steinbach LS, Schnarkowski P, et al. Ganglia and cysts around joints. Radiol Clin North Am. 1996;34:395–425.

Szkudlarek M, Court-Payen M, Strandberg C, et al. Power Doppler ultrasonography for assessment of synovitis in the metacarpophalangeal joints of patients with Rheumatoid Arthritis: a comparison with dynamic magnetic resonance imaging. Arthritis Rheum. 2001;44(9):2018–23.

Taljanovic MS, Sheppard JE, Jones MD, Switlick DN, Hunter TB, Rogers LF. Sonography and sonoarthrography of the scapholunate and lunotriquetral ligaments and TFC: initial experience and correlation with arthrography and magnetic resonance arthrography. J Ultrasound Med. 2008;27(2):179–91.

Teefey SA, Middleton WD, Patel V, et al. The accuracy of high-resolution ultrasound for evaluating focal lesions of the hand and wrist. J Hand Surg. 2004;29:393–9.

Hesham El Sheikh, Mohamed H. Faheem, Ahmed K. Abdelmoeim. Role of ultrasonographic examination of the knee in evaluation of meniscal injury in correlation with magnetic resonance imaging. BMFJ. 2021;38:90–7.

Van Holsbeeck MT, Introcaso JH. Musculoskeletal ultrasound. 2nd ed. Maryland Heights: Mosby; 2001.

Van Holsbeeck M, Strouse PJ. Sonography of the shoulder: evaluation of the subacromial-subdeltoid bursa. AJR. 1993;160:561–4.

Walsh DA. Angiogenesis and arthritis. Rheumatology. 1999;38:103–12.

Wang SC, Chen RK, Cardinal E, Cho KH. Joint sonography. Radiol Clin North Am. 1999;37:653–68.

Tendons and Ligaments

3

Davide Orlandi, Umberto Viglino,
and Elena Massone

Contents

3.1 Sonographic and Doppler Normal Anatomy

Tendons are critical biomechanical units in the musculoskeletal system, the function of which is to transmit the muscular tension to mobile skeletal segments. They are extremely resistant to traction, almost like bone. A tendon with a 10 mm^2 transverse section can bear a maximum of 600–1000 kg. On the other hand, tendons are not very elastic, and can only tolerate a maximum elongation of 6% before being damaged.

Tendons have very slow metabolism, even during action. This can be significantly increased only by inflammatory conditions and traumas. When a reparative process occurs, a proliferation of fibrocytes is observed with deposition of collagen cells.

Tendons macroscopically appear as ribbon-like structures, with extremely variable shape and

D. Orlandi (✉)
Department of Radiology, Ospedale Evangelico Internazionale, Genova, Italy

U. Viglino
Postgraduate School of Radiology, Genoa University, Genova, Italy

E. Massone
Department of Radiology, Ospedale Santa Corona, Pietra Ligure (SV), Italy

F. Martino et al. (eds.), *Musculoskeletal Ultrasound in Orthopedic and Rheumatic disease in Adults*,
https://doi.org/10.1007/978-3-030-91202-4_3

dimensions, characterized by the presence of dense fibrous tissue arranged in parallel bundles.

More specifically, they consist of about 70% of type I collagen fibers that form primary bundles. Among the primary bundles are fibrocytes endowed with large laminar protrusions, named tenocytes or alar cells. Among the collagen fibers of tendons, elastic fibers (about 4%) can also be found; their role is not different from that of a "shock absorber" when muscular contraction begins. The collagen and elastic fibers both have the same direction as the main lines of force and lie in a gel consisting of proteoglycans and water. The primary bundles are assembled to form secondary bundles (representing the tendon's functional unit), which are clustered in tertiary bundles.

The endotenon is a thin connective strip surrounding the primary, secondary, and tertiary bundles, and separating them. Vessels and nerves run within the endotenon thickness. The epitenon is a stronger connective covering, surrounding the whole tendon (Fig. 3.1).

From a functional and anatomical point of view, tendons can be divided into two types: supporting tendons (or anchor tendons) and sliding tendons. Anchor tendons (such as the Achilles and the patellar tendon) are typically bigger and stronger than sliding tendons; they are not provided with a synovial sheath, but they are surrounded by a connective lamina external to the epitenon, called peritenon; the two connective sheaths (epitenon and peritenon) form the paratenon together with highly vascularized adipose and areolar tissue (Fig. 3.2).

Sliding tendons are wrapped in a covering sheath (tenosynovial sheath) whose function is to guarantee better sliding and protection to the tendons when they run adjacent to irregular osseous surfaces, sites of potential friction. The tenosynovial sheath consists of two layers: a visceral layer, and a strictly connected synovial "fold" named mesotenon. A closed cavity, nearly virtual, containing a very small amount of synovial fluid, is found between the two layers (Fig. 3.3a).

The tenosynovial sheath of sliding tendons corresponds anatomically and functionally to the peritenon of anchor tendons and, similarly, the tenosynovial sheath and the epitenon together constitute the paratenon of the sliding tendon.

The vascularization varies according to the type of tendon. In sliding tendons, the vessels run within the mesotenon, the mentioned synovial "fold," which connects the parietal and visceral layers.

The vessels pass therefore along the tendon's surface, where some arterioles arising from the vessels penetrate into the tendon following the course of connective laminae (Fig. 3.3b).

On the other hand, the vessels of the anchor tendons constitute a thick and irregular anastomotic net within the paratenon. Arteriolar vessels arise from this net and penetrate inside the tendon to different levels, following the course of the connective laminae. The arterioles, within these connective structures, form vascular arcades with the nearby arterioles. Tendons may present with less vascularized zones, named critical areas, which are extremely important in the pathogenesis of several tendon diseases. Examples include the pre-insertional area of the supraspinatus tendon of the shoulder, or the central part of the Achilles tendon, which typically constitutes highly susceptible sites of degenerative disease and tendon rupture.

The points of union between the tendons and the muscle or the bone are named myotendinous junction and osteotendinous junction (enthesis), respectively. The myotendinous junction is usually well defined: at this level the tendon fibers are intertwined with the endomysium fibers. The osteotendinous junction has a more complicated structure: its nature may be either fibrous or fibrocartilaginous according to the tendon mobility, the angle formed between the tendon fibers and the bone, and the presence of an underlying retinaculum. The tendons moving in a single spatial plane and whose insertion on the bone occurs with an acute angle (e.g., flexor tendons of the toes) have a fibrous enthesis. The same situation occurs for tendons whose course is modified and kept in position by a retinaculum—for example the peroneal tendons—and whose insertion on the bone once again forms an acute angle.

The tendons controlling multiplanar movement (e.g., Achilles tendon) and whose insertion

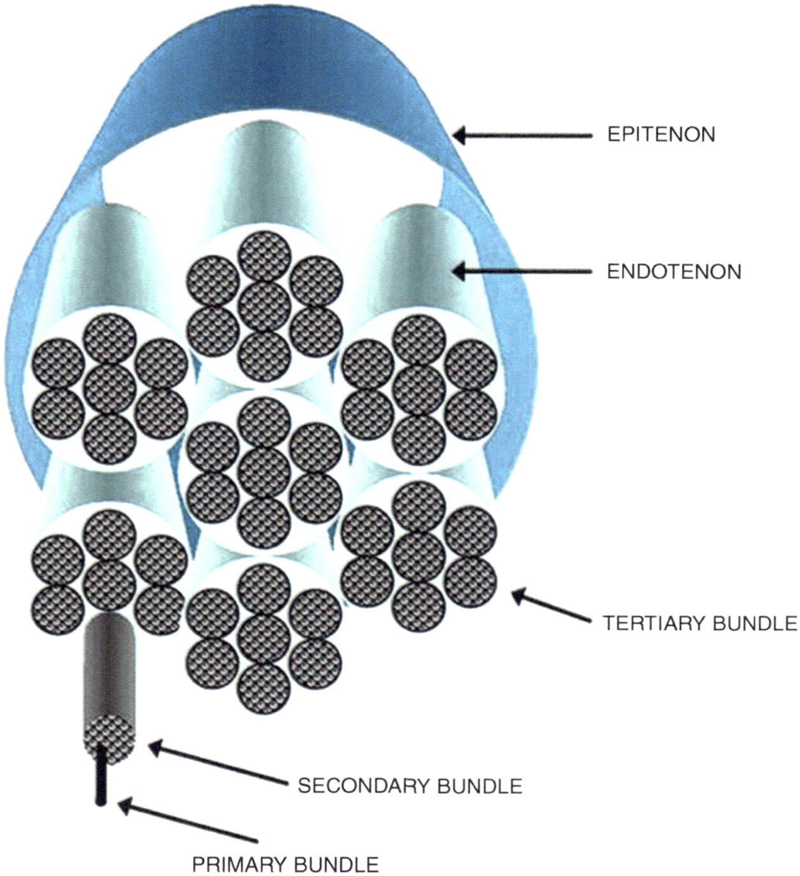

Fig. 3.1 Anatomical drawing of a tendon

on the bone surface is orthogonal have a thick fibrocartilaginous enthesis that minimizes the risk of tendon tear. This more complicated type of osteotendinous junction consists of four layers in quick succession, represented—from the most superficial to the deepest one—by tendinous tissue, fibrocartilage, calcified fibrocartilage, and bone. The osteotendinous junction is well vascularized and the paratenon vascular net is anastomosed with that of the periosteum.

A retinaculum is a transversal thickening of the deep fascia attached to a bone's eminence. The biomechanical function of a retinaculum is to keep the tendons in position as they pass underneath it, in order to avoid their dislocation during muscular action. Retinacula therefore guarantee that tendons are correctly deviated and kept in position in their respective osteofibrous canals, allowing their efficient action; the synovial sheath, which always covers these types of tendons, makes the sliding of a tendon easy, and reduces friction. Retinacula are typically found in the wrist and ankle. Some examples are the transverse carpal ligament, which defines the superior aspect of the carpal tunnel, where the flexor digitorum tendons and the median nerve run, and the ankle retinacula, which stabilize the flexor and extensor tendons in their deflection points. Some specific types of retinacula are found in the fingers, where the flexor digitorum tendons, wrapped in the synovial sheath, run along osteofibrous canals extending from the palm of the hand to the distal phalanx. The superior aspect of these osteofibrous canals (the "vault") consists of archlike fibers running over the tendons, in points where more stabilization is needed. For their peculiar biomechanical function, these structures are named flexor annular pulleys. On the contrary,

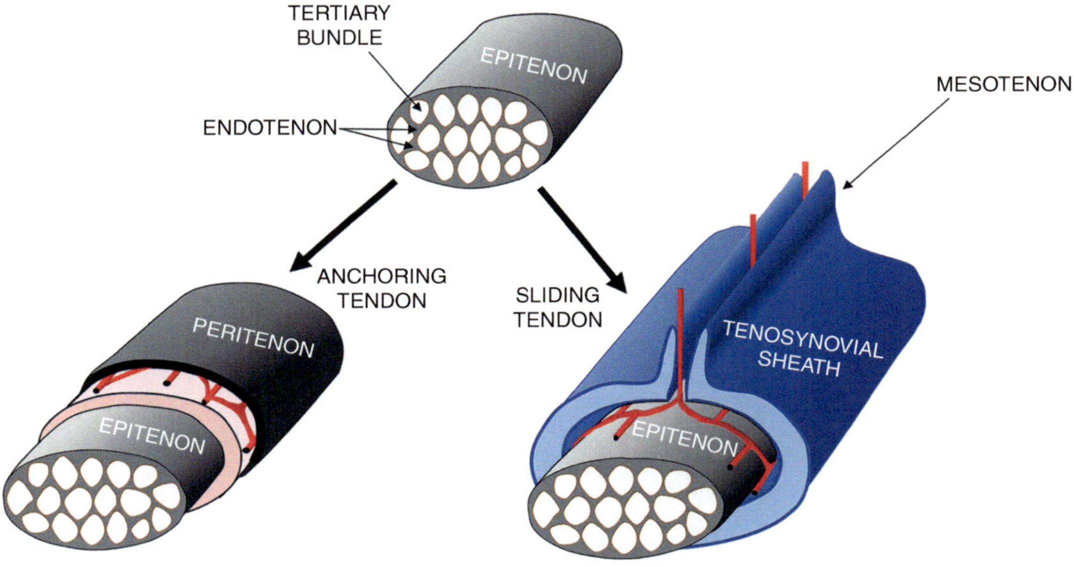

Fig. 3.2 Schematic drawing of the tendon sheaths. The tendons are differentiated into anchoring tendons and sliding tendons, depending on the structure of the sheath enclosing it. The sheath of the anchor tendon is named epitenon, while that of the sliding tendon is called tenosynovial sheath. The epitenon is constituted by a strong superficial covering, of dense fibrous connective tissue, under which the vascular network runs, embedded in loose connective tissue (colored pink in the figure). The synovial sheath is made up of two serous sheaths that delimit the synovial space, containing the synovial fluid that guarantees slipping. The blood vessels are distributed around the tendon below the synovial sheath, with vascular peduncles afferent through the mesotenon

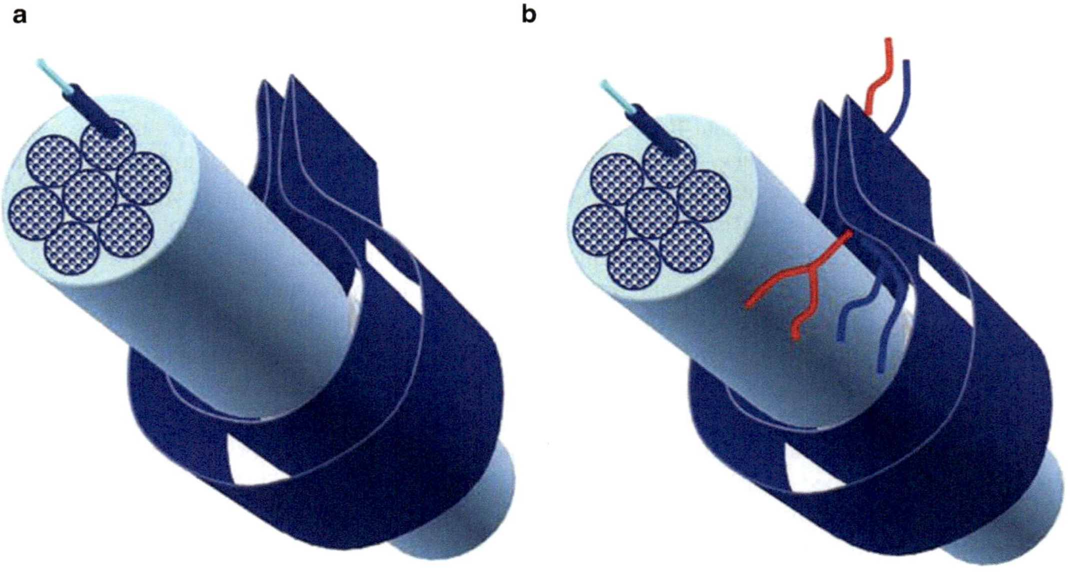

Fig. 3.3 Anatomy (**a**) and vascularization (**b**) of a sliding tendon. Vessels arise from mesotenon

in regions where the canal needs to be more flexible, in order to allow the flexion of joints, a device consisting of loose plaited fibers is present, providing support to the tendon sheath without fixing it.

Ligaments have an analogous structure to that of tendons; however, they are thinner and they contain a higher amount of elastin, which is a necessary element to supply these structures with some degree of elasticity for their very important biomechanical role in the stabilization of joints.

There are two types of ligaments: the intrinsic capsular ligaments, which appear as localized thickenings within the capsule with a strengthening function, and the extrinsic ligaments, which are independent from the fibrous capsule and can be further classified as extracapsular and intracapsular ligaments.

Nowadays US represents the gold standard technique for the assessment of tendons. With the advent, for clinical purposes, of high-resolution transducers and specific image processing software, it became possible to make detailed analysis of the shape and structure of tendons. In addition, US is the only technique that allows the radiologist to perform a dynamic study of tendons, which is extremely important for the diagnosis of tendon pathology. In longitudinal ultrasound views (long axis), the tendons appear as echoic ribbon-like bands, defined by a marginal hyperechoic line corresponding to the paratenon and characterized by a fibrillar internal structure.

The fibrillar echotexture is represented by a succession of thin hyperechoic parallel bands, slightly wavy, which tend to grow apart from one another when the tendon is released and to move closer when the tendon is tense. This fibrillar echostructure is caused by the specular reflections within the tendon determined by the existing acoustic interface between the endotenon septa (Fig. 3.4a).

The number and thickness of such structures change depending on the frequency of the transducer. In transversal views (short axis) tendons appear as round or oval shaped structures, characterized by several homogeneously scattered spotty echoes (Fig. 3.4b).

In transverse views the Achilles tendon thickness (anteroposterior diameter) can be best assessed. In transverse section the Achilles tendon is elliptical, with its major axis following an oblique anteromedial direction. The sonographer must be aware of the risk of overestimating tendon thickness when assessed on longitudinal scans. When evaluating a tendon by US, it is extremely important to apply a correct orthogonal direction to the US beam, both for longitudinal and axial views. When the US beam is not orthogonal to the tendon course, both a decrease of the reflected echoes and an increase of the diffracted ones occur, resulting in a significant or partial reduction of the tendon echotexture (tendon anisotropy). This artifact is more frequently found when assessing the rotator cuff tendons of the shoulder, the quadriceps femoris, the patellar and Achilles tendons, the osteotendinous junctions, and the flexor and extensor tendons of the ankle, hand, and wrist. In these regions a less experienced sonographer can risk making an incorrect diagnosis (Fig. 3.5).

The sliding and anchor tendons present some differences regarding their US appearance. Sliding tendons, as already described, are wrapped in a synovial sheath which contains, even in physiological situations, a minimum amount of synovial fluid acting as a lubricant. This slight film of fluid can be easily recognized, both in axial views and in longitudinal views, as a thin anechoic halo surrounding the tendon. The pathological increase in synovial fluid inside the tendon sheath often allows the mesotenon to be identified. On the other hand, anchor tendons are surrounded by the peritenon, a layer of dense connective tissue leaning on the epitenon, which contributes to constitute the paratenon. The paratenon appears as an echoic line surrounding the tendon, without the possibility of distinguishing, in normal conditions, between peritenon and epitenon. High-resolution ultrasound is performed to study the inflammatory pathology of tendons in order to depict the morphological and structural variety of tendons and the synovial sheath expansion. The grayscale ultrasound technique is still not able to recognize indirect signs

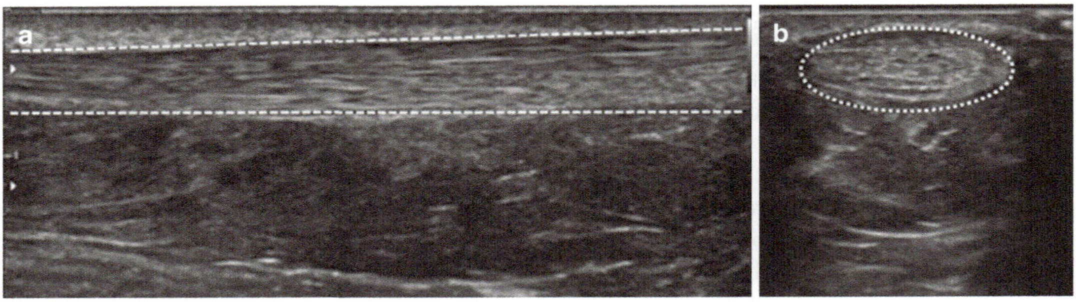

Fig. 3.4 Ultrasound anatomy of normal tendon: (**a**) long axis; (**b**) short axis

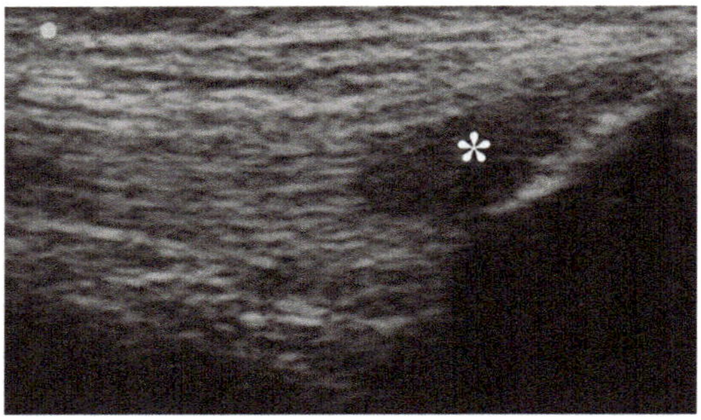

Fig. 3.5 Longitudinal US scan of relaxed quadriceps tendon in a healthy man. The hypoechoic spot (*) (tendon anisotropy) corresponds to the pre-insertional area

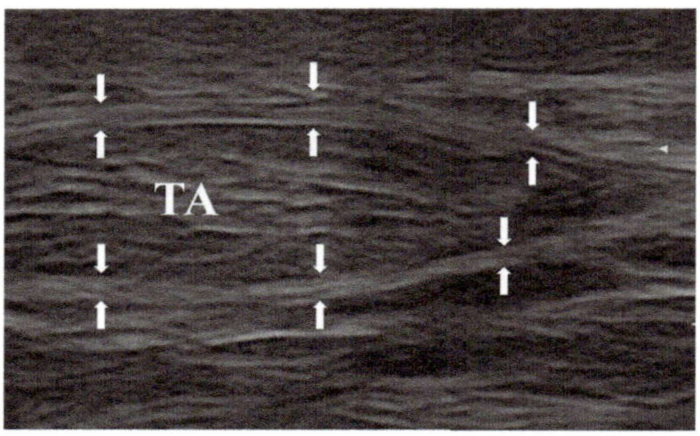

Fig. 3.6 Transverse anterior US scan (22 MHz) of the ankle. The retinaculum (white arrows) is the thin hyperechoic line that lies around the tendon. *TA* tibialis anterior tendon

of inflammation and needs to be implemented by power Doppler evaluation.

Retinacula at ultrasound appear as thin hyperechoic structures located more superficially than the sliding tendons, in very critical areas from a biomechanical point of view (Fig. 3.6).

Annular pulleys are biomechanical devices made of fibrous connective tissue, which keep the flexor digitorum tendons in position during flexion-extension movements. For this reason, the sonographic assessment of the pulleys has to be performed with a dynamic method; the US dynamic analysis should be obtained during flexion-extension movements of the fingers and, if a tendon tear is suspected, it should be supplemented with contrasted flexion. The transducer should always have a perpendicular and transverse position over the flexor tendons, with a high amount of gel used as a spacer in order to avoid any pressure on the tissue. In longitudinal views of flexor tendons, the pulley appears as a thin oval structure lying superficially compared with the tendon sheath (Fig. 3.7).

The structure of ligaments is very similar to that of tendons; the main differences are reduced thickness and a less regular arrangement of structural elements; for this reason, it is harder to study ligaments with US than tendons. The US examination of ligaments, unlike tendons, is mainly performed using long-axis views, the transducer being aligned on the ligament's major axis. Transverse views (short axis) have poor diagnostic value.

With US, ligaments appear as homogeneous, hyperechoic bands, 2–3 mm thick, lying close to the bone (Fig. 3.8a, b).

The easiest ligaments to assess with US are those of the medial and lateral compartments of the ankle (deltoid, anterior talofibular, and fibulocalcaneal), the collateral ligaments of the knee, the collateral and annular ligaments of the elbow, the coracoacromial and coracohumeral ligaments of the shoulder, and the ulnar collateral ligament of the thumb. The medial collateral ligament of the knee (MCL) has a very complicated structure that deserves detailed description. The MCL is a flattened, large structure extending from the distal extremity of the medial femoral condyle to the proximal tibial extremity; it is about 9 cm long and it is divided into two components, deep and superficial, which are separated by a thin layer of loose connective tissue. The deep component is then divided into two small ligaments that fix the medial meniscus, respectively, to the femur (menisco-femoral ligament) and to the tibia (menisco-tibial ligament). Sonographically the MCL appears as a trilaminar structure consisting of two hyperechoic layers, separated by a central interleaved hypoechoic area. The hyperechoic bands correspond to deep and superficial fiber bundles, whereas the loose areolar tissue constitutes the hypoechoic central area that divides the superficial component from the deep one (Fig. 3.9).

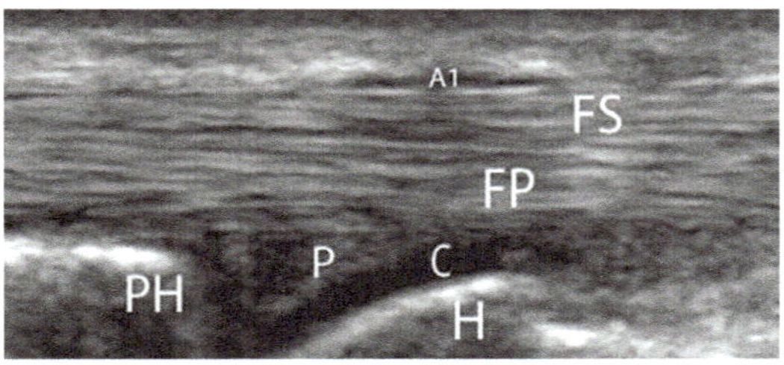

Fig. 3.7 Longitudinal US scan of flexor digitorum tendons at the metacarpophalangeal joint. The first (A1) out of five pulleys is clearly shown over the tendons. *FP* flexor digitorum profundus; *FS* flexor digitorum superficialis; *PH* proximal phalanx; *H* metacarpal head; *P* palmar plate; *C* cartilage

By implementing the information obtained from a grayscale ultrasound examination with that obtained from a power Doppler study, the sonographer is able to identify functional parameters regarding the vascularization of the tendons for a better clinical evaluation. In standard conditions, tendons have low metabolic activity and the blood supply is given by high-resistance arteries and small veins, too thin to be studied with the Doppler technique. In such cases, weak flow signals can be observed near small arterial structures afferent to the cortical bone. These vascular structures are usually arteries with a high resistance index, corresponding to the periosteal vessels. Several conditions such as inflammatory, post-traumatic, and infectious are responsible for the activation of vascular hyperemia with an increase in blood flow and a drop in vascular resistance. In this way the tendon vessels become easy to assess with color or power Doppler technique and it is also possible to perform a semiquantitative flow analysis of pulsed-wave Doppler ultrasound spectrum (Fig. 3.10).

A recently developed imaging technique, sonoelastography (SEL), allows for qualitative visual or quantitative measurements of the mechanical properties of tissues. It is based on the principle for which, applying an extrinsic (mechanical or physical) stress, it is possible to induce changes in a determined tissue, depending on the elastic properties of the tissue itself; hence, qualitative and/or quantitative measurements of the elastic changes induced through

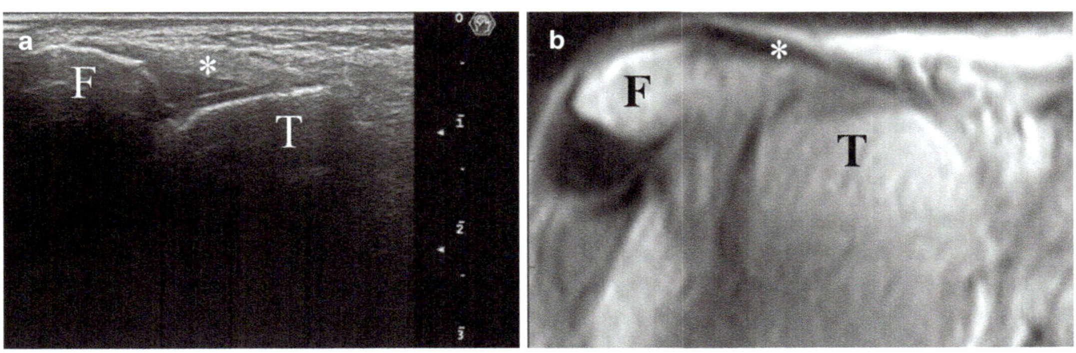

Fig. 3.8 (**a**, **b**) Transverse fusion US-MR scan of the lateral ankle compartment showing the course of the anterior talo-fibular ligament (*) *F* fibula; *T* talus

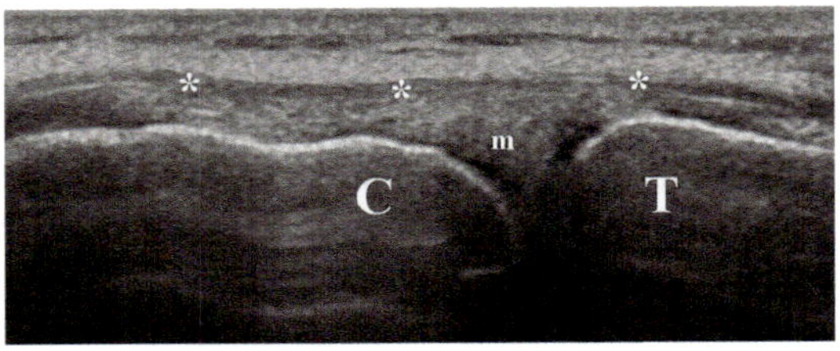

Fig. 3.9 Longitudinal US scan of the medial side of the knee: medial collateral ligament; asterisks = superficial component; *C* femoral condyle; *T* tibial plateau; *m* meniscus

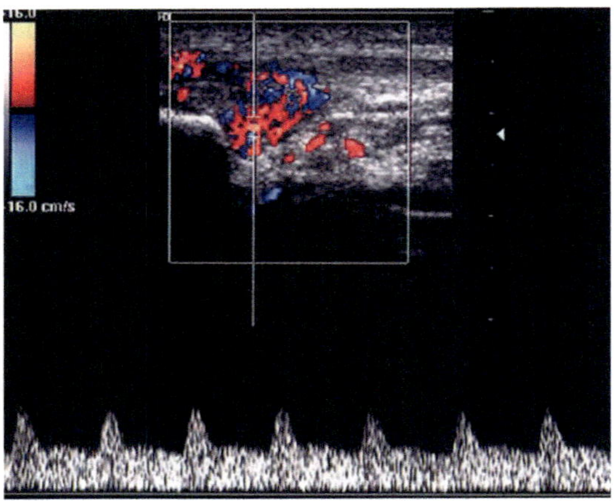

Fig. 3.10 Color Doppler scan in jumper's knee. Peri- and intratendinous hypervascularization of the proximal third of the tendon is clearly shown. The spectral analysis shows arteries with low resistance and high diastolic flow

the tissue could be obtained, usually by means of an ultrasound transducer in clinical practice. EUS could detect or differentiate an early-stage alteration which could progress to higher stages of tendinopathy, providing supplementary information useful for diagnostic, therapeutic (ultrasound-guided procedures), and follow-up purposes.

Two main types of SEL have become established in clinical practice, in particular for musculoskeletal evaluation:

- *Strain elastography*: It is also described as "quasi-static elastography," "compression elastography," and "real-time elastography." The stress is applied by repeated manual compression of the transducer, and the amount of tissue deformation (strain) relative to the surrounding normal tissue is measured, usually with a tracking algorithm working on the radiofrequency data. The resulting data can then be used to form an image that is coded in color or grayscale to show the pattern of strain, which is inversely related to tissue stiffness and can be assessed subjectively. These are qualitative data; however, regions of interest (ROIs) can be positioned over target areas in the screen in order to obtain semiquantitative analysis (Fig. 3.11).
- *Shear-wave elastography*: It is a very potential technique for the noninvasive quantification of tissue stiffness. Shear waves in the body can be induced by various methods, including physiological motion, external mechanical excitation, or acoustic radiation force (by a focused ultrasound beam). Shear waves are transverse; they are rapidly attenuated by tissue, they travel much more slowly (between 1 and 10 m/s), and they are not supported by liquids of low viscosity. Using a real-time imaging modality such as ultrasound (but also magnetic resonance), the underlying tissue stiffness can be estimated measuring the produced shear-wave speeds. Their speed is commonly expressed in meters per second (m/s); it is closely related to the modulus of elasticity of the tissue, and there is a simplified formula for converting between the shear-wave speed and the elastic modulus of the tissue to locally quantify its stiffness in kilopascals (kPa). In contrast to strain elastography, this technique allows for the performance of quantitative analysis of the tissue stiffness (Fig. 3.12).

In strain elastography, data acquisition and interpretation of elasticity images are largely dependent on the "operators'" experience and skills. In contrast, the quantitative nature of shear-wave elastography is an advantage and seems to let this technique be more reproducible; the fact that the system displaces the tissue could improve consistency since the examiner does not need to move the transducer.

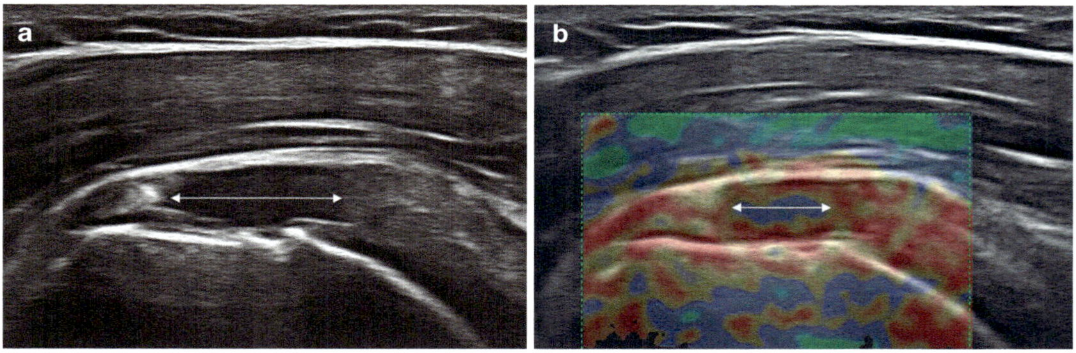

Fig. 3.11 Strain elastography. Qualitative analysis: the modulus of elasticity of the soft tissue scanned in the B-mode image (**a**) is represented by a superimposed color-coded map (**b**) in which (in this case) the lower values are depicted in green and the higher ones in red; in this case the elastogram helps in a more precise quantification of a supraspinatus tendon tear (double-headed arrow)

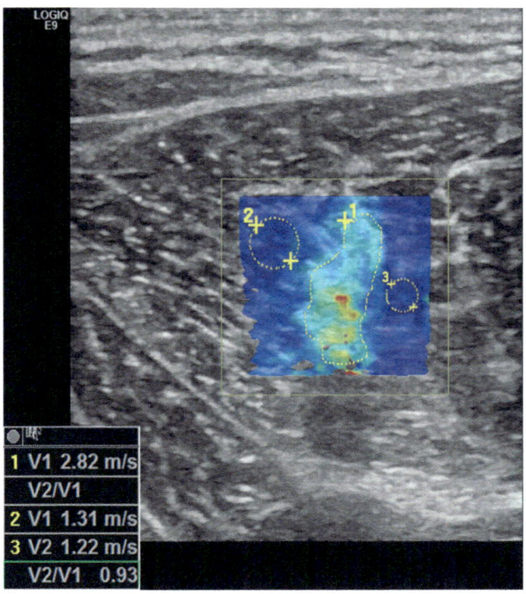

Fig. 3.12 Shear-wave elastography of rectus femoris muscle: after the generation of the "pushing" beam by the transducer, the values of the shear modulus in the targeted area are represented by means of a color-coded map set. It is possible to get also a quantitative analysis of the investigated tissue by placing some ROIs (with modifiable dimensions) over the map and get the corresponding value at the left bottom angle of the screen

3.2 Paratenonitis

Nowadays, US is the imaging tool of first choice for the study of tendons. Compared to other imaging techniques, such as MR, US allows static evaluation, with a highly detailed representation of the intrinsic anatomic structure of tendons and a dynamic evaluation, which is an extremely important element for an accurate diagnosis. Tendons are divided, from an anatomic and functional point of view, into two types: (1) ***supporting tendons*** and (2) ***sliding tendons***.

This distinction is extremely important in order to understand the most common pathological conditions, both rheumatological and traumatic. In inflammatory tendinopathies all the layers of the tendons are involved (paratenonitis), while the tendon's parenchyma (collagen fibers, proteoglycans) is usually only affected in degenerative conditions (tendinosis), where the two pathologic conditions often coexist.

Moreover, paratenonitis can be distinguished in tenosynovitis and peritendinitis, according to the specific involvement of sliding tendons or supporting tendons. Inflammatory and degenerative involvement of the osteotendinous junction is called enthesopathy and is very common in seronegative spondyloarthritis, but it can also be the expression of a microcrystalline arthropathy, or the result of chronic functional overuse of the osteotendinous junction. Tendon tears and dislocations usually follow mechanical overload which exceeds the resistance threshold of the system, the latter being the final expression of a potential instability of sliding tendons lying in critical areas.

Tendon cysts represent quite a common condition, frequently found in the hand and causing painful swelling.

3.2.1 Tenosynovitis

Tenosynovitis is an inflammatory process affecting the tenosynovial sheath. Tenosynovitis can be classified as *acute, subacute, or chronic*, while from a pathologic point of view they are distinguished in exudative, proliferative, and mixed forms. Even though the clinical diagnosis of tenosynovitis may seem easy, the distinction between the different pathologic forms can instead be difficult without US examination, which allows an easy and quick diagnosis to be made.

A peculiar form of tenosynovitis is the chronic stenosing tenosynovitis, affecting biomechanically critical anatomic regions. An exudative tenosynovitis can be easily diagnosed by means of US. In this case, an increase of fluid is seen within the tenosynovial sheath appearing as an anechoic halo surrounding the tendon in axial views, and lying along the tendon course in longitudinal views, frequently with a fusiform appearance (Fig. 3.13a, b).

Sometimes increased echogenicity of the tenosynovial fluid collection may be observed, due to the presence of clusters of leukocytes, fibrin, cholesterol, uric acid, calcium pyrophosphate, or hydroxyapatite crystals. This hyperechoic appearance may create doubts about the diagnosis of exudative tenosynovitis and, in such cases, compression made with the transducer may help to confirm the liquid nature of the finding. Power Doppler analysis gives no evidence of vascular signal; therefore it can be used to complement the information obtained with grayscale US. It should be pointed out that in some anatomical locations, the tenosynovial sheath may be in communication with the joint cavity. For example, the tenosynovial sheaths of the flexor hallucis longus tendon at the ankle and the long head of biceps tendon at the shoulder are in communication with the tibiotalar and glenohumeral joint. In these cases, when the sheath is expanded with fluid the presence of a joint fluid collection must be considered. In proliferative tenosynovitis hypertrophic proliferation of the synovial tissue is observed, showing various degrees of echogenicity (Fig. 3.14).

Dynamic ultrasound examination and compression of the transducer performed by the operator are helpful to assess the solid nature of the finding. In these cases the power Doppler analysis is very useful to confirm the diagnosis by detecting vascular signals within a thickened tenosynovial sheath (Fig. 3.15a, b).

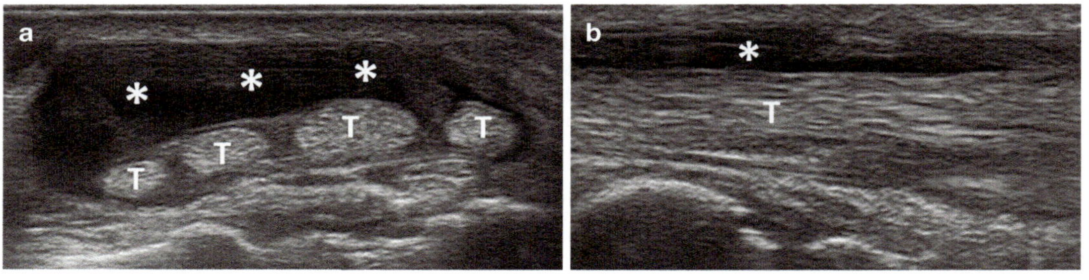

Fig. 3.13 (**a**) Transverse scan, dorsum of wrist: synovial effusion (asterisk) into IV compartment extensor tendons (T); (**b**) longitudinal view

The degree of vascularization is strictly related to the severity of the inflammation and to the "activity" of the synovial proliferation. These forms of tenosynovitis are often an extra-articular expression of some rheumatic diseases such as rheumatoid arthritis. Mixed tenosynovitis is the most common form of tenosynovitis. It is characterized by the simultaneous presence of both synovial fluid and proliferative thickening of the synovial membrane within the sheath. The US pattern shows several echoic spots of synovial tissue jutting from the sheath expanded by anechoic fluid (Fig. 3.16).

In order to differentiate fluid from the proliferating tissue it is very useful to apply compression with the transducer. In dubious cases the two components can also be distinguished with power Doppler, because vascular signals exclusively occur within the solid tissue.

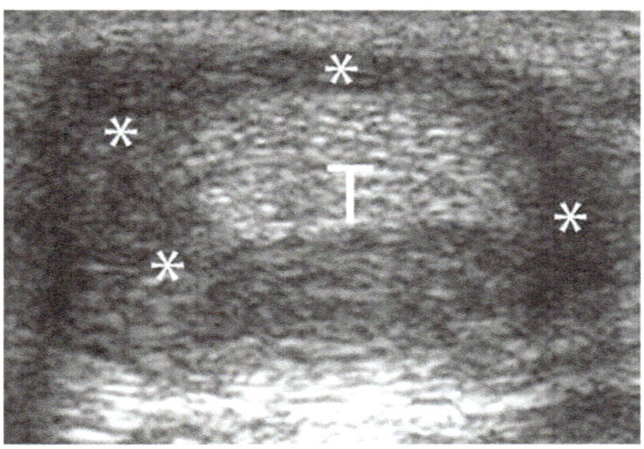

Fig. 3.14 Transverse scan, finger flexor tendons. Expansion of the tendon sheath with hyperechoic synovial proliferation (*) is shown. *T* tendon

In all cases where inflammatory involvement of the tenosynovial sheath is observed, US evaluation of the tendon's morphology and intrinsic structure should be performed. Tendons presenting with an alteration of their echotexture express concomitant pathologic involvement of its parenchyma (Fig. 3.17).

Chronic stenosing tenosynovitis occurs in peculiar anatomical regions, where the tendons run through fibro-osseous canals. The most common US pattern is that of a mixed tenosynovitis, accompanied by thickening of the corresponding retinaculum and consequent stenosis of the canal (Fig. 3.18).

From a functional point of view, the dynamic US examination may demonstrate a defective sliding of the tendon within the sheath which could be easily seen on long-axis scans (Fig. 3.19).

Notta-Nelaton's disease, also known as "trigger finger," and De Quervain's disease are the most common forms of chronic stenosing tenosynovitis.

3.2.2 Peritendinitis

The term peritendinitis refers to inflammation of the paratenon of anchor tendons, especially involving the highly vascular loose areolar connective tissue that is found between epitenon and peritenon.

In practice, peritendinitis of anchor tendons corresponds to tenosynovitis of sliding tendons,

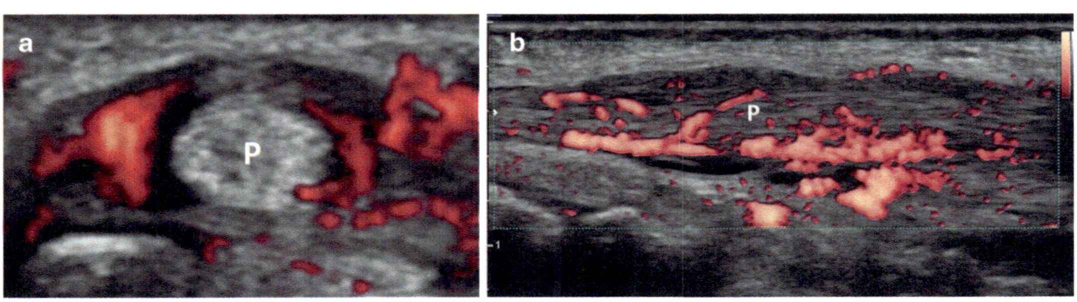

Fig. 3.15 (**a**) Finger flexor tendon, transverse power Doppler scan; proliferative tenosynovitis with diffuse hypervascularization is shown; *P* flexor profundus tendon; (**b**) longitudinal view

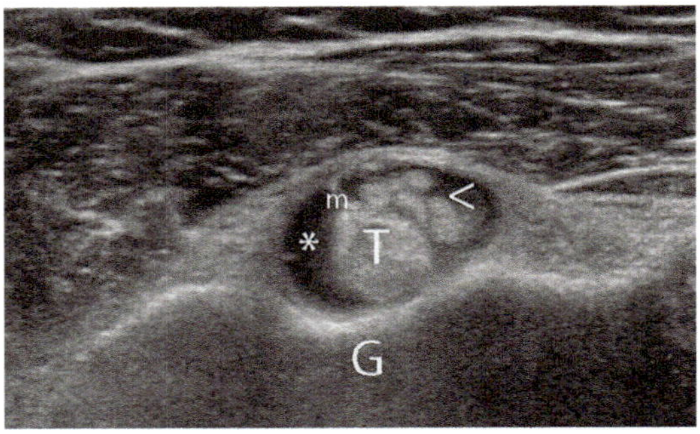

Fig. 3.16 Long head of biceps tendon of the shoulder, transverse scan. Fluid expansion (*) of the synovial sheath with synovial proliferation (arrowheads) is shown (mixed tenosynovitis); *m* mesotenon; *G* intertubercular groove; *T* tendon

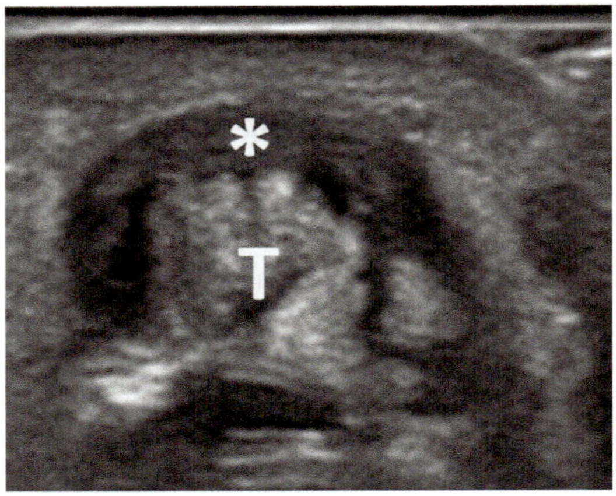

Fig. 3.18 Chronic stenosing tenosynovitis of first extensor compartment tendons (T). 18 MHz US shows synovial tendon sheath enlargement (*)

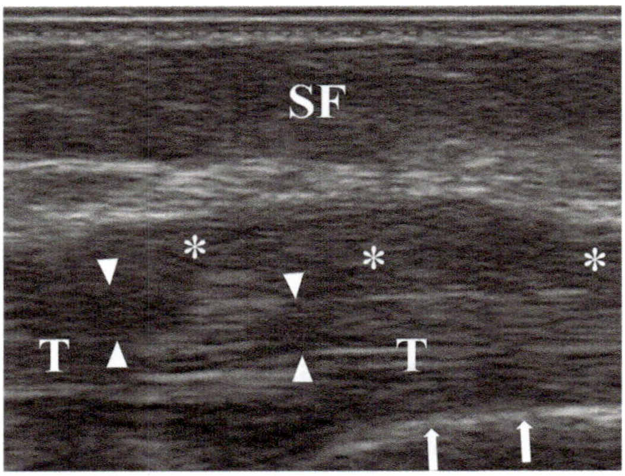

Fig. 3.17 Wrist US dorsal longitudinal scan; extensor tendons of fingers (T): tenosynovitis with inflammatory expansion of the sheath (asterisks); inhomogeneous echotexture of tendons (arrowheads), subcutaneous fat (SF), bone surface (white arrows)

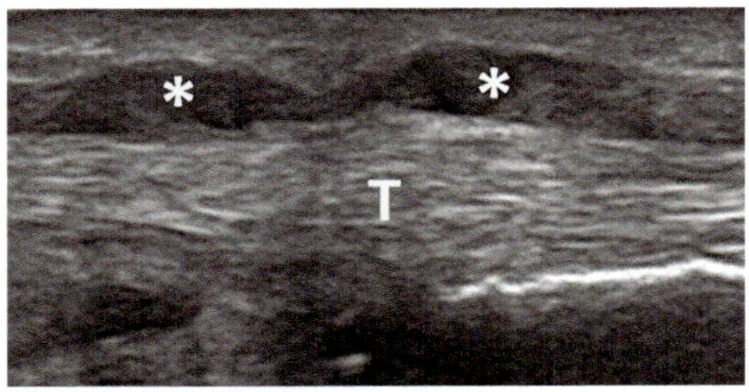

Fig. 3.19 Longitudinal scan of first extensor compartment. Tendon (T) sliding could be seen during dynamic maneuvers under synovial sheath enlargement (*)

for they both represent a paratenonitis. Peritendinitis often affects tendons of the lower limbs, particularly the patellar and Achilles tendons. Like tenosynovitis, peritendinitis can be classified as acute, subacute, or chronic. The most common cause of peritendinitis is repeated microtrauma. US highlights the inflammatory edema, a hypoechoic thickening of the peritendinous wrapping layers (Fig. 3.20) with a hypoechoic ring-like appearance in short-axis views. In the classic pattern of peritendinitis, the fibrillar tendon echotexture does not appear altered; it is altered instead in mixed forms where peritendinitis and tendinosis coexist.

The information obtained with grayscale US can be usefully integrated with an accurate color and power Doppler analysis that can add further information regarding the presence of peritendinous inflammation and hyperemia. It should also be mentioned that in standard conditions the vascularization of tendons is very poor with low-speed flow, invisible on Doppler analysis. When hyperemia is detected, a typical hypervascular pattern is observed; this is characterized by several signal spots and typically located in the peritendinous area.

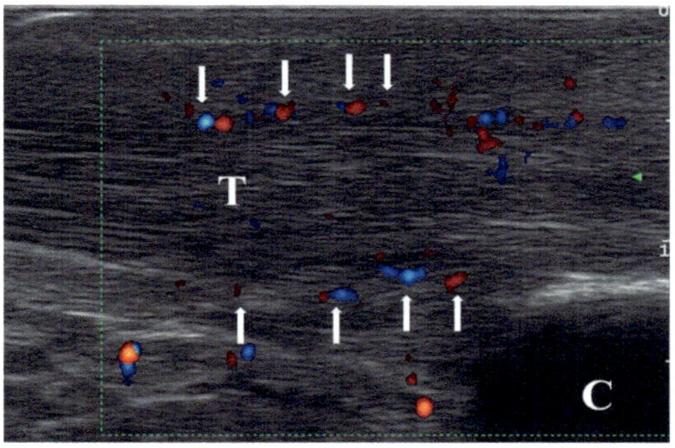

Fig. 3.20 Peritendinitis of the Achilles tendon (T); the power Doppler scan shows some peritendineal vascular signals (arrows), expression of hyperemia, and inflammation. C: calcaneus

3.3 Tendinosis

Tendinosis is a degenerative pathology affecting both anchor and sliding tendons, presenting with mild pain or with no symptoms at all. Consequently, US plays a fundamental role in diagnosis, because the patient's history and clinical examination alone cannot accurately implicate the involved tendon. From a histopathologic point of view, fibroblasts are activated with the production of high-molecular-weight collagen and proteoglycans, causing diffuse edema. Necrosis and fibrinous exudation occur with a probable consequent fibrocartilaginous metaplasia and calcium deposition. US is able to detect tendon alteration in early phases. The earliest US sign of tendinosis, in long-axis views, is a disarray of tendon echotexture and its fusiform thickening corresponding, in short-axis views, to the rounded appearance with loss of the typical ventral concavity. In early US patterns of tendinosis, fragmentation of the fibrillar echotexture is observed (Fig. 3.21).

In later phases, focal hypoechoic areas related to mucoid degeneration can be observed (Fig. 3.22). Collagen fibers show a lack of organization; several hyperechoic spots can be detected, suggesting the presence of micro- and macro-calcification.

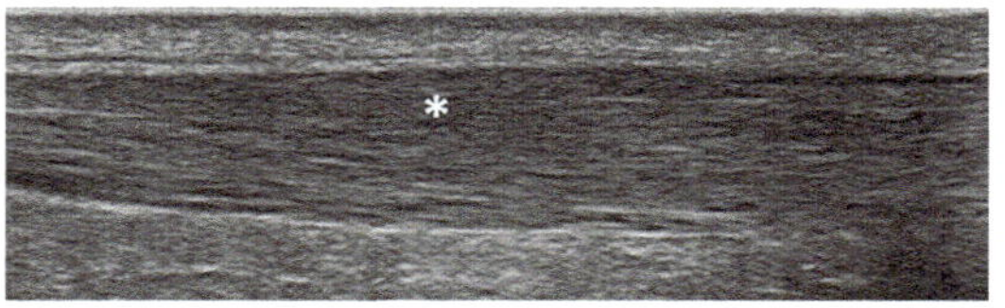

Fig. 3.21 Low-grade tendinosis. The characteristic fragmentation of the fibrillar echotexture is shown (asterisk)

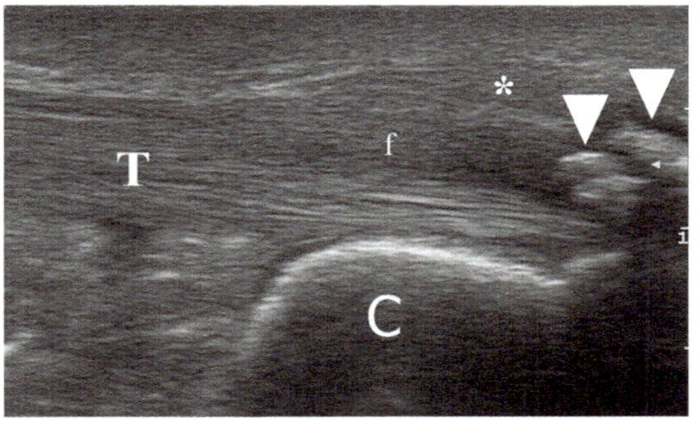

Fig. 3.22 Longitudinal scan of Achilles tendon (T) enthesopathy; diffuse fibrillar echotexture disarray (f), calcifications (arrowheads), and peri-calcaneal soft-tissue thickening (asterisk). C: calcaneus

The largest hyperechoic spots show posterior acoustic shadowing, representing areas of calcific metaplasia within the tendon (Fig. 3.23).

Further assessment of intratendinous hypoechoic focal areas using color or power Doppler techniques can be useful to detect vascular signals within the degenerative spots, a finding suggestive of the presence of angiogenesis, with a potential consequent substitution of the degenerate area. The absence of vascular signals within the degenerate areas of the tendon suggests necrotic evolution of the degenerative focus. It should be mentioned that in clinical practice it is common to find cases in which an overlap between degenerative (tendinosis) and inflammatory (paratenonitis) tendon conditions occurs, and in these cases the complex color and power Doppler images can be integrated with grayscale US to give a more precise assessment (Fig. 3.24a–c).

It should also be considered that some anatomical regions present peculiar biomechanical characteristics that promote the onset of tendinosis. For instance, the presence of a prominent posterosuperior calcaneal tubercle (Haglund's disease) may cause friction with the pre-insertional portion of the Achilles tendon. In these cases, ultrasound shows the presence of inflammatory and degenerative tendon involvement, especially located at the pre-insertional portion, which appears thickened and inhomogeneous and is often associated with a precalcaneal and retrocalcaneal bursitis (Fig. 3.25a, b). Sonoelastography shows increased stiffness in symptomatic enlarged Achilles tendons in comparison to normal ones.

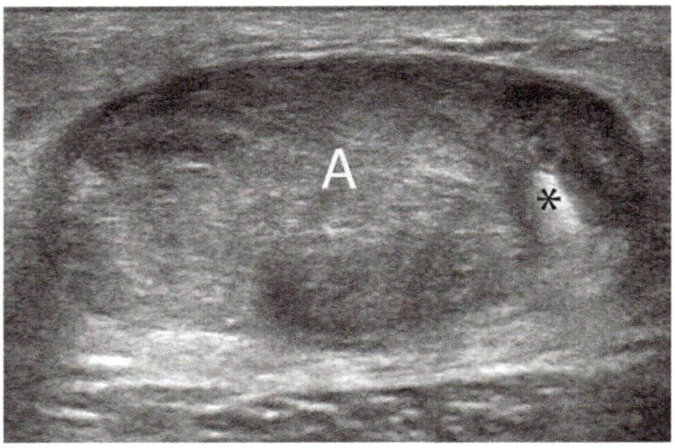

Fig. 3.23 Transverse scan of Achilles tendinosis (A). The tendon is thickened and inhomogeneous with a small focus of calcification (*)

3.4 Degenerative and Inflammatory Enthesopathy

Enthesopathy, also known as insertional tendinopathy, is an inflammatory-degenerative pathology involving the osteotendinous junction, usually caused by functional overload. It typically affects anchor tendons submitted to continual and intense mechanical stress. The affected anatomical region, therefore, varies according to the athletic task, resulting in the onset of typical pathologies associated with specific sports, such as tennis elbow and jumper's knee.

In standard conditions the enthesis consists of intertwined tendon fibers and fibrocartilage, with slow-flowing vessels that cannot be visualized on

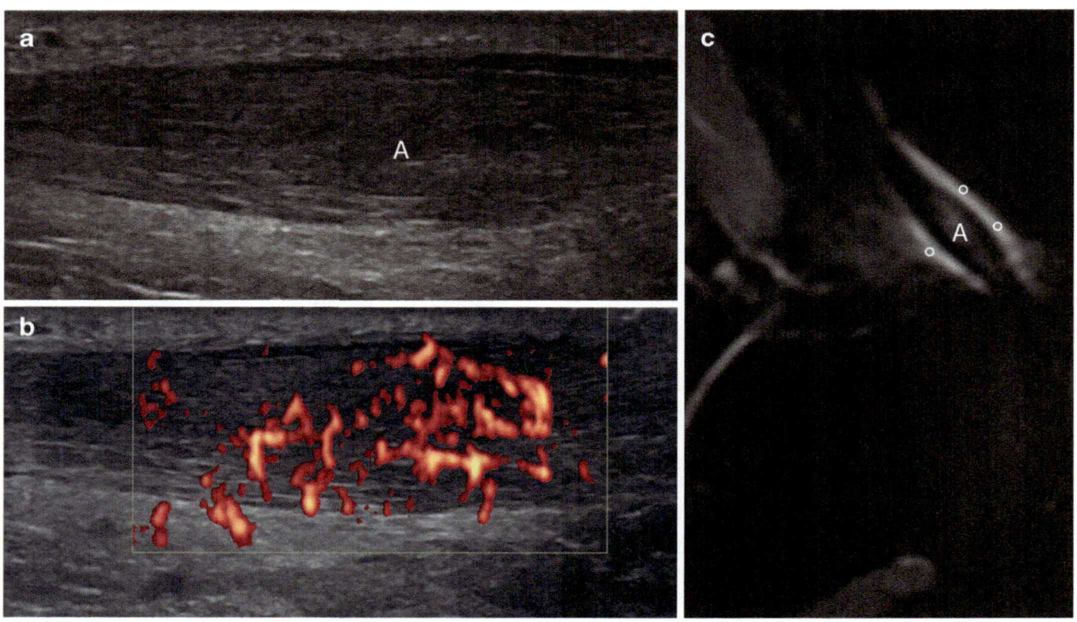

Fig.3.24 (a) Longitudinal scan of Achilles tendinosis (A). The tendon is thickened and inhomogeneous and devoid of its characteristic fibrillar echotexture. (b) The power Doppler scan shows some intratendinous vascular signals. (c) An MR STIR longitudinal scan of Achilles tendinosis (A) and peritendinitis (circles)

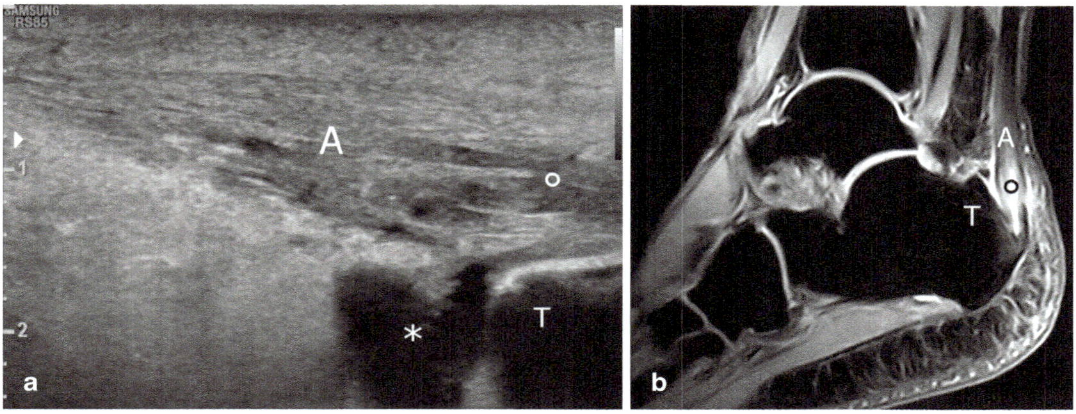

Fig. 3.25 Haglund's disease. (**a**) Longitudinal scan. The pre-insertional segment of Achilles tendon (A) appears inhomogeneous and thickened, with a longitudinal tear and inflammation of the retrocalcaneal bursa (*). (**b**) MR scan of the same patient (gradient echo (GE) T2W sequence) demonstrating a prominent posterosuperior calcaneal tubercle. **T** = tubercle

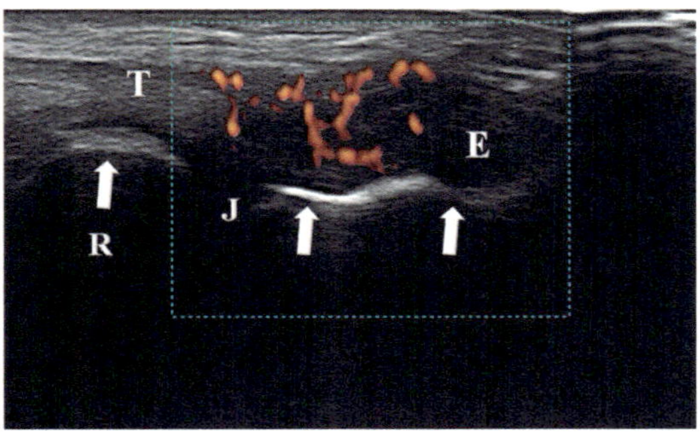

Fig. 3.26 Longitudinal US scan of epicondylitis. The power Doppler scan shows some intratendinous vascular signal; enthesis (E), extensor tendons (T), bone surface (white arrows), joint space (J), radial head (H). R: radius.

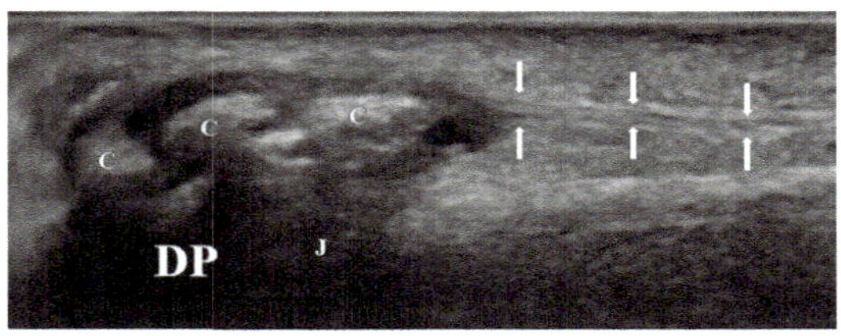

Fig. 3.27 Longitudinal scan of terminal extensor slip of digitorum tendon; diffuse disarray of the fibrillar echotexture, calcifications, and thickening; tendon slip (white arrows), distal phalanx (DP), calcifications (C), joint (J)

Doppler analysis. In enthesopathies, the earliest pathologic finding is local hyperemia and angiogenesis; with Doppler techniques the increase of vascular signals can be identified early (Fig. 3.26).

US is a highly sensitive technique for identifying and quantifying the tendon insertional thickening, the hypoechoic pattern, and the inhomogeneous echotexture. Insertional calcification and hypoechoic focal areas, corresponding to myxoid degeneration within the tendon, may be observed (Fig. 3.27).

An inflammatory reaction of the adjacent serous bursa and the presence of erosions and of an irregular cortical bone outline at the insertion are often associated. On US, erosions appear as interruptions of the hyperechoic cortical bone outline. In advanced cases, an MR examination should be performed, because it represents the only technique capable of determining the insertional bone involvement appearing as medullary edema within the bone in high-contrast sequences (Fig. 3.28).

A peculiar form of enthesopathy is that affecting patients in adolescence. During growth, the tendon insertion does not occur on the bone, but on the growth plate cartilage, which represents a weaker structure of the enthesis compared to bone and tendon, and is less resistant to mechanical stress. Impact is therefore mostly absorbed by the growth plate cartilage, and the corresponding bone and tendon are relatively spared. Typical

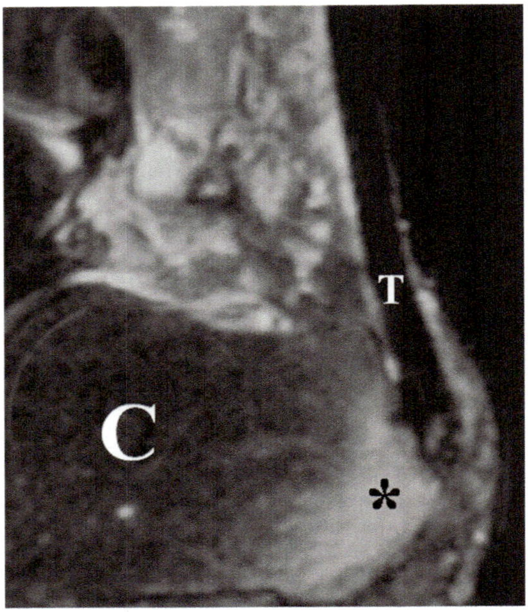

Fig. 3.28 MR of the ankle, sagittal scan (fat suppression technique). Reactive hyperemia (asterisk) of calcaneus (C) at the Achilles tendon (T) insertion

clinical conditions that follow this situation are some juvenile osteochondrosis, such as Osgood-Schlatter's disease (affecting the patellar tendon at its distal insertion), Sinding-Larsen-Johansson disease (affecting the patellar tendon at its proximal insertion), and Haglund-Sever's disease (affecting the Achilles). All these patients present with pain at the enthesis level and functional loss. The typical US pattern shows thickened growth plate cartilage and fragmented nucleus of ossification, suggestive of irregular endochondral ossification (Fig. 3.29a, b).

3.5 Entheseal Tear and Tendon Rupture

A tendon tear may be observed after an acute injury or as a poor outcome of tendinosis, with a spontaneous rupture. Mechanical overload, especially when excessive and repetitive, may eventually cause partial or total tears within a degenerative tendon structure. Such tears are often incomplete, but they still alter the tendon continuity and consequently its integrity. Histological samples show degenerative involution of the collagen fibers, with necrotic foci. On US scans, a tear appears as a hypo- to anechoic spot that interrupts the fibrillar structure of the tendon (Fig. 3.30a, b).

In complete tears, US allows the discontinuity of the fibers, the two tendon stumps, and the hemorrhagic collection within the retraction gap to be visualized (Fig. 3.31).

In these cases it is important to perform a dynamic US examination for a more accurate evaluation of the tear location. In some regions, the US signs of tendon tears can be very complicated. A clear example is represented by the rotator cuff tendons and particularly by the supraspinatus tendon in which tears are classified, according to the site and extension of the lesion, into the following:

1. *Partial lesions*: These can be further divided into ***bursal***, when the involved aspect of the tendon is in contact with the subacromial-deltoid bursa (Fig. 3.32); ***articular***, when the involved aspect is in contact with the humeral head; and ***intratendinous***. A partial intratendinous tear appears as an anechoic line within the tendon substance (Fig. 3.33).
2. *Complete lesions*, which correspond to full-thickness tears of the tendon (small, intermediate, wide, total) (Fig. 3.34), with possible retraction of the two stumps.

In complete lesions of the rotator cuff, the humeral head appears uncovered with a tendency to articulate with the acromion (subacromial impingement). Hypoanechoic fluid collection is observed between the two tendon stumps with a consequent expansion of the subacromial-deltoid bursa (Fig. 3.35a, b).

3.6 Tendon Dislocation

Along their course, sliding tendons may undergo flexion and consequent spatial misalignment from the corresponding muscle's functional axis.

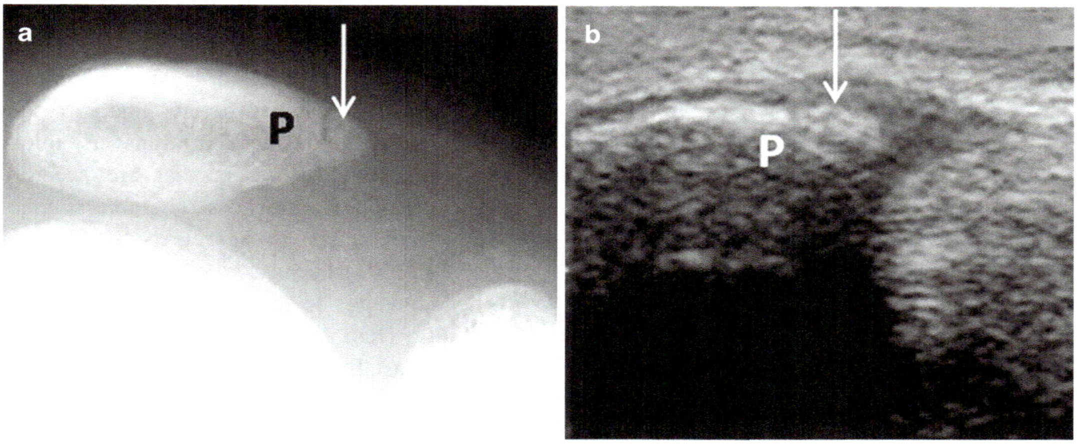

Fig. 3.29 Sinding-Larsen-Johansson syndrome in a young patient. (**a**) The plain film shows fragmented appearance of the ossification center (arrow) of the lower patellar (P) pole. (**b**) The US scan shows an irregular bone outline (arrow) and swelling at the patellar tendon insertion

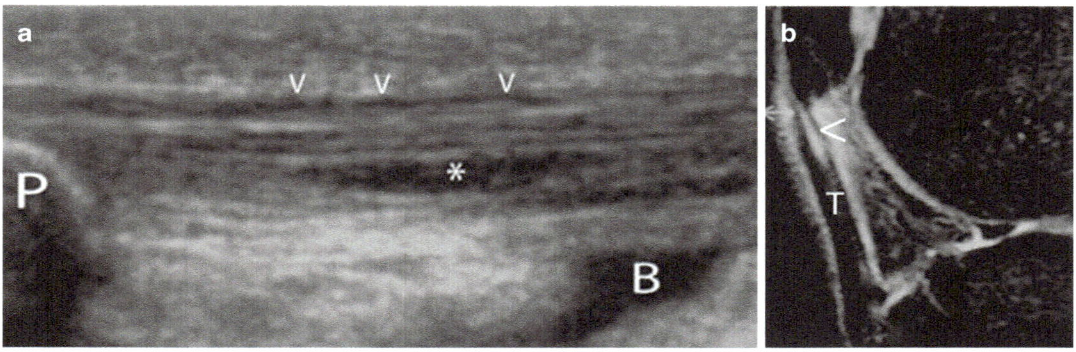

Fig. 3.30 (**a**) This longitudinal scan at the proximal third of patellar tendon shows a partial tear (*) with inflammatory involvement of peritenon (arrowheads). *P* lower patellar extremity; *B* deep pretibial bursa. (**b**) The MR scan of the same patient (sagittal scan, fat suppression technique) confirms the US findings and highlights the inflammation of peritendinous tissues. *T* patellar tendon; *arrowheads* partial tear

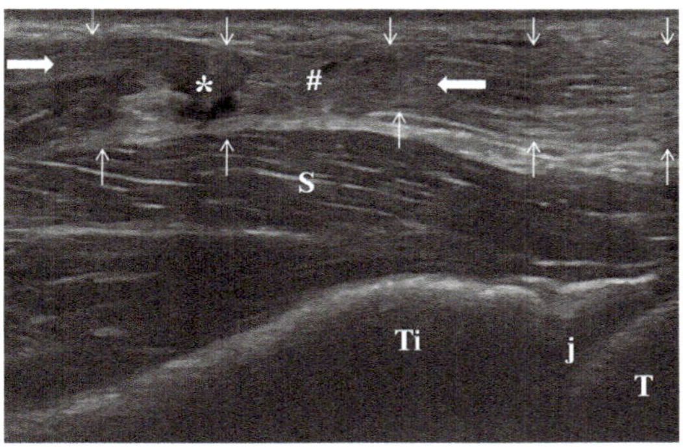

Fig. 3.31 Longitudinal scan of complete Achilles tendon tear; soleus muscle (S), posterior aspect of tibiotalar joint (j), tibia (Ti), talus (T), Achilles tendon (thin white arrows), tear area (thick arrows), hemorrhagic (#) and fluid (*) collection

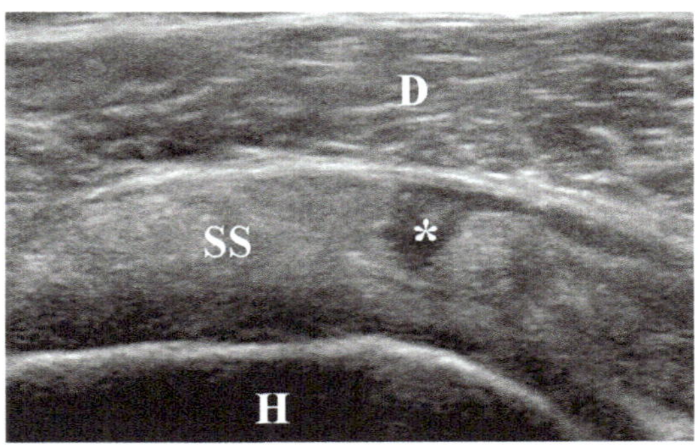

Fig. 3.32 Transverse scan of the shoulder: partial tear (asterisk) of bursal side of supraspinatus tendon (SS); humerus (H), deltoid muscle (D)

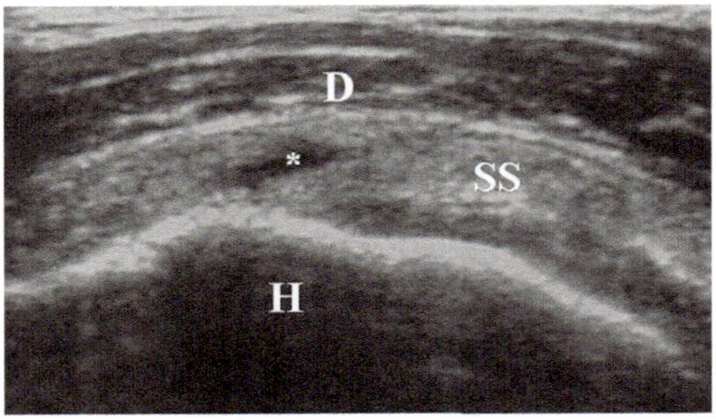

Fig. 3.33 Transverse scan of the shoulder: partial tear (asterisk) of supraspinatus tendon (SS); humerus (H), deltoid muscle (D)

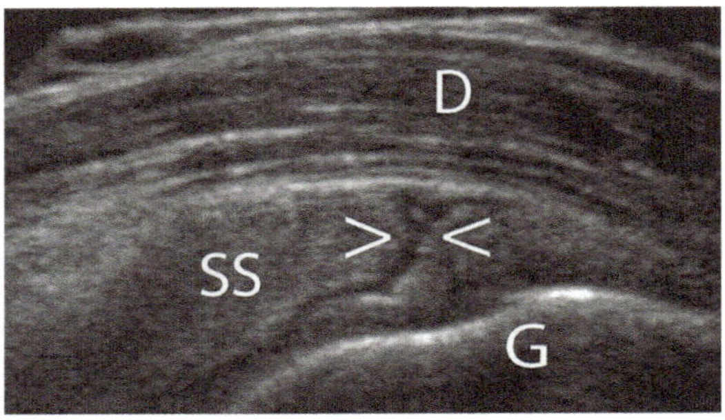

Fig. 3.34 Complete tear of supraspinatus tendon (arrowheads) is clearly shown as a full-thickness rupture in this US scan. *SS* supraspinatus tendon; *D* deltoid; *G* greater humeral tubercle

In order for correct biomechanical function, the angular points and lever fulcra of the tendon must be kept in their physiological osteofibrous grooves. The anatomic structures that carry out this task are the retnacula: focal transverse thickenings of the deep fascia that are securely anchored to bone eminences. The correct functioning of their stabilizing role is therefore of great importance because whenever it is lacking, the tendon tends to dislocate, with consequent instability. There are several degrees of severity in tendon instability: in moderate lesions the tendon tends to dislocate only when a specific movement is performed, while in more severe lesions subluxation and luxation can be observed. The possibility of performing dynamic examination makes US the gold standard technique when tendon instability is suspected. Even though tendon instability is not very common, it should always be considered when deriving a differential diagnosis, because an early diagnosis is fundamental to avoid the onset of tendinosis or of a tendon tear. The most commonly affected tendons are the long head of the brachial biceps at the shoulder and the fibular tendons at the ankle. Dislocation of the long head of biceps may follow a transverse ligament tear or a coracohumeral

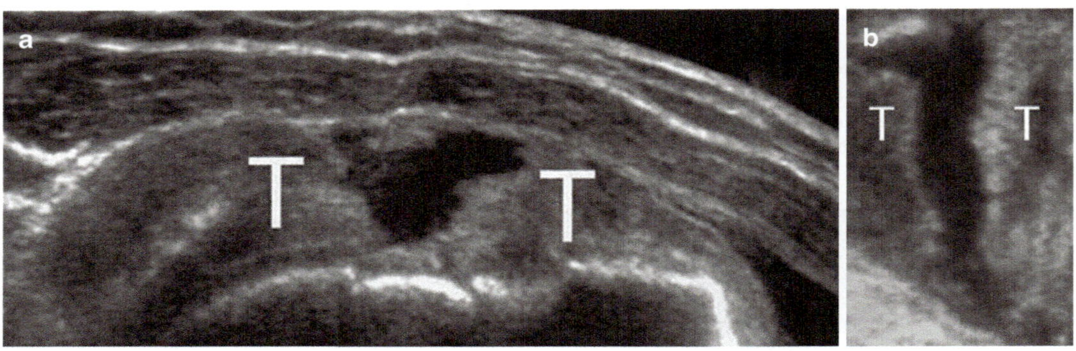

Fig. 3.35 (**a**) Complete tear of a degenerative supraspinatus tendon with retraction of the two tendon stumps. (**b**) MPR reconstruction on a coronal plane (view from the top). *T* tendon stumps

ligament tear, with or without an associated tear of the subscapularis tendon. It should be mentioned that there are several congenital conditions that promote instability, such as the presence of a flat intertubercular groove. When dislocation occurs, US shows an empty groove and a medially dislocated tendon (Fig. 3.36).

The application of dynamic maneuvers with external rotation of the arm, with 90° flexion of the elbow, can be useful because they reproduce the stressing action. At the ankle, the fibular tendons are kept in site by the fibular retinacula, superior and inferior, that are, respectively, located over and under the angular flexion point, at the lateral malleolus. Instability is caused by a lesion of the superior fibular retinaculum with subsequent tendency of the fibular tendons to dislocate anteriorly over the lateral malleolus. In short-axis views, with the transducer on the angular flexion point and performing a dynamic maneuver of dorsal flexion of the foot, dislocation of the fibular tendons over the lateral malleolus can be observed (Fig. 3.37a, b).

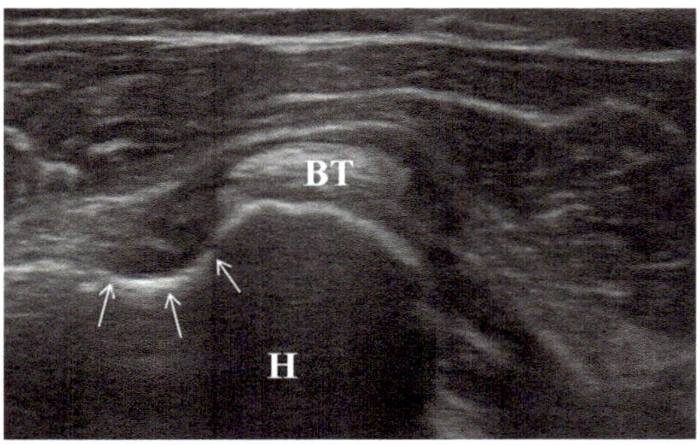

Fig. 3.36 Transverse scan of the anterior aspect of the shoulder: complete medial dislocation of long head of biceps tendon; humerus (H), bicipital groove (arrows), long head of biceps tendon

3.7 Tendon Cysts

Tendon cysts occur more frequently in the palmar aspect of fingers, along the flexor tendons' course, strictly in contact with the tenosynovial sheath from which they arise. The US diagnosis is simple because they usually appear as round, anechoic, formations with well-defined walls. They should always be evaluated in long- and short-axis views (Fig. 3.38a, b); short-axis views allow the relation between cyst and tenosynovial sheath to be demonstrated. A dynamic examination can be performed during flexion of the fingers.

3.8 Ligament Tears

Compared to tendons, ligaments are thinner and contain a higher amount of elastin, to give a better stabilization of the joints with the necessary

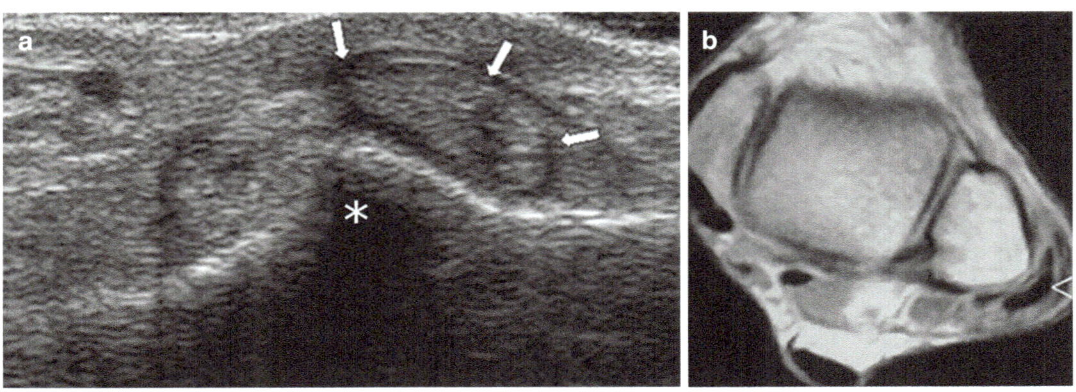

Fig. 3.37 (**a**) Lateral compartment of ankle, transverse scan. Dislocation of fibular tendons (arrows) over the fibular malleolus (*) is shown. (**b**) MR scan in the same patient (axial scan, SE T1W sequence) confirms the fibular tendon luxation (arrowhead)

elasticity. There are two different types of ligaments: *intrinsic capsular ligaments*, consisting of focal thickenings of the articular capsule with a strengthening function, and *extrinsic ligaments*, which do not depend on the capsule and can be further divided into extracapsular and intracapsular. US can easily assess the ligaments of the medial and lateral compartments of the ankle (deltoid, anterior talofibular, and calcaneofibular), the collateral ligaments of the knee, the collateral and annular ligaments of the elbow, the coracoacromial and coracohumeral ligaments of the shoulder, and the ulnar collateral ligament of the first metacarpophalangeal joint.

When assessing a ligament tear, it should always be remembered that US, unlike MR, is limited by its small field of view that does not allow an overview of the joint compartments. US, therefore, is not able to detect a possible concomitant lesion of the joint, which is a fundamental diagnosis in order to plan correct therapy. Ligaments are mainly affected by traumatic injuries that can be classified as *first degree* (stretching lesions), *second degree* (partial lesions), and *third degree* (complete lesions). They can be divided into acute, subacute, and chronic. It should be kept in mind that the US assessment of a ligament injury can be more accurate when performed a few days after the trauma, in a subacute phase. Only then does the enzymatic lysis of figurative elements cause a progressive reduction of the echoes and of the corpuscular appearance of the hemorrhagic effusion. Finally, the collection appears anechoic and it is used as acoustic window to visualize the ligament lesion. In first-degree injuries, US shows a thickened ligament with a relatively hypoechoic appearance, depending on the interstitial edema; the ligament is continuous with a regular outline (Fig. 3.39).

In second-degree injuries the normal echotexture appears altered. The ligament is thickened and inhomogeneous and shows an irregular outline; a minimal discontinuity of the ligament can be observed. In third-degree injuries, US allows a full-thickness lesion to be detected, with possible retraction of the fibers and the hemorrhagic collection filling the gap (Fig. 3.40).

A dynamic examination is always useful in doubtful cases.

To assess subacute and acute ligament injuries, power Doppler analysis allows the presence of diffuse perilesional hyperemia to be detected.

In the presence of fibrous and scar tissue resulting from a post-traumatic ligament lesion, US shows typically focal hypoechoic tissue. In some cases, minute calcification can also be found.

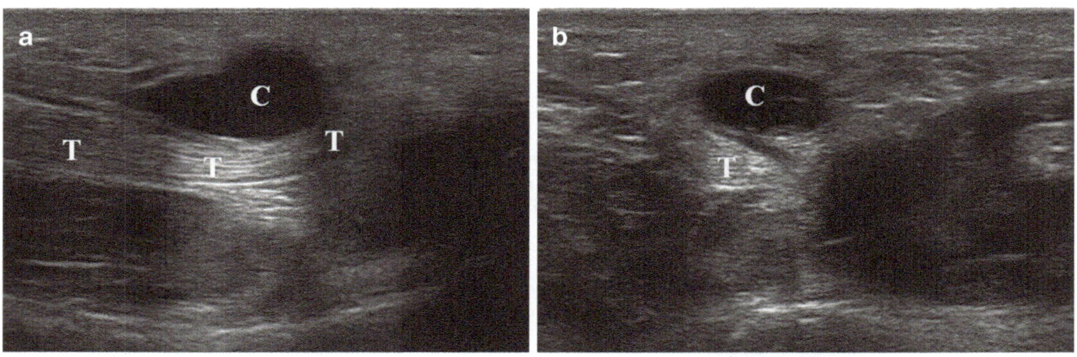

Fig. 3.38 (**a**) Longitudinal and (**b**) transverse scans of first foot finger. Anechoic cyst (C) of flexor tendon (T) synovial sheath

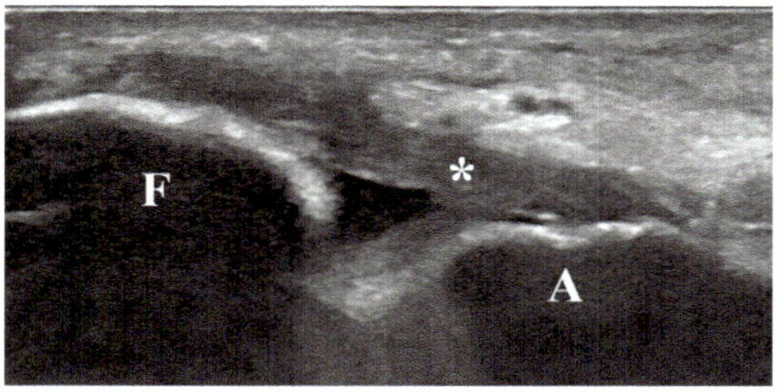

Fig. 3.39 US scan of the lateral compartment of the ankle. The anterior talofibular ligament is continuous but thickened and inhomogeneous for a first-degree lesion. *F* fibula; *T* talus

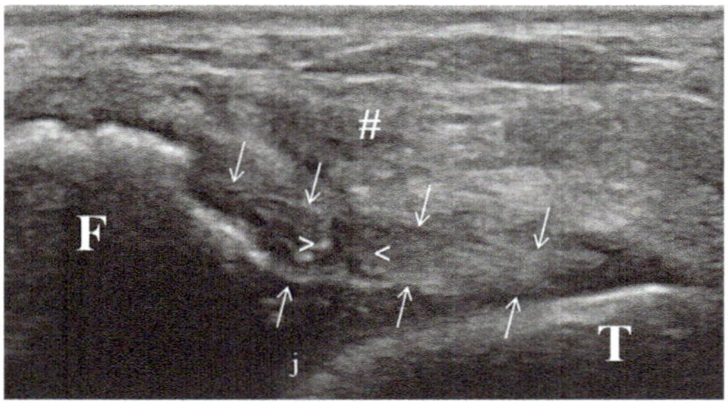

Fig. 3.40 US scan of the lateral side of the ankle. The anterior talofibular ligament is completely torn with minimal effusion; talofibular joint (j), fibula (F), talus (T), anterior talofibular ligament (arrows), tear area (arrowheads), soft-tissue thickening (#)

Further Readings

Bruce RK, Hale TL, Gilbert SK. Ultrasonographic evaluation for ruptured Achilles tendon. J Am Pediatr Med Assoc. 1982;72:15–7.

Davis WH, Sobel M, Deland J, et al. The superior peroneal retinaculum: an anatomic study. Foot Ankle Int. 1994;15:271–5.

Dillehay GL, et al. The ultrasonographic characterization of tendons. Invest Radiol. 1984;19:338–41.

Grechenig W, Clement H, Bratschitsch G, et al. Ultrasound diagnosis of the Achilles tendon. Orthopade. 2002;31:319–25.

Jozsa L, Kannus P, Balint JB, Reffy A. Three-dimensional ultrastructure of human tendons. J Anat. 1995;142:306–12.

Ling SC, Chen CF, Wang SC. A study on the vascular supply of the supraspinatus tendon. Surg RadiolAnat. 1990;12:161–5.

Martinoli C, Derchi LE, Pastorino C, et al. Analysis of echotexture of tendons with US. Radiology. 1993;186:839–43.

O'Brien M. Functional anatomy and physiology of tendons. Clin Sports Med. 1992;11:505–20.

Silvestri E, Biggi E, Molfetta L, et al. Power Doppler Analysis of tendon vascularization. Int J Tissue React. 2003;25:149–58.

Stolinski C. Disposition of collagen fibrils in human tendons. J Anat. 1995;186:577–83.

Muscles

4

Davide Orlandi, Enzo Silvestri,
and Matteo De Cesari

Contents

4.1 Sonographic and Doppler Normal Anatomy

Muscle is made of bundles of contractile elementary units—the striated muscle fibers—with their major axis lying along the contraction direction. The muscular fibers are multinuclear cellular units derived, during embryonal development, from mesodermal cells of the primitive segments. The fibers have a cylindrical or polyhedral shape with smoothed angles; they have a considerable length, varying from a few millimeters to several centimeters, and a width between 10 and 100 mm. Considerable differences between different muscle fibers can be observed and, even within the same muscle, the fibers' diameter can vary according to work, nutritional conditions, and other causes.

Muscular fibers are arranged parallel to one another and they are supported by a structure of connective tissue. Muscle is externally surrounded by a thick connective sheath called the epimysium; from the internal aspect of this sheath several septa depart to constitute the perimysium, which surrounds diverse bundles of muscular fibers, named fascicles. Blood vessels and nerves run within the perimysium, which also contains neuromuscular spindles. Very light and thin septa arising from the perimysium spread into the fascicles to surround every single muscular fiber and thus form the endomysium. The endomysium, a network made of reticular fibers, blood capillaries, a few connective cells together with some small nervous bundles, constitutes the framework found right around the striated muscle fibers, and it represents the site of

D. Orlandi (✉)
Department of Radiology, Ospedale Evangelico Internazionale, Genova, Italy

E. Silvestri
Radiology, Alliance Medical, Genova, Italy

M. De Cesari
Department of Radiology, Ospedali del Tigullio, Lavagna, Italy

F. Martino et al. (eds.), *Musculoskeletal Ultrasound in Orthopedic and Rheumatic disease in Adults*,
https://doi.org/10.1007/978-3-030-91202-4_4

metabolic exchange between striated muscle fibers and blood (Figs. 4.1 and 4.2).

The epimysial, perimysial, and endomysial coverings come together converging where muscles merge with adjacent structures: the extremity of the muscle may continue as a tendon or insert onto the periosteum, aponeurosis, or dermis; this structure is extremely resistant, since the tensile forces turn into tangential forces that are more easily born. At a submicroscopic level, the muscular fibers end in a conical shape and adapt to the connective tissue just like fingers adapt to a glove; at the two endpoints of the muscular fiber, the myofibrils are attached to the sarcolemma. The muscular myofibers, and mostly the connective framework, are strongly connected to the terminal insertion and the force developed by contraction does not lose any efficiency at the passage from muscle to tendon and there is no risk of detachment. From a clinical point of view, such detachments occur only in rare situations, for it is much easier for a tendon to detach from a bone fragment at its insertion, in the case of an exceptionally strong contraction.

Each muscle presents at least one muscular belly and two tendons, one at the origin and the other at the distal insertion. The physical arrangement of fibers inside the muscle defines the muscle architecture, which determines a muscle's mechanical function, particularly affecting the force–velocity relationship. The main types of muscle architecture include the parallel type and the pennate one. The parallel type corresponds to muscle in which fibers with length close to that of the whole muscle run almost parallel to each other and to the muscle line of action. It includes the flat muscles and the fusiform one (Fig. 4.3), e.g., the sartorius and biceps brachii muscles, respectively.

In pennate-type muscles, e.g., the gastrocnemius and deltoid muscles, short fibers are oriented at an angle relative to the muscle's line of action. In fact, in pennate muscles, from each side the tendon penetrates far into the muscle, as thick superficial fascia (in unipennate muscles) or deeply as central tendon (in bipennate and multi-pennate muscles). Relatively short muscle fibers attach diagonally onto the central tendon at an oblique angle. The arrangement of fibers and tendons in these muscles resembles the shape of a bird feather, leading to the designation of such muscles as pennate (from Latin "penna" or feather). If all the fascicles of a pennate muscle are on the same side of the tendon, the pennate muscle is called unipennate. If the fascicles lie to either side of the tendon, the muscle is called

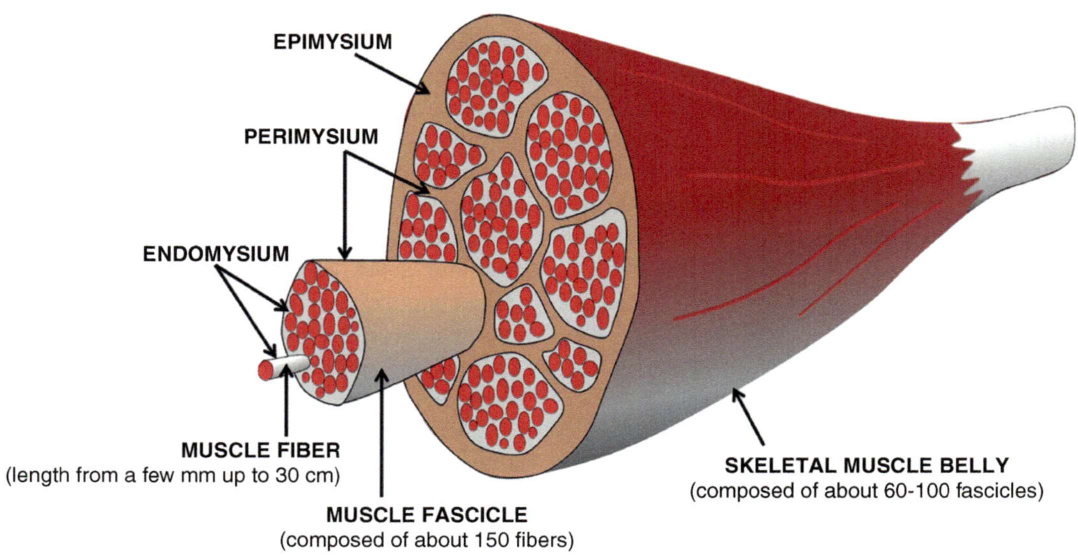

Fig. 4.1 Schematic drawing of the gross organization of skeletal muscle

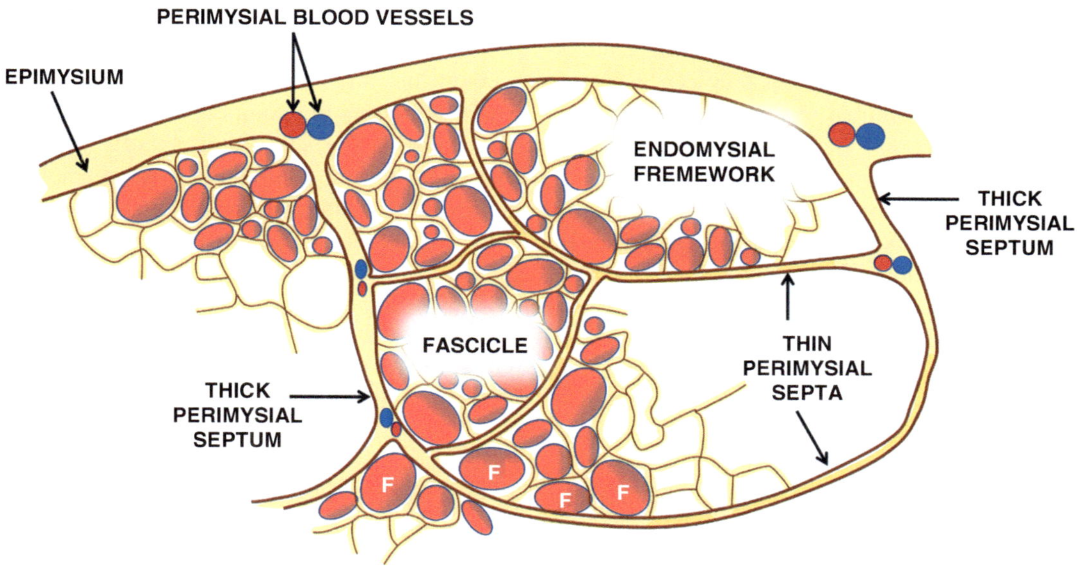

Fig. 4.2 Architectural arrangement of muscle fascicles. Muscle fibers (F) are grouped into fascicles, and bundles of fascicles comprise the entire muscle. The skeletal muscle is enclosed externally in a thick connective tissue envelope (epimysium). From the inner side of the epimysium, loose connective septa (perimysium) divide the muscle in fascicles, surrounding each one, and also between the individual muscle fibers (endomysium). Blood vessels run within the connective framework

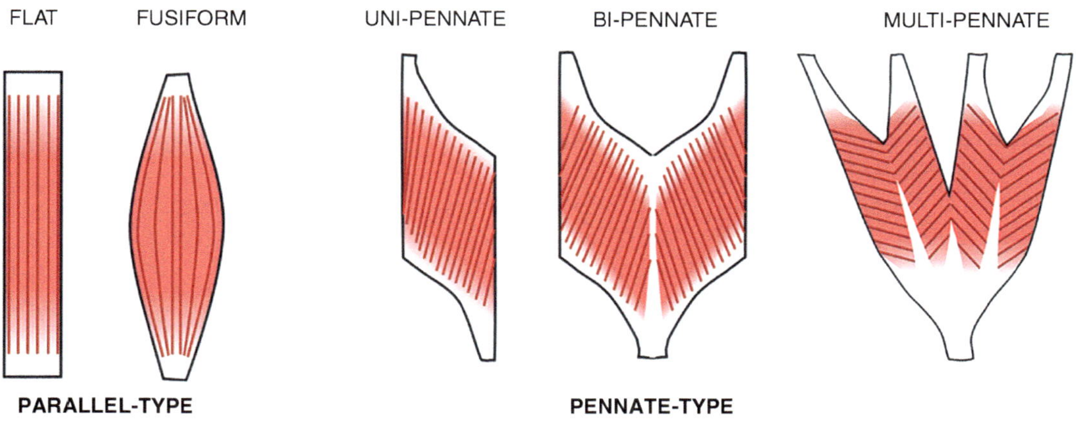

Fig. 4.3 Skeletal muscle architecture

bipennate. If the central tendon branches within a pennate muscle, the muscle is called multipennate (Fig. 4.3).

Skeletal muscle architecture, defined by the length and the arrangement of fascicles relative to the axis of force generation, influences strongly the muscle functional properties. This is because the degree of muscular shortening depends on the fibers' length and the energy of contraction depends on the number of fibers constituting the muscle. The parallel-type muscles, such as the biceps brachii, are composed of relatively long fibers lying nearly parallel to each other. Since muscle fibers can contract about one-third of their resting length, this arrangement is suitable to an extensive and quick movement. Then, these muscles have a long excursion (% of shortening), but they are only moderately strong in terms of the whole muscle force that they can generate, due to the low number of fibers constituting the muscle. Conversely, the pennate muscles, e.g., the rectus femoris muscle, have a greater thickness and many more muscle fibers than similarly sized parallel-type muscle, due to angled disposition of fibers, thus allowing the muscle to produce more force. In fact, the fiber quantity that makes up a muscle is expressed by the **physiological cross-sectional area** (**PCSA**), which is measured perpendicular to the axis of the fibers at muscle largest point, not to the axis of the whole muscle (Fig. 4.4).

The muscle bundles are directed obliquely from tendon to tendon, and the shorter and more numerous they are, the wider the tendon insertion is. This setting influences biomechanics, because the degree of muscle shortening depends on the fibers' length and the energy of contraction depends on the number of fibers that make up the muscle; two muscles with the same length, width, and thickness, and therefore the same volume, but with different number, length, and slope of the fibers, will also have different shortening capability and contraction energy. Therefore, when assessing the biomechanical characteristics of a muscle, whose internal structure varies according to its specific function, not only the volume should be taken into account, but also the type of insertion, whose width influences the number, length, and slope of the fibers. The speed and extent of muscle shortening during contraction depend a lot on the fibers' direction with respect to the longitudinal axis of the muscle itself. These are the greater the smaller the inclination of the fibers, as in the case of parallel muscles; conversely, they progressively decrease as the angle of inclination of the fibers increases. The obliquity of the muscle fibers is defined by the pennation angle, which refers to the angle that the muscle fibers run across the load axis of the muscle; it varies from 0° to 30°. In pennate muscles the load axis (line of action) corresponds to that of the central tendon (Fig. 4.5).

The muscle morphology, internal structure, and architecture can be easily assessed by ultrasound imaging. The external connective sheath of the muscle (epimysium) appears as a hyperechoic external band measuring a maximum of 2–3 mm of thickness and, on longitudinal US sections, continues without interruption along the corresponding tendon profile.

The fibro-adipose septa (perimysium) are seen as hyperechoic lines separating the contiguous

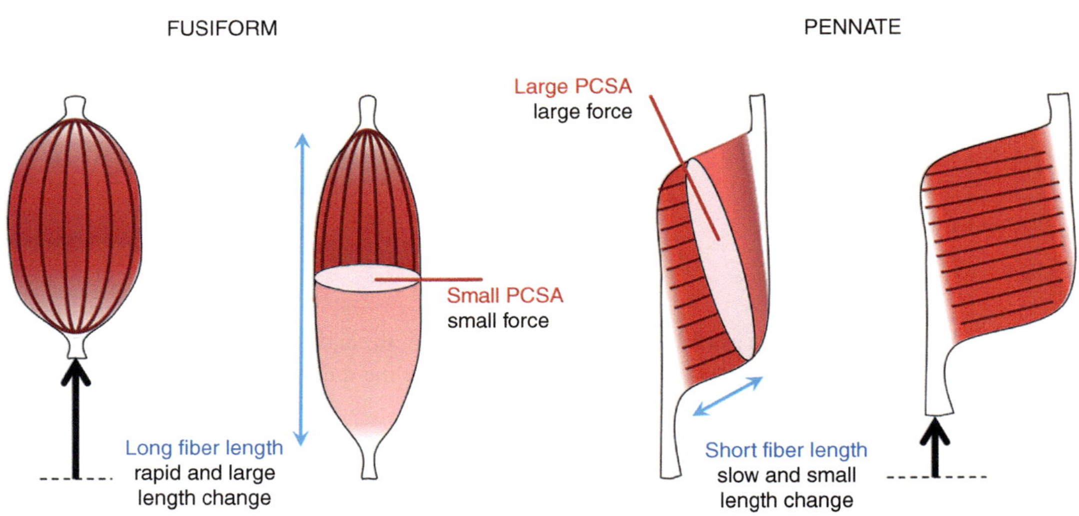

Fig. 4.4 Physiological cross-sectional area (PCSA) measured perpendicular to the axis of the fibers at muscle largest point

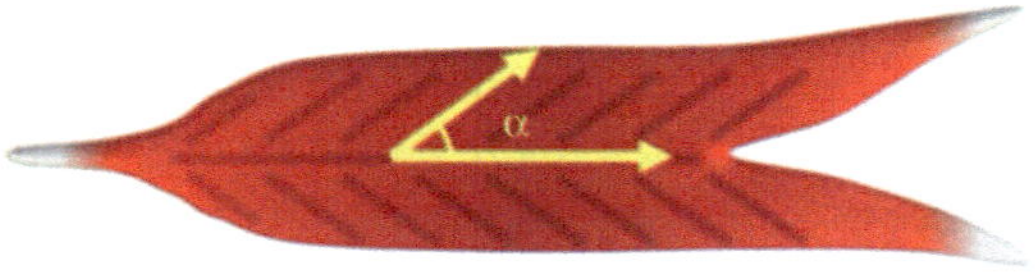

Fig. 4.5 Pennation angle evaluation

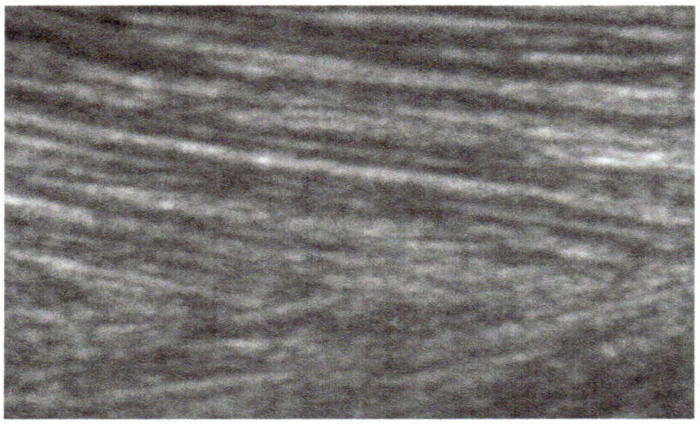

Fig. 4.6 Longitudinal US scan of a pennate muscle. The characteristic pennate appearance is given by the convergence of perimysial septa

hypoechoic muscular bundles (fascicles) from one to another (Fig. 4.6).

In transverse views, the muscle is sectioned according to a plane that is orthogonal to the muscular longitudinal axis, with a typical US structure appearance; the first- and second-order fascicles show an irregular polygonal shape, defined by thin, hyperechoic septa corresponding to the perimysial fibro-adipose framework (Fig. 4.7). Using color or power Doppler, vascular flow in normal resting muscles is usually not observed.

There is proven relationship between performance and muscle architecture, which main components are muscle thickness, fascicle length, and pennation angle.

The most common method of assessing muscle architecture is by ultrasound, acquiring longitudinal images of the muscle. By orienting the ultrasound probe in the plane of the fascicles, the thickness of the muscle, fascicle lengths, and pennation angle can be accurately measured (Fig. 4.8). Manual measurement of muscle architecture parameters takes time and subjective; various semiautomatic or automatic methods are

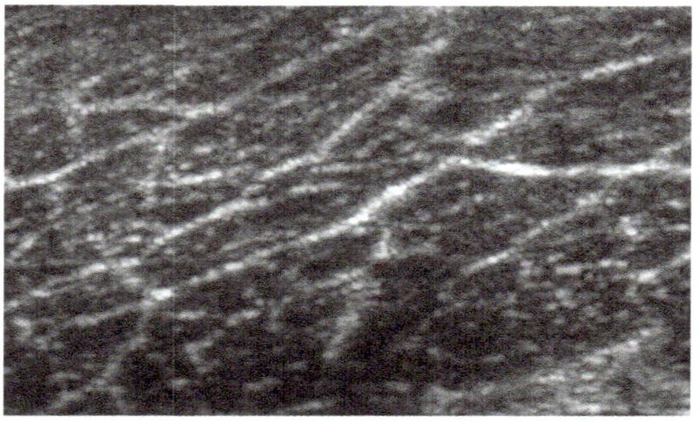

Fig. 4.7 The transverse echographic scan of a muscle shows the polygonal arrangement of the hyperechoic perimysial framework, which separates the hypoechoic fascicles

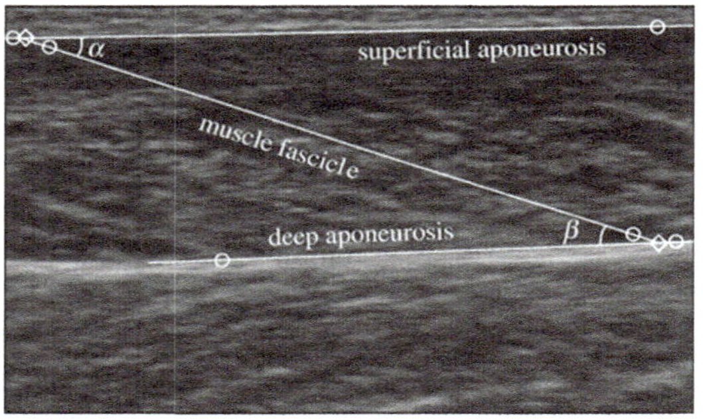

Fig. 4.8 Muscle architecture US evaluation. The fascicle length is measured as the distance between the two intersection points, while the pennation angle refers to the angle between the fascicle line and line passing along the deep aponeurosis (usually corresponding to central tendon)

also proposed in the literature, using digitizing software.

The muscle thickness in the longitudinal plane is defined as the orthogonal distance between the superficial and deep aponeuroses.

After drawing of two guidelines on the muscle contours with the aim to highlight the superficial and deep aponeuroses, a line is drawn as an extension of the fascicle using a linear path until it intersects both aponeuroses. The fascicle length is measured as the distance between the two intersection points, while the pennation angle refers to the angle between the fascicle line and line passing along the deep aponeurosis (usually corresponding to central tendon). The value of the angle is 12°–20° in mean and can vary between the nearly 0° of parallel-type muscles, e.g., biceps brachii, and at most the 30° of large pennate-type muscles. It has been demonstrated that the muscle size, determined as anatomical or physiological cross-sectional area (PCSA), is closely and directly related to the maximal muscle strength: the larger the PCSA, the greater the strength. In addition, the muscle pennation angle also influences maximal isometric strength, with negative correlation: the higher the degree, the lower the strength (Fig. 4.9). The relationship between the force of the muscle effectively transmitted to the tendon and the pennation angle is regulated by the equation:

$$F_{\text{tendon}} = \cos\ \alpha\ \text{pennation angle} \times F_{\text{muscle}}$$

Ultrasound evaluation of muscle architecture parameters should always be performed as a comparative technique with the contralateral muscle and in an active and passive dynamic way, both at rest and during muscle contraction. The muscle thickness and the pennation angle are not static values, but adapt to the different functional conditions of the muscle. Their values increase linearly as the intensity of contraction increases. It has been shown that muscle training, particularly the resistance training, causes certain changes in muscle architecture parameters. In literature it has been referred that the quadriceps muscle of subjects experienced to intensive training (already after a month) first shows changes in muscle architecture and, subsequently, hypertrophy. On average, the following can be observed: increase in fascicle length (+10% approximately), increase in pennation angle (+8% approximately), and increase in muscle thickness (approximately +7%), due to the overall increase in the diameter of the fascicles. Some authors reported that in the elite sprinters' leg muscles (LV, MG, and LG), a greater fascicle length and a lower pennation angle have been detected, compared to what is found in the elite distance runners' muscles. If the training is performed at speed and without load, the elongation of the fascicles is prevalent with respect to the increase in the pennation angle. The sedentary lifestyle and aging induce a shortening of the fascicles and a lower pennation angle. Therefore, the architecture parameters allow a functional evaluation of the muscle. Hypertrophy of the muscular bundles, typically observed in athletes, can be associated with increased muscular hypoechogenicity.

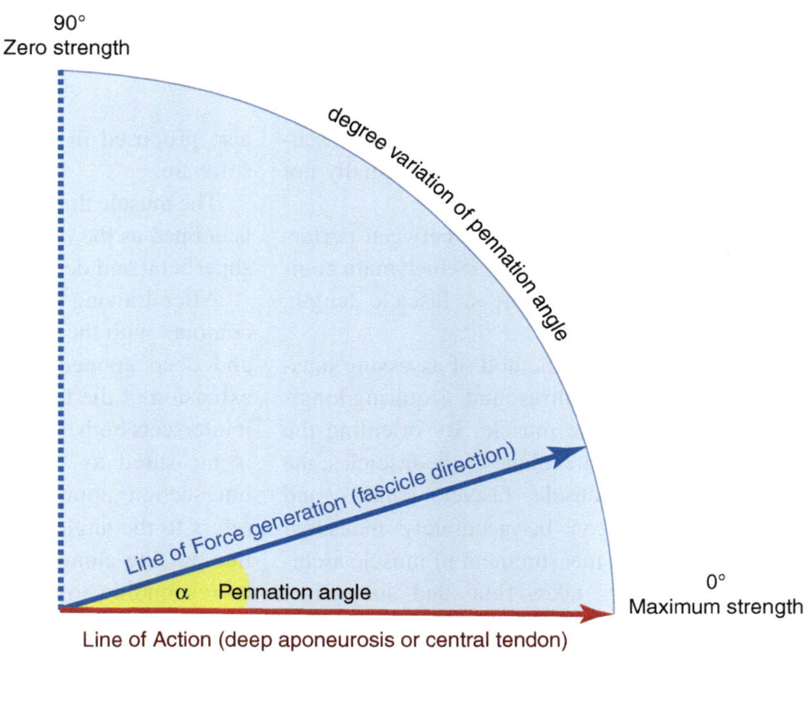

Fig. 4.9 Graphical representation of the relationship between the pennation angle and muscle strength

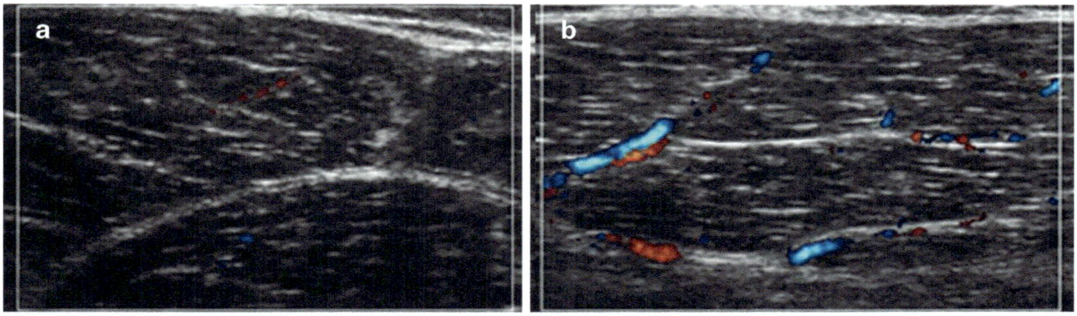

Fig. 4.10 (**a**, **b**) Color Doppler ultrasound of the quadriceps (vastus lateralis) before (**a**) and after exercise (**b**). A diffuse intramuscular hypervascularization is shown after intense activity. This is related to the physiological hyperemia

Finally, physical exercise is also associated with an increase in muscle vascularization (blood flow is 20 times higher than in standard conditions) and a consequent increase of the muscular mass volume, up to 10–15%. The muscular volume gets back to standard conditions after about 10–15 min of rest. Doppler techniques and, more specifically, power Doppler can demonstrate the physiological muscular hyperemia after contraction (Fig. 4.10a, b). Typically, blood vessels run in the septa of the perimysium.

When studying both muscles and tendons, it is fundamental that the ultrasound beam is correctly tilted so that it is always perpendicular to the examined muscular plane, in order to avoid the appearance of hypoechoic artifactual zones that can be misinterpreted by inexperienced operators. In some body regions the sonographer can observe accessory muscles, not to be misinterpreted as pathologic masses. The most commonly described "pseudomasses" are the palmaris longus muscle at the wrist, and the accessory soleus and the peroneus quartus at the ankle.

Ultrasound has a very important role in the diagnosis of muscle pathology and should be considered the first-choice imaging technique for traumatic pathology. When an inflammatory, degenerative, or a malignant pathology is in progress, US must be complemented with magnetic resonance (MR) and sometimes with computed tomography (CT).

According to etiology, muscular pathology can be divided into:

1. Inflammatory and degenerative
2. Malignant
3. Traumatic (major and minor lesions)

Rheumatology mostly deals with inflammatory and degenerative pathology, but a deep knowledge of the other lesions is necessary for a correct differential diagnosis. Degenerative muscular pathology does not show any specific features within the echotextures, but it is possible to detect some characteristic ultrasound signs of degeneration in several inflammatory pathologies.

4.2 Inflammatory and Degenerative Diseases

Muscular inflammatory pathology can be divided into:

1. Nonspecific myositis (serous, purulent, and chronic)
2. Specific myositis (syphilitic, tubercular, and viral)
3. Focal myositis ossificans (post-traumatic, post-inflammatory, and chronic)
4. Interstitial granulomatous myositis of unknown origin
5. Polymyositis

Serous myositis has a traumatic, toxi-infective, or viral origin. It is characterized by interstitial inflammatory, hyperemia, and serous infiltration

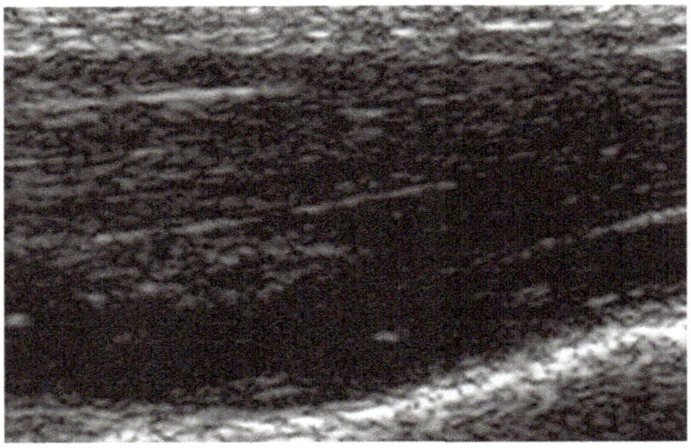

Fig. 4.11 Serous myositis. The muscle appears thickened and hypoechoic in relation to an extensive perimysial edema

of the perimysium. The thickening of the muscle fascicles is a typical degenerative aftereffect. In the earlier stages, the muscular structure can be easily assessed with US and it appears thickened and diffusely hypoechoic, due to the perimysial edema, with hazy muscular fascicles that appear interrupted and spaced (Fig. 4.11).

In the later stages, fibro-adipose involution has an inhomogeneous appearance. Purulent myositis, usually caused by deep and infected wounds or by blood flow-derived bacteria, is characterized by several scattered abscessed foci. With US, the abscess appears as a hypo-anechoic rounded mass, with hazy margins and inhomogeneous echoes. This kind of examination allows the size and the site of the abscess to be precisely described and a percutaneous drainage of the purulent material to be performed. In the later stages, the echogenicity of the abscess either further reduces or, if they become chronic, increases according to the inner organization of the collection (filaments, fibrous branches, or sediments) with a consensual hyperechoic appearance of the wall (pseudocapsular appearance). Chronic myositis follows an acute nonspecific myositis and is characterized by fibrosclerotic substitution of the normal echotexture with an increase of the interstitial connective tissue that can also involve large parts of the muscle belly. Tubercular myositis is usually the result of direct propagation of bone, articular or lymphoglandular granulomas; the caseous exudate spreads through the interstitium to the muscular tissue, producing complex and extensive fistulous tracts. Hematogenous tubercular dissemination in patients affected by miliary tuberculosis is extremely rare. The most common viral myositis is caused by Coxsackie B virus (Bornholm's disease) and is characterized by necrotic and degenerative lesions of the muscle fibers.

Myositis ossificans may have different forms: focal myositis ossificans can represent the fibrocalcific involution following violent trauma, chronic inflammatory processes, or suppurative lesions, or it can be the direct consequence of central or peripheral nervous system diseases. Sometimes, it can represent natural evolution of an intramuscular hematoma that calcifies and leads to an ossification process (Fig. 4.12); the development of these lesions occurs over a 5–6-month period. In earlier phases, the lesion has an inhomogeneous architecture and may mimic neoplasia; afterwards, the first calcification appears, mostly on the margins, which is then followed by true ossification.

Progressive myositis ossificans (PMO) or progressive ossificans fibrodysplasia of Munchmeyer is a rare and incurable genetic disease with autosomal dominant transmission, characterized by a progressive ossification of skeletal muscles until a complete substitution with a mineralized osseous matrix has occurred. The early histopathologic alterations of connective tissue (particularly aponeurosis, fascias, tendons, and ligaments) represent the basics of the disease, while skeletal muscle is involved last. At first, US shows typical muscular inflammation, with reduced echoes within the involved areas; then the consequent fibrous involution causes a hypoechoic appearance (Fig. 4.13) until several ossified foci can be observed in later stages. In these cases, other imaging techniques are necessary to understand the exact origin of the bony growths.

Polymyositis consists of a group of muscular disorders of unknown origin characterized by an inflammatory process of the skeletal musculature. Polymyositis is classified among the systemic rheumatic diseases, more precisely among the connective tissue diseases, and can be idiopathic, juvenile, or tumor related. The main symptom is muscular weakness that mainly

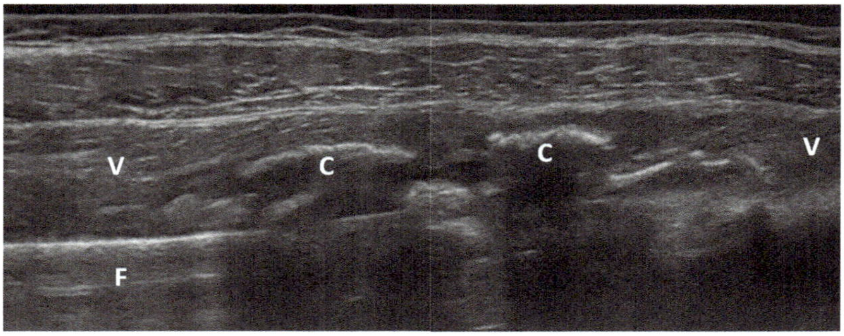

Fig. 4.12 Ultrasound longitudinal view of the thigh showing myositis ossificans, with blurred calcified spots within the muscle

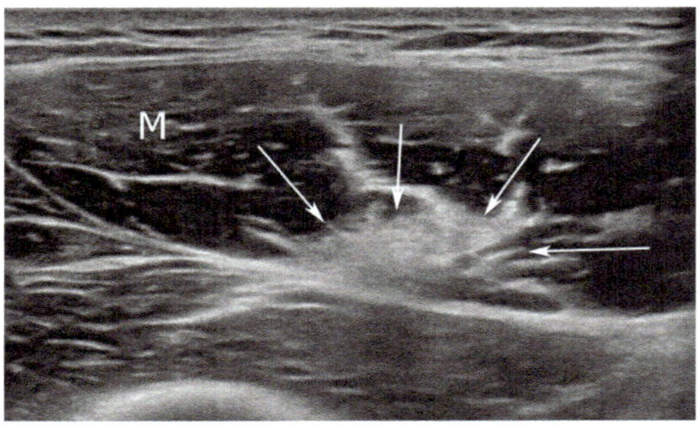

Fig. 4.13 Extensive muscular fibrosis with multiple fibrocalcific areas (arrows) within the muscle; muscle (M)

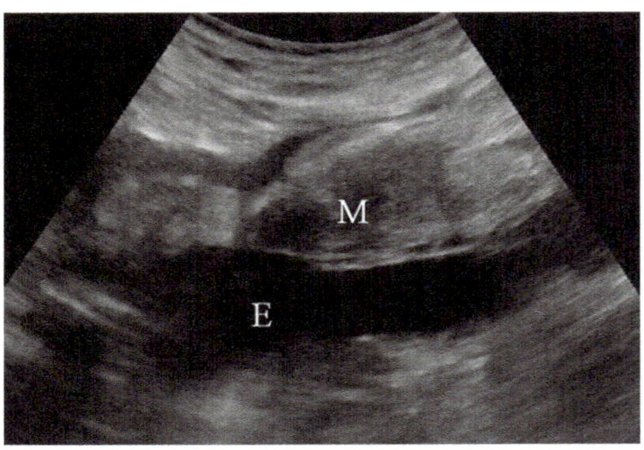

Fig. 4.14 Longitudinal scan of the posterior side of the thigh: hamstrings tear with bell-clapper aspect (M) and extensive effusion (E)

affects the proximal muscles of the limb girdle musculature. Several cutaneous symptoms are typically associated with this disease. US is helpful both as a diagnostic tool, detecting the muscular degeneration areas and the intramuscular calcific foci, and as a guide to muscular biopsy, which is necessary to definitively confirm the diagnosis.

4.3 Traumatic Injury

US is extremely helpful in the field of muscular trauma. Within minor traumatic lesions, muscular contractures and contusions are difficult to detect with US, unless complemented with an accurate comparative examination. They are characterized by slight widening of perimysial partitions with hypoechoic post-traumatic edema. Major traumatic lesions are represented by intramuscular hematoma and muscle rupture. Muscular hematoma is the typical sign of a muscular tear and its dimensions usually indicate the extension of the tear (excluding some hematological conditions). The formation of a hematoma creates dissection of the fascial planes, and if the collection exceeds 100 ml of fluid—as in case of a complete rupture—it must be drained quickly to avoid any compression on the surrounding muscular and neurovascular structures (Fig. 4.14).

The evolution of an intramuscular hematoma is not dissimilar to that which occurs in other sites of the human body. A recent hemorrhage has a hyperechoic appearance (Fig. 4.15) but becomes hypoechoic after a couple of hours until a separation between the liquid and the corpuscular phase occurs.

When the hematoma is resolving, it appears as a homogeneous anechoic collection (Fig. 4.16) that can be more or less organized.

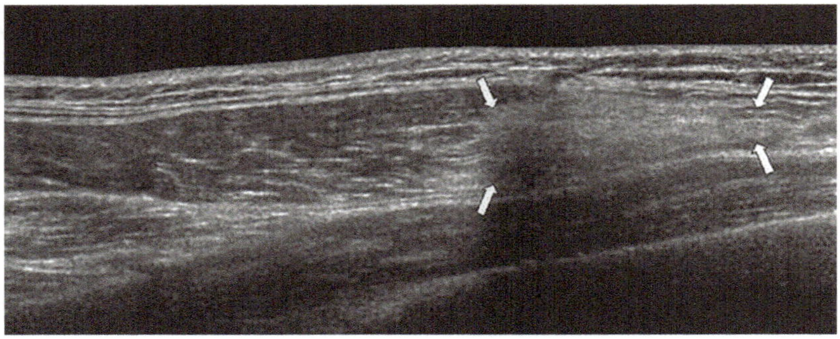

Fig. 4.15 Diffusely hyperechoic hematoma (arrows) following recent muscle trauma

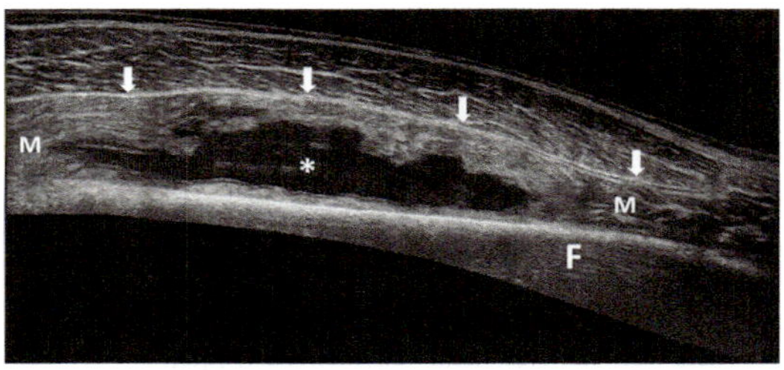

Fig. 4.16 Extended field of view: (*) muscular hematoma, (F) femur, (M) vastus intermedius muscle; white arrows = fascia

Muscular ruptures can be caused by compression (direct trauma) or by a distraction of the muscular extremities. If direct trauma occurs, the muscle is directly compressed against the underlying bone. US demonstrates an irregular cavity with rough borders followed, a few hours after the trauma, by a hematoma. As the lesion heals, US can detect extensive scar tissue that appears hyperechoic and calcific (post-traumatic myositis ossificans). Indirect trauma is caused by a sudden and violent contraction of the muscle and is more frequent in the lower limbs, especially in those muscles that connect two bone segments. Distraction traumas can be basically divided into three groups, according to their ultrasound features: strain (grade I), partial rupture (grade II), and complete rupture (grade III). More detailed muscle tear classifications are also available (see Chap. 24).

Muscle strain occurs when it is stretched beyond its elastic limit. The patient reports acute pain that cannot be distinguished from cramp. The lesions are mostly microscopic but the macroscopic exam can detect several small sero-hemorrhagic collections up to 6–7 cm long and

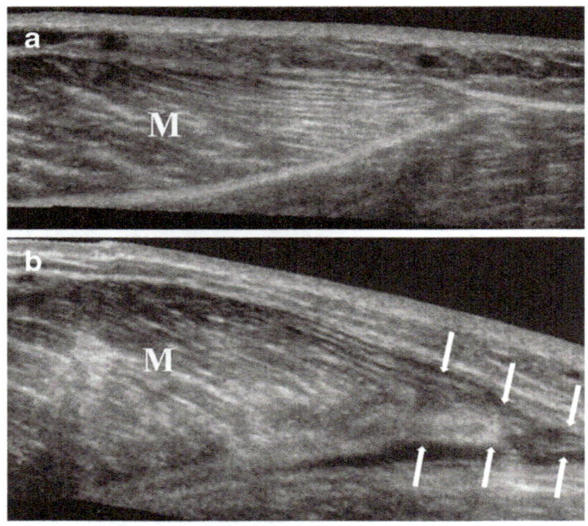

Fig. 4.17 Normal appearance of medial gastrocnemius (M) myotendinous junction (**a**). Partial tear (arrows) of medial gastrocnemius (M) at the myotendinous junction (**b**)

from 2 to 10 mm of diameter. On US, these collections have a stretched and irregular hypoechoic appearance. Healing occurs in about 2 weeks. Partial rupture (grade II) is a lesion that occurs when the muscle is stretched over its maximal elastic potential. It involves more than 5% of the muscular tissue but not the whole transverse section. In acute cases, the patient reports a "snap" with localized sharp pain and a complete loss of muscle function that is usually recovered in a couple of days. US clearly shows the discontinuity of the muscle with interruption of the fibro-adipose septa, in particular at the myotendinous junction, as in the gastrocnemius (Fig. 4.17a, b).

A partial rupture shows three different US findings: a hypoechoic cavity within the muscular tissue, a thick hyperechoic cavity border, and

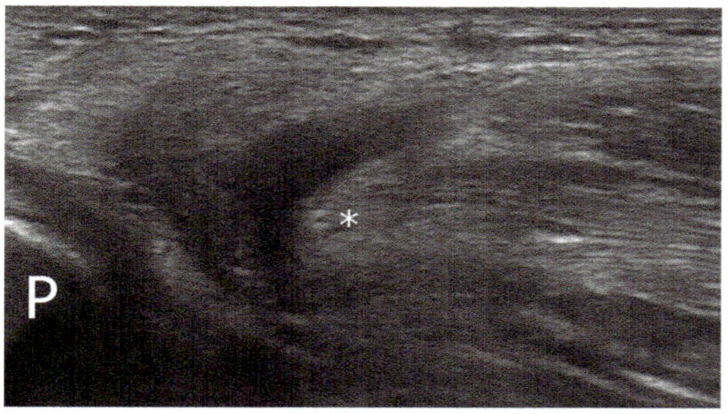

Fig. 4.18 Bell-clapper (asterisk) appearance of muscular stump. P pubis

the "bell-clapper" sign, due to small shreds of muscular tissue floating in the hematoma (Fig. 4.18).

Complete ruptures (grade III) are far less common than the other lesions. The initial clinical presentation is very similar to the partial rupture but the functional loss persists longer and, if the muscle is superficial, the lesion can be appreciated on palpation. US shows complete dislocation of the muscular ends with a hematoma filling the gap (Fig. 4.19).

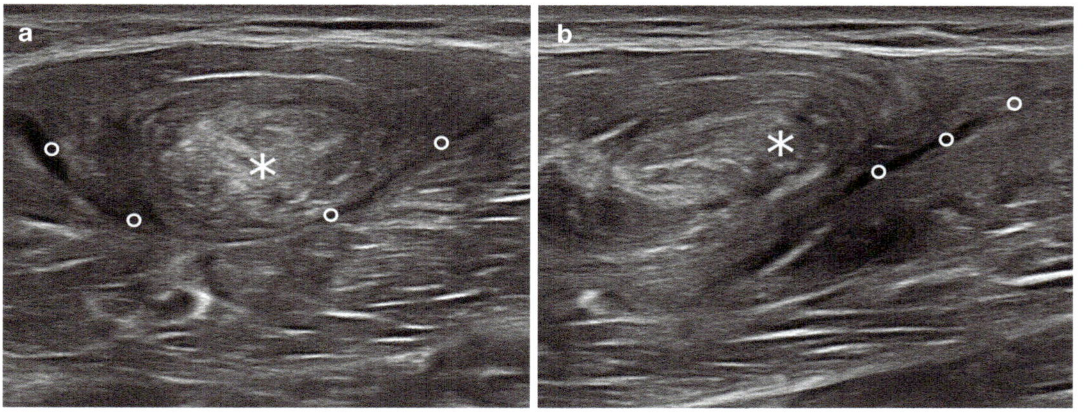

Fig. 4.19 Transverse (**a**) and longitudinal (**b**) US scans of a severe rupture of rectus femoris with retraction of muscular stumps (*) and wide sero-hemorrhagic collection filling the resulting gap (circles)

Further Readings

Abe T, et al. Fascicle length of leg muscles is greater in sprinters than distance runners. Med Sci Sport Exerc. 2000;32(6):1125–9.

Bianchi S, Martinoli C, Sureda D, Rizzatto G. Ultrasound of the hand. Eur J Ultrasound. 2001;14:234.

Blazevich OJ. Effects of physical training and detraining, immobilisation, growth and aging on human fascicle geometry. Sports Med. 2006;36(12):1003–17.

Bureau NJ, Chhem RK, Cardinal E. Musculoskeletal infections: US manifestations. Radiographics. 1999;19:1585–92.

Chau CL, Griffith JF. Musculoskeletal infections: ultrasound appearances. Clin Radiol. 2005;60:149–59.

de Oliveira FTM, de Oliveira CG, Farinatti P. Pennation angle of vastus lateralis during isometric contractions performed at two knee angles. Fisioter Mov. 2017;30(Suppl 1):S75–83.

Erickson S. High resolution imaging of the musculoskeletal system. Radiology. 1997;205:593–618.

Narici MV, Maganaris CN, Reeves ND, Capodoglio P. Effect of aging on human muscle and architecture. J Appl Phisiol. 2003;95:2229–34.

Park A, Lehnerdt G, Lautermann J. Myositis of the sternocleidomastoid muscle as a result of arthritis of the sternoclavicular joint. Laryngorhinootologie. 2006;86(2):124–7.

Peetrons P. Ultrasound of muscles. Eur Radiol. 2002;12:35–43.

Reimens K, Reimens CS, Wagner S, et al. Skeletal muscle sonography: a correlative study of echogenicity and morphology. J Ultrasound Med. 1993;2:73–7.

Scott JE. High resolution imaging of the musculoskeletal system. Radiology. 1997;205:593–618.

Seynnes OR, et al. Early skeletal muscle hypertrophy and architectural changes in response to high-intensity resistance training. J Appl Physiol. 2007;102(1):368–73.

Van Holsbeeck M, Introcaso JH. Musculoskeletal Ultrasonography. Radiol Clin North Am. 1992;5:907–25.

Peripheral Nerves

5

Enzo Silvestri, Davide Orlandi,
and Elena Massone

Contents

5.1 Sonographic and Doppler Normal Anatomy

Peripheral nerves are usually made of nervous fibres (containing axons, myelin sheaths and Schwann cells) grouped in fascicles and loose connective tissue (containing elastic fibres and vessels). Each fascicle is encased by a proper connective sheath called perineurium. Inside the fascicle are a group of axons bathed in endoneurial fluid. Each axon has an insulating lining of myelin: a fatty material inside the Schwann cells. Between the fascicles and the outer nerve sheath, there is a fatty material called the interfascicular epineurium which houses the nerve vascular structure. The nerve is then wrapped in the main outer epineurium—an external sheath. Clinical experience with ultrasound and improvements in technology have been helpful in the evaluation of peripheral nerve, and the improvements in Doppler sensitivity and power Doppler have made it possible to assess vascular changes within major nerve segments. Peripheral nerve ultrasound, when compared to electrodiagnostic testing, adds the possibility to provide anatomic detail of the affected site without any discomfort. In fact, ultrasound is a low-cost, quick and non-invasive imaging method, providing an excellent view of peripheral nerve anatomy as well as of surrounding structures. US provides high spatial resolution and the ability to explore long segments of nerve trunks in a single study, also allowing nerve examination in both static and dynamic conditions, during passive or active movements of the extremities. US enables the identification of post-traumatic changes of nerves, neuropathies secondary to compression

E. Silvestri
Radiology, Alliance Medical, Genova, Italy

D. Orlandi (✉)
Department of Radiology, Ospedale Evangelico Internazionale, Genova, Italy

E. Massone
Department of Radiology, Ospedale Santa Corona, Pietra Ligure (SV), Italy

F. Martino et al. (eds.), *Musculoskeletal Ultrasound in Orthopedic and Rheumatic disease in Adults*,
https://doi.org/10.1007/978-3-030-91202-4_5

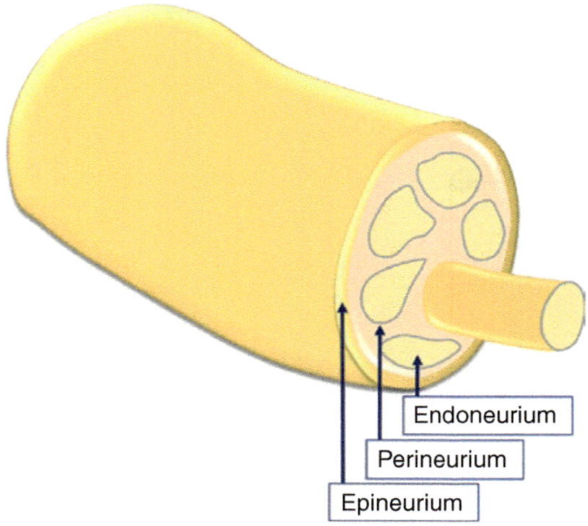

Fig. 5.1 Scheme of peripheral nerve illustrating its inner structure

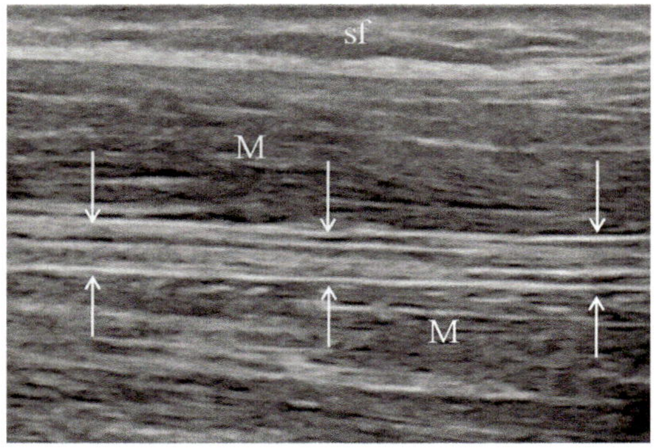

Fig. 5.2 Peripheral nerves. Longitudinal 3–16 MHz US image obtained over the median nerve (white arrows) at the middle third of the forearm. The nerve is made of parallel linear hypoechoic areas, the fascicles, separated by hyperechoic bands, the interfascicular epineurium; muscles (M), subcutaneous fat (sf)

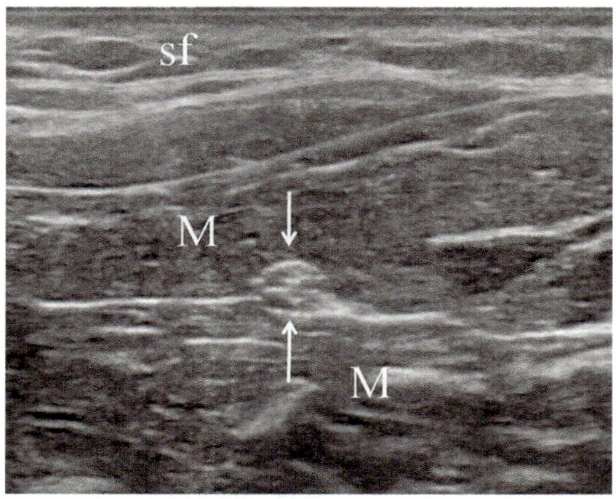

Fig. 5.3 Nerve echotexture. Transverse US image of the median nerve at the middle third of forearm. The nerve (white arrowhead) is characterized by a honeycombing appearance made of round hypoechoic areas in a homogeneous hyperechoic background; subcutaneous fat (sf), muscles (M)

syndromes and inflammatory or neoplastic nerve lesions as well as the evaluation of post-operative complications, and it is increasingly used in anaesthesiology for regional anaesthesia. Nerves present cable-like structures and have a distinct architecture consisting of fascicles and surrounding epineurium (Fig. 5.1).

In the transverse plane, the echo pattern is described as a 'honeycomb' aspect because tiny round and hypoechogenic areas representing the nerve bundles with hyperechogenic rims of the epineurium are visible. In the longitudinal plane, nerves present as long, slim structures with a mixture of parallel hyperechogenic lines, representing the perineurium, between two more prominent and also hyperechogenic layers of the epineurium. This image resembles that of an electric cable (Figs. 5.2 and 5.3).

The transverse image is much more frequently used in clinical practice, as it allows for the nerve to be examined by the so-called elevator technique which consists of finding the set nerve at a characteristic anatomic point and 'tracking it' either proximally or distally. In this way, it is possible to assess the nerve's shape, echogenicity and thickness and its relation to the surrounding tissues, the surface area of the nerve and its vasculature. If an abnormality is seen in the transverse view, the nerve should be examined in the longitudinal view. The US aspect of nerves changes from hypo- to hyperechogenic as they are followed more peripherally for an increasing amount of connective tissue between the nerve bundles. It has been assumed that nerves are not anisotropic even if the property of anisotropy is seen in cases of nerves with large cross sections.

The shape of a nerve may also be different and vary between individuals, round, oval, triangular or irregularly shaped, which may change under compression by the probe or with the movement of a neighbouring muscle. Nerve may change its shape along its course, for example, from a triangular to a round cross section, or may present anatomic variants (e.g. bifid or trifid variants of the median nerve).

Motor and motor-sensory nerves may be evaluated indirectly analysing the skeletal muscles which they innervate: we can evaluate muscular atrophy in case of chronic denervation as a decrease of the muscle's volume and fatty infiltration, which increases its echogenicity.

Ultrasound measurement of nerve size is very important because nerve enlargement is the most important diagnostic marker of an abnormal nerve: cross-sectional area and swelling ratio (the ratio between the cross-sectional area of the nerve at the site of maximal enlargement and that at an unaffected site) can be measured on transverse images, and diameter can be measured on longitudinal images. For correct measurement, the transducer should be perpendicular to the nerve, with minimal pressure, and the site of maximal enlargement should be selected for the measurement of nerve size. Variability within a measurement can be reduced doing multiple measures. Measuring just inside the echogenic rim of the nerve is the preferred technique.

Placing the power Doppler box over the nerve and slowly increasing the gain can be useful to evaluate the vascularity of the peripheral nerves.

No colour Doppler signal will be observed in the normal nerve.

Nerve mobility can be routinely assessed to exclude nerve entrapments.

5.2 Compressive Chronic Involvement

Nerve compressive syndromes are relatively common pathologies. They can occur acutely or chronically anywhere in the body; however, they develop more frequently at certain anatomic sites where the nerve passes through fibro-osseous tunnels or at the level of anomalous bony, muscular or connective structures. Nerve conduction study and US examination provide complementary assessment in evaluating nerve entrapment syndromes; in particular, US can be very helpful for the detection of the site of compression and for the identification of abnormal findings in the nerve surroundings. Ultrasound can directly demonstrate morphologic changes in the nerve appearance, and, sometimes, it can identify secondary causes (i.e. accessory muscle, thickened fibrous band, cyst, bony prominence, vascular or neoplastic mass, foreign body, orthopaedic implants); this is especially true for larger and more superficial nerves. In case of nerve compression, a focal flattening with reduction of nerve cross-sectional area (CSA) at the compression point can be appreciated. Proximal to the level of compression, a fusiform enlargement of the nerve could be observed: it usually extends 2–4 cm in length and presents maximum diameter immediately before the compression point, where the nerve suddenly flattens. In combination to such morphologic changes, also the normal US echotexture is altered: the nerve appears homogeneously hypoechoic with loss of the typical fascicular pattern, reflecting the substanding venous congestion and consecutive epi/endoneurial oedema; consequently the outer lining of the nerve becomes well delineated from the hyperechoic perineural fat. Furthermore, intraneural microcirculation can be assessed with colour or power Doppler US examination: in cases of acute compression, a local interruption in the microcirculation can occur with possible venous congestion; on the other hand, an increase in intraneural blood flow signals can be appreciated in chronic compressive neuropathies. Long-standing nerve compression leads to fibrosis and eventually to damage to the myelin sheath and to axonal degeneration. At this stage, a diffuse hyperechogenicity and reduction of volume of the innervated muscles can be assessed because of muscular atrophy.

Carpal tunnel syndrome is the most common entrapment neuropathy. It results from the compression of the median nerve in the fibro-osseous tunnel between the carpal bones and flexor retinaculum (or carpal transverse ligament). US may demonstrate the homogeneously hypoechoic enlargement of the median nerve proximal to the

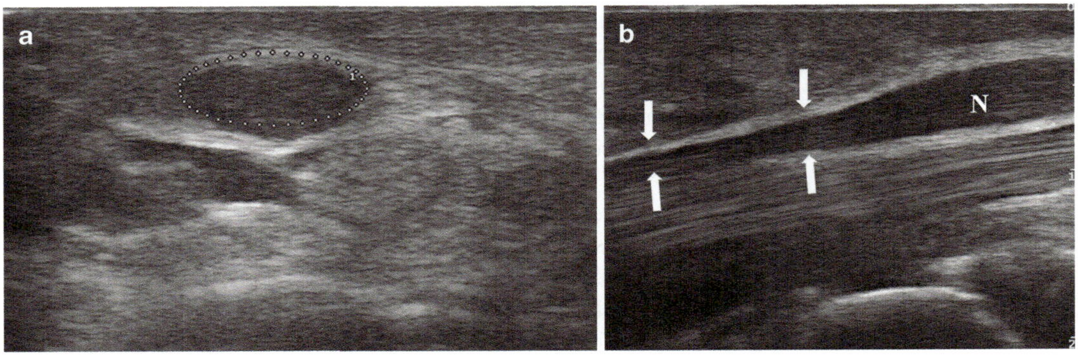

Fig. 5.4 Carpal tunnel syndrome. (**a**) axial view, median nerve (dots) with hypoechoic appearance and loss of the typical fascicular pattern; (**b**) Longitudinal view, flattened (arrows) median nerve (N)

carpal tunnel, with sudden flattening through the fibro-osseous tunnel (Fig. 5.4a and b); palmar bowing of the flexor retinaculum and hypomobility of the nerve during dynamic manoeuvres (opening and closing of fingers) may be associated. However, in few cases, the median nerve may appear normal even in the presence of positive clinical and electrophysiological findings.

5.3 Acute Traumatic Injuries

Three different types of traumatic or iatrogenic nerve damage have been described based on the mechanism of injury: traction, contusion and penetrating trauma (multiple mechanisms may coexist), which could result in neurapraxia, axonotmesis or neurotmesis. Ultrasound examination, being able to evaluate and differentiate fascicles, perineurium, epineurium and surrounding tissues, can be used to assess the site of injury, discriminate nerve injury in continuity from nerve transection and identify foreign bodies, neuroma and scarring. It is very useful in the case of traumatic nerve injury and could help clinical examination and nerve conduction studies to provide information about the condition of the injured nerve and, consequently, possible surgical indications.

Nerve-stretching syndromes can occur from sprain or strain injuries and, less frequently, from overuse. A typical injury is the avulsion of the nerve roots of the brachial plexus during motor vehicle accidents. Another typical injury is the peroneal nerve traction at the popliteal fossa during high-grade sprain traumas. Neurapraxic injury can be appreciated as a swollen nerve with hypoechoic appearance. The outer nerve sheath may be intact. In cases of partial nerve tear, a so-called traction neuroma can be seen along the course of the stretched nerve without discontinuity: it appears as an irregular focal thickening of hypoechoic tissue (Fig. 5.5).

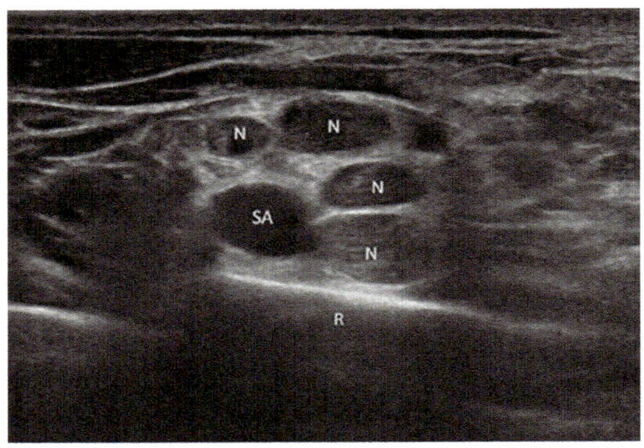

Fig. 5.5 Brachial plexus stretching. Supraclavicular region, oblique view: subclavian artery (SA), enlarged cords (N), rib (R)

In mild traumas, the neuroma may involve only one or few fascicles without resulting in nerve cross-sectional enlargement. In complete nerve lesions, US demonstrates the retraction of the fascicles with a wavy appearance of the nerve ends.

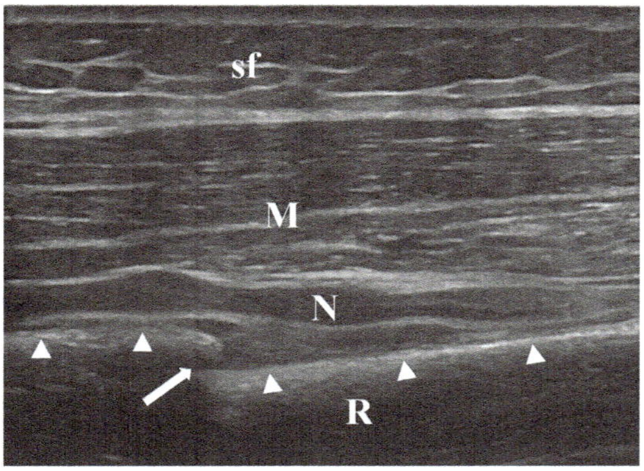

Fig. 5.6 Radial nerve injury; US longitudinal scan: radius (R), bone surface (arrowheads), fracture (arrow), subcutaneous fat (sf), thickened radial nerve (N) with irregular shape and loss of fascicular aspect

Contusion traumas typically occur where nerves run in proximity of bony surfaces. In most cases, they do not cause morphologic changes detectable with US, and the pathologic process is self-resolving. Nevertheless, in some cases repeated minor traumas could lead to a focal fusiform thickening of the nerve at the site of repetitive contusions (e.g. peroneal nerve neuritis in soccer players and ulnar nerve friction neuritis in cubital tunnel instability). In penetrating wounds or in bone fracture such as radial bone fracture, where the radial nerve runs in proximity of bony surfaces, US can detect shape alteration, loss of normal echostructure and thickening (Fig. 5.6), a partial tear or a complete transection of the nerve fascicles.

In the last two cases, the regenerative process leads to the formation of a hypoechoic fibrous mass in the attempt to restore the continuity of the nerve, but in different ways. In partial tears, the hypoechoic neuroma may develop from the resected fascicles preserving the healthy fascicles, and its size would be smaller than the CSA of the nerve, or it may encase both the resected and the unaffected fascicles determining a fusiform swelling of the nerve. In complete tears, the so-called stump neuromas or terminal neuromas appear as hypoechoic mass-like lesions at the resected nerve edges with a CSA slightly larger than the nerve itself. The detection of terminal neuromas is of additional help when the resected nerve ends are retracted from the site of injury (Fig. 5.7).

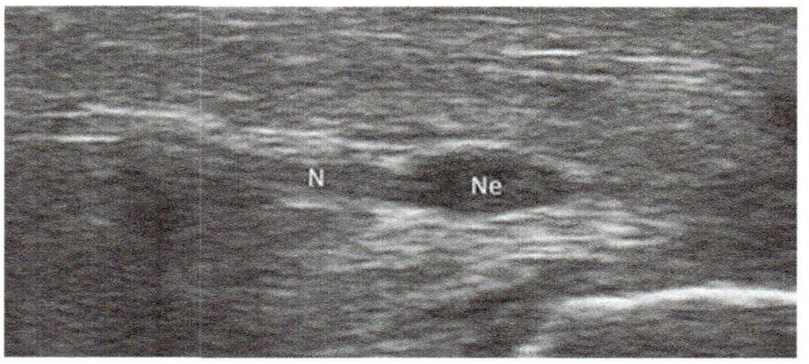

Fig. 5.7 Terminal post-traumatic neuroma. Longitudinal view of a digital nerve (N) and traumatic neuroma (Ne)

Further Readings

Beekman R, Visser LH. High-resolution sonography of the peripheral nervous system: a review of the literature. Eur J Neurol. 2004;11:305–14.

Martinoli C, Bianchi S, Derchi LE. Tendon and nerve sonography. Radiol Clin N Am. 1999;37(691–711):41.

Martinoli C, Bianchi S, Gandolfo N, et al. US of nerve entrapments in osteofibrous tunnels of the upper and lower limbs. Radiographics. 2000;20:199–217.

Silvestri E, Martinoli C, Derchi LE, et al. Echo-texture of peripheral nerves: correlation between US and histologic findings and criteria to differentiate tendons. Radiology. 1995;197:291–6.

Dermis and Hypodermis

6

Davide Orlandi, Enzo Silvestri,
and Alessandro Muda

Contents

6.1 Sonographic and Doppler normal anatomy

Assessment of skin and subcutaneous tissue is possible using high-frequency transducers (up to 30 MHz) that are able to differentiate skin from subcutaneous tissue (Fig. 6.1).

Specific skin diseases are usually diagnosed by clinical examination, sometimes followed by skin biopsy.

D. Orlandi (✉)
Department of Radiology, Ospedale Evangelico Internazionale, Genova, Italy

E. Silvestri
Radiology, Alliance Medical, Genova, Italy

A. Muda
Department of Radiology, IRCCS Policlinico San Martino-IST, Genova, Italy

6.2 Main Pathological Findings

Currently US has no role in the diagnosis of skin lesions but can be very helpful in assessing and following up several systemic pathologies with cutaneous involvement. In dermatopolymyositis, cutaneous lesions can be easily found: for example, the characteristic Gottron's papule, erythematous or violaceous plaques, slightly thickened over bony eminences, often detected on the extensor aspect of finger joints. With US they appear as small nodular iso-hyperechoic areas with characteristic calcification if the disease occurs in childhood. Involvement of adipose tissue is observed as moderate thickening that appears as a homogeneous hyperechoic line affecting the fibrous connective tissue bands that lose their linear architecture.

On US, liposclerosis is characterized by hypoechoic micro- and macronodules of fibrous tissue that progressively replace the subcutaneous tissue. Rheumatic nodules have a hypoechoic appearance with smooth margins and can be sometimes mistaken for gout tophi; the incidental finding of calcific intralesional foci (hyperechoic

F. Martino et al. (eds.), *Musculoskeletal Ultrasound in Orthopedic and Rheumatic disease in Adults*,
https://doi.org/10.1007/978-3-030-91202-4_6

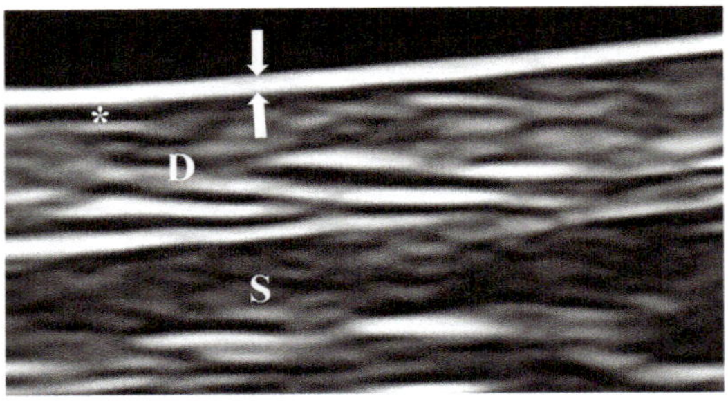

Fig. 6.1 Normal dermis and hypodermis (22 MHz transducer): skin (arrow), superficial dermis (asterisk), hypodermis (D), subcutaneous fat (S)

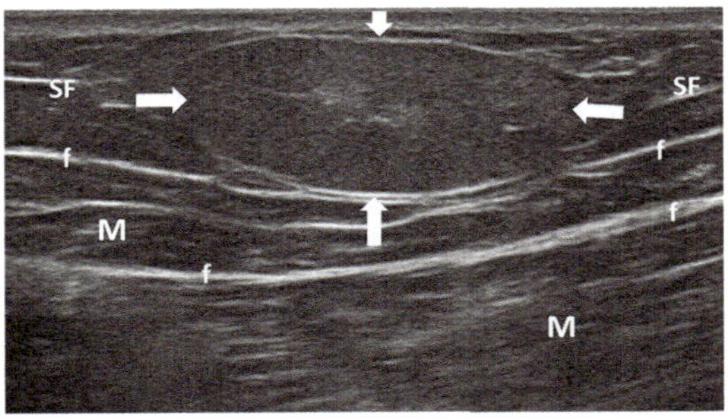

Fig. 6.2 Superficial lipoma (white arrows), subcutaneous fat (SF), muscle (M), muscle fascia (f)

with posterior acoustic shadow) makes the diagnosis easier. In systemic sclerosis, sclero-atrophic hypo-isoechoic alteration of the subcutaneous tissue can be seen, especially in the fingertips. Subcutaneous edema is characterized by a large mesh hypoechoic net with a characteristic "cobblestone" appearance.

Panniculitis is an inflammatory phenomenon of the subcutaneous tissue with a probable vasculitic origin. It can be divided into lobular and septal panniculitis and appear as hypo-hyperechoic inhomogeneous areas, rich in calcific nodules of various dimensions (1 cm up to 15 cm in erythema nodosum). Moreover, in the acute phases, marked surrounding edema and thickening of the septa can be seen.

Lipomas and angiomas are common findings and are characterized by specific US vascular pattern (Figs. 6.2 and 6.3a, b).

There are several pathologies—less important but not less common—involving the overloaded fat pads in specific anatomical sites, such as the fibro-adipose subcalcanear sole, that may be affected in overload syndromes that involve the nearby plantar fascia (Fig. 6.4).

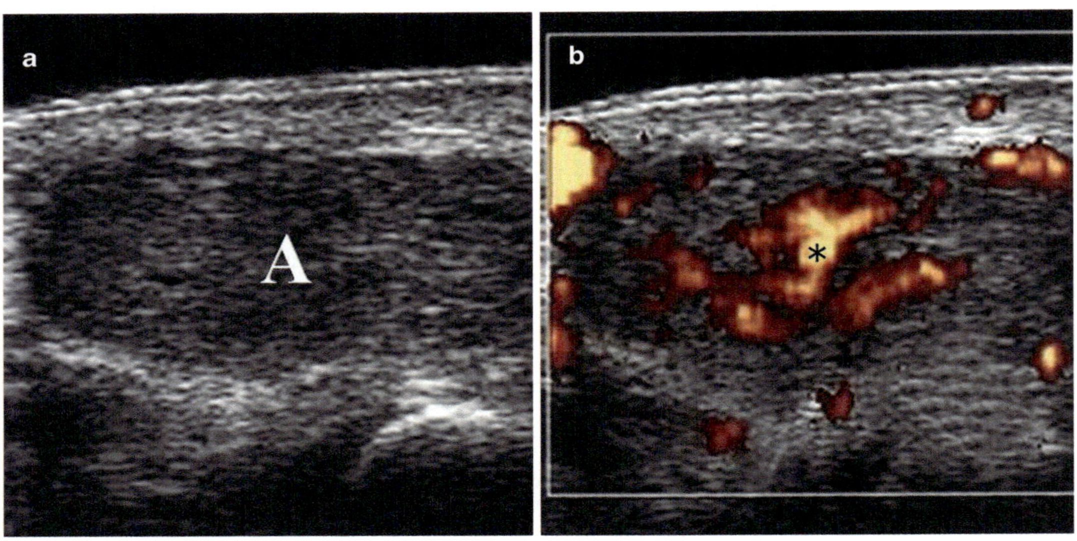

Fig. 6.3 (**a**) Hypoechoic, ovoid, well-defined mass typical of an angioma (A). (**b**) The corresponding power Doppler scan shows the typical vascular pattern with a single pedicle (*)

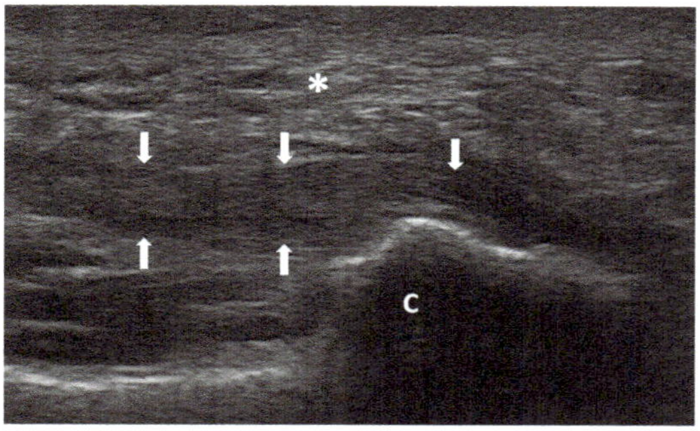

Fig. 6.4 Plantar fasciitis: inhomogeneous appearance of subcutaneous planes (*); plantar fascia thickening (white arrows); calcaneus (C)

Plantar fibromatosis (Ledderhose disease) is a pathological condition characterized by nodularity along the aponeurosis course which appears homogeneously hypoechoic (Fig. 6.5a, b) and shows no vascular signals at color and power Doppler analysis.

A similar condition, sometimes connected with plantar fibromatosis, is Dupuytren's contracture, in which the hypoechoic nodules are found in longitudinal bundles of the palmar fascia along the course of the flexor tendons.

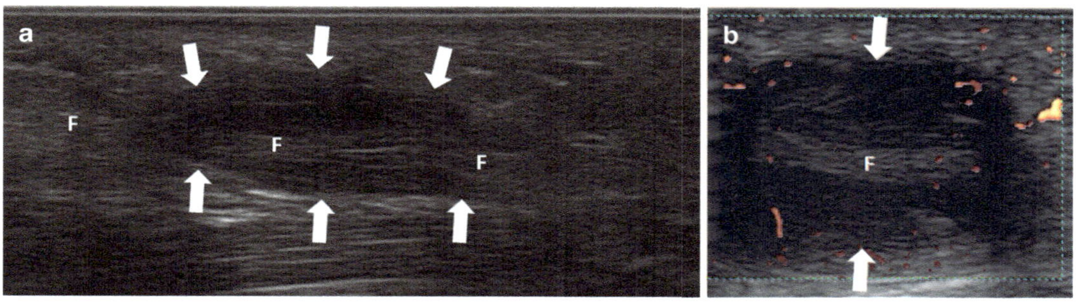

Fig. 6.5 Ledderhose disease; (**a**) plantar fascia longitudinal scan, fibrous nodule (white arrows), plantar fascia (F); (**b**) power Doppler showing mild nodule vascularity

Further Readings

Grassi W, Cervini C. Ultrasonography in rheumatology: an evolving technique. Ann Rheum Dis. 1998;57:268–71.

Grassi W, Lamanna G, Farina A, Cervini C. Sonographic imaging of normal and osteoarthritic cartilage. Semin Arthritis Rheum. 1999;28:398–403.

Sheperd DET, Seedhom BB. Thickness of human articular cartilage in joints of the lower limb. Ann Rheum Dis. 1999;58:27–34.

Wortsman X, Jemec GBE. Dermatologic ultrasound with clinical and histological correlations. New York: Springer ed; 2018.

Wortsman X. Atlas of Dermatologic ultrasound with clinical and histological correlations. New York: Springer ed; 2013.

Xu H, Guo L, Wang Q. Diagnostic ultrasound in dermatology. Shangai: Springer ed; 2022.

Part II

Ultrasound Pathologic Findings in Rheumatic Diseases

Osteoarthritis

7

Marco Di Carlo, Edoardo Cipolletta, Emilio Filippucci, and Fabio Martino

Contents

7.1 Introduction

Osteoarthritis (OA) is the most common joint disease in the world and its prevalence is rising with the growing ageing population of Western countries. Knee or hip OA has a prevalence of 40% in people over 65 years of age. Pain with movement, limited mobility, and consequent disability are the main features of this disease.

The early detection of the clinical expressions of the disease is fundamental to start adequate therapeutic interventions before the development of irreversible joint damage. In this perspective, imaging techniques have been indicated as important tools to help in the diagnosis and follow-up of OA. Conventional radiography remains the most widely used imaging technique for the diagnosis of OA. It allows the detection and assessment of two main pathological findings, joint space narrowing and osteophytes, which are fundamental to determine the extent of the OA process. In fact, the Kellgren-Lawrence score, the most widespread composite index allowing the assessment of OA severity, is based on these two pathological findings. In particular, joint space narrowing represents in daily clinical practice the "gold standard" to estimate the OA severity. However, conventional radiography is able to detect joint space narrowing only in advanced stages of joint damage and it is therefore not sensitive to early degenerative cartilaginous changes, which start largely earlier than the radiographic evidence of joint space narrowing and/or osteophytes which appear only in established OA. Joint

M. Di Carlo · E. Cipolletta · E. Filippucci
Clinica Reumatologica, Dipartimento di Scienze Cliniche e Molecolari, Università Politecnica delle Marche, Jesi (Ancona), Italy

F. Martino (✉)
Radiology, Sant'Agata Diagnostic Center, Bari, Italy

F. Martino et al. (eds.), *Musculoskeletal Ultrasound in Orthopedic and Rheumatic disease in Adults*,
https://doi.org/10.1007/978-3-030-91202-4_7

space narrowing, in particular, continues to be widely applied as an indirect indicator of tibiofemoral cartilage thinning, even in the more recent Kellgren-Lawrence scoring methods. However, the reduction of articular space in conventional radiography does not necessarily identify cartilage damage, being detectable also in case of meniscal extrusion.

Over the years, the imaging technique that has probably gained the most importance in OA is magnetic resonance imaging (MRI). This technique is currently considered the "gold standard" for the evaluation of OA, allowing a detailed visualization of articular cartilage and other intra-articular structures. However, MRI is not applicable on a large scale as a first-line imaging technique due to the high costs, scarce availability, and high prevalence of OA in the general population.

Over the last few years, musculoskeletal ultrasound (US) has been increasingly investigated, mainly in research areas, but also with interesting applications in daily clinical practice. A great advantage is US ability to reveal subclinical inflammatory features such as intra-articular effusion or synovitis. Moreover, US allows the detection and assessment of morpho-structural changes involving the joint cartilage reachable by the US beam, the outer profile of the bony cortex, and the external portions of the menisci. Compared to MRI it is a cheaper and more available method and overall there are no contraindications to perform an US examination. In light of these aspects, there is increasing evidence to support the use of US as the first imaging technique in OA together with conventional radiography.

This chapter focuses on the basic US pathological findings that are commonly detected in patients with OA.

7.2 Synovitis

OA is classically considered as a degenerative disease; however, it is frequently associated with a low degree of joint inflammation. In order to avoid diagnostic mistakes, it is essential to distinguish joint inflammation resulting from OA from the one that may be a consequence of joint inflammatory disease.

Conventional radiography is of limited help in assessing soft tissue inflammatory involvement. Conversely, US and MRI are the imaging methods of choice for assessing the joint inflammation.

According to the recent redefinition of the terminology proposed by the Outcome Measures in Rheumatology (OMERACT) US Working Group, US synovitis is defined by the "presence of a hypoechoic synovial hypertrophy regardless of the presence of effusion or any grade of Doppler signal" (Fig. 7.1).

Power Doppler (PD) US provides an estimation of synovial tissue hyperemia and measures the degree of synovial inflammation. In patients

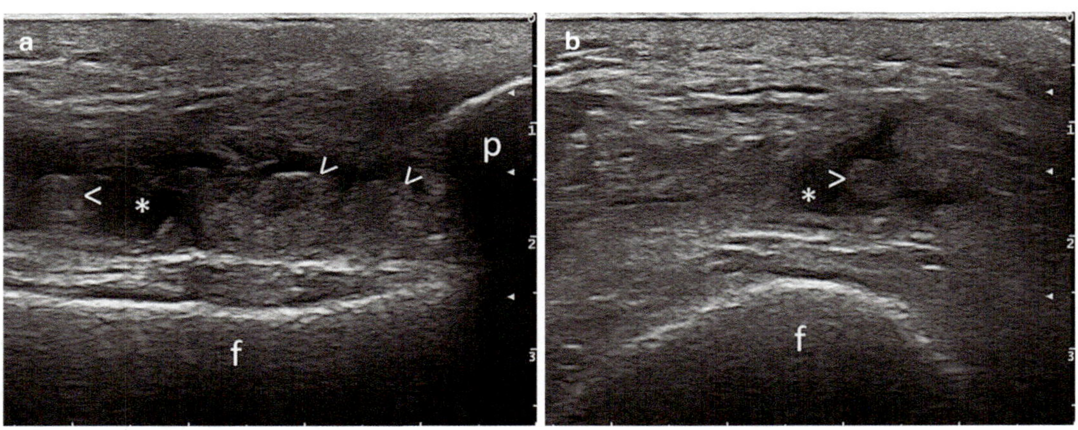

Fig. 7.1 Osteoarthritis. Knee synovitis. Suprapatellar views obtained using longitudinal (**a**) and transverse (**b**) scans show areas of synovial hypertrophy (arrowheads) and fluid collections (*). *f* femur; *p* upper pole of the patella

with chronic inflammatory arthritis, intra-articular PD signal represents the US finding indicative of "active" synovitis.

In the course of OA, synovitis, when present, is usually of low grade. However, its detection is important because, at the knee level, it is a predictor of future joint replacement. Of note, in OA patients the presence of US synovitis (i.e., intra-articular PD signal) has shown to have a greater correlation with histopathological findings than MRI signs of joint inflammation.

In patients with painful OA of the thumb carpometacarpal joint, intra-articular PD signal is a relatively common finding (Fig. 7.2).

7.3 Synovial Fluid

In the preliminary definition of the OMERACT Special Interest Group on US dating back to 2005, synovial fluid was defined as an "intra-articular anechogenic or hypoechogenic material that is displaceable and compressible (Fig. 7.3) but does not exhibit power Doppler signal." The degree of echogenicity of synovial fluid depends on several factors, and it is increased by the presence of high-protein material and/or calcified material in the liquid itself.

As a general rule, the more abundant the joint effusion, the greater the degree of inflammatory activity in the joint itself. At knee level, the presence of joint effusion is in most cases documented in the suprapatellar recess. To increase the sensitivity of US examination in the detection of even small amount of synovial fluid, the suprapatellar recess can be assessed during active contraction of quadriceps muscle. Nevertheless a comprehensive US examination should also

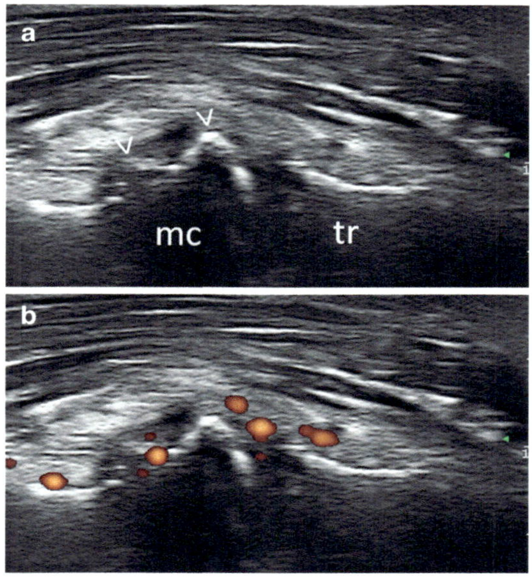

Fig. 7.2 Osteoarthritis. Trapeziometacarpal joint. Longitudinal scan through the thenar eminence shows osteophytes (arrowheads) at the base of the first metacarpal bone (**a**) and "active" synovitis (**b**). *mc* base of the first metacarpal bone; *tr* trapezius

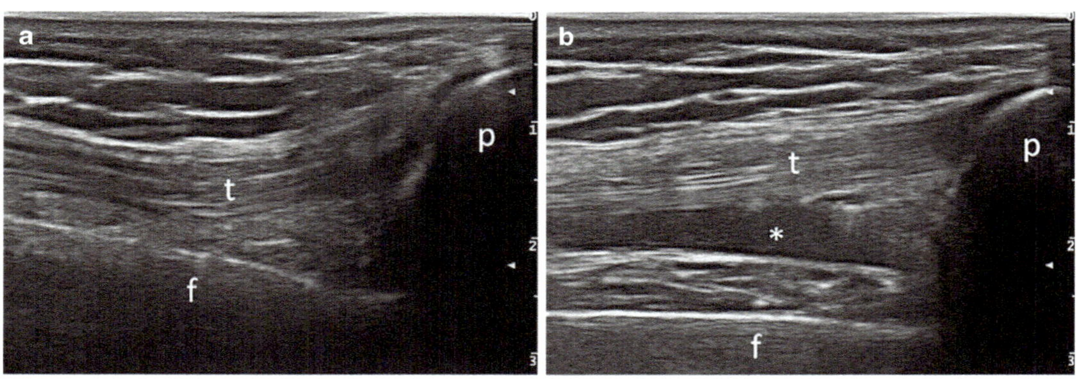

Fig. 7.3 Osteoarthritis. Knee effusion. Suprapatellar longitudinal scan with quadriceps muscle relaxed (**a**) and during active contraction (**b**). Quadriceps contraction reveals synovial effusion. *synovial fluid; *f* femur; *p* upper pole of the patella; *t* quadriceps tendon

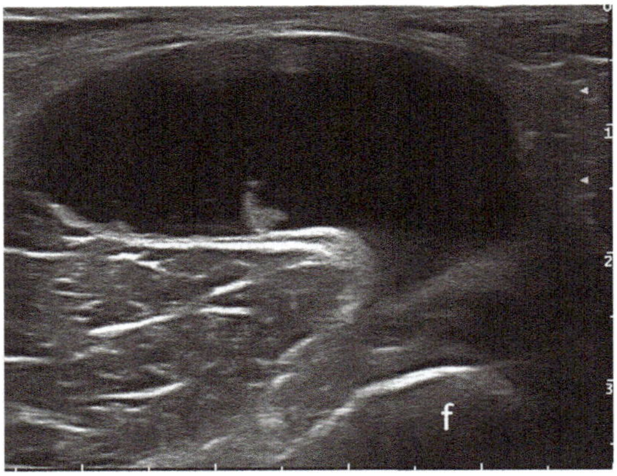

Fig. 7.4 Osteoarthritis. Popliteal cyst. Transverse posterior view showing mainly anechoic enlargement of the semimembranosus gastrocnemius bursa. *f* femur

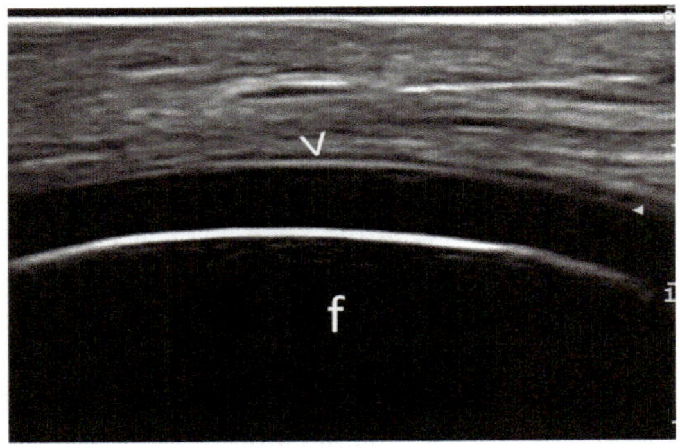

Fig. 7.5 Healthy subject. Knee. Longitudinal scan of the medial femoral condyle (f) with knee in 90° flexion. Note the ultrasound features of the normal hyaline cartilage when perpendicularly insonated: sharply defined continuous hyperechoic margins with the chondro-synovial interface (arrowhead) thinner than the osteochondral interface; homogeneously anechoic echotexture of the cartilage layer

include other potential sites of synovial fluid collection, such as popliteal cysts (Fig. 7.4). US examination of the popliteal cavity can document the presence of a cyst more frequently than clinical examination, even in the absence of symptoms at this level.

When joint effusion is small in size or deeply located, US facilitates synovial fluid aspiration guiding the needle placement at the target area.

7.4 Cartilage Damage

US appearance of the normal hyaline cartilage is characterized by a homogeneously anechoic layer delimited by two hyperechoic, regular, and continuous margins: the superficial margin (the chondro-synovial interface) and the deep margin (osteochondral interface). The superficial margin is typically thinner than the deep one (Fig. 7.5).

The US features of cartilage damage include the loss of normal anechogenicity, the loss of sharpness of the superficial margin, the thinning of the cartilage layer which can be partial or complete, and the subchondral bone erosions (Fig. 7.6).

The main limit of US in the assessment of cartilage is in the limited acoustic window. Taking the knee joint as an example, the hyaline cartilage of the femoral condyles requires the flexion of the knee to be visualized using a supra or medial para-patellar view, and a large portion of the tibial and patellar cartilage is not accessible by US.

From a technical point of view, the correct US visualization of the hyaline cartilage requires an insonation angle of 90° which is obtained when the US beam direction is perpendicular to the cartilage surface.

The thickness of the cartilage is an important parameter to detect and possibly monitor the progression of OA. At least in the early stages of OA, the typical injury is a reduction in hyaline cartilage thickness. With respect to healthy controls, a reduction in tibiofemoral cartilage thickness has been documented during knee OA and measurement of cartilage thickness in the middle of the medial femoral condyle could be a useful parameter to assess early morphological changes. Comparing US and MRI in the measurement of cartilage thickness in the medial femoral condyle, the correlation between the two methods is significantly positive. US can therefore be used as a reliable examination to assess cartilage thickness in the medial femoral condyle.

Moreover, US allows the visualization of the meniscal fibrocartilage (Fig. 7.7). At knee level the normal menisci appear as homogenous echogenic triangular structures located between femoral and tibial epiphysis (Fig. 7.7a). Only outer portions of the menisci can be clearly visualized,

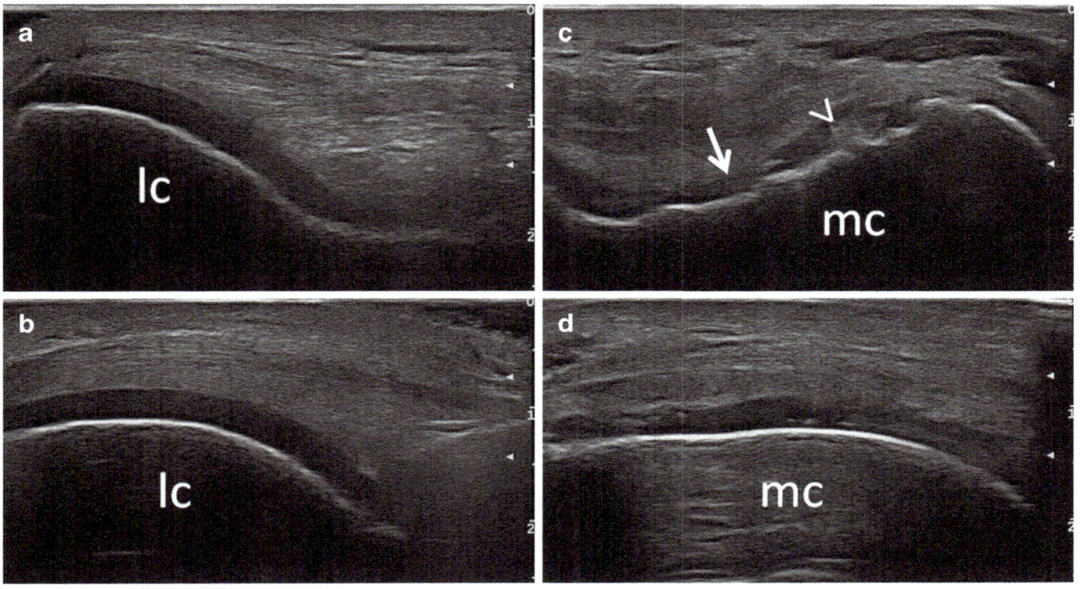

Fig. 7.6 Osteoarthritis. Knee. Suprapatellar views obtained with knee in 90° flexion using transverse (**a** and **c**) and longitudinal (**b** and **d**) of the lateral (**a** and **b**) and medial (**c** and **d**) facets of femoral trochlea showing osteoarthritic changes of the hyaline cartilage. Note the focal thinning (arrow) and the loss of the homogeneous echotexture of the cartilage layer (arrowhead). *lc* lateral condyle; *mc* medial condyle

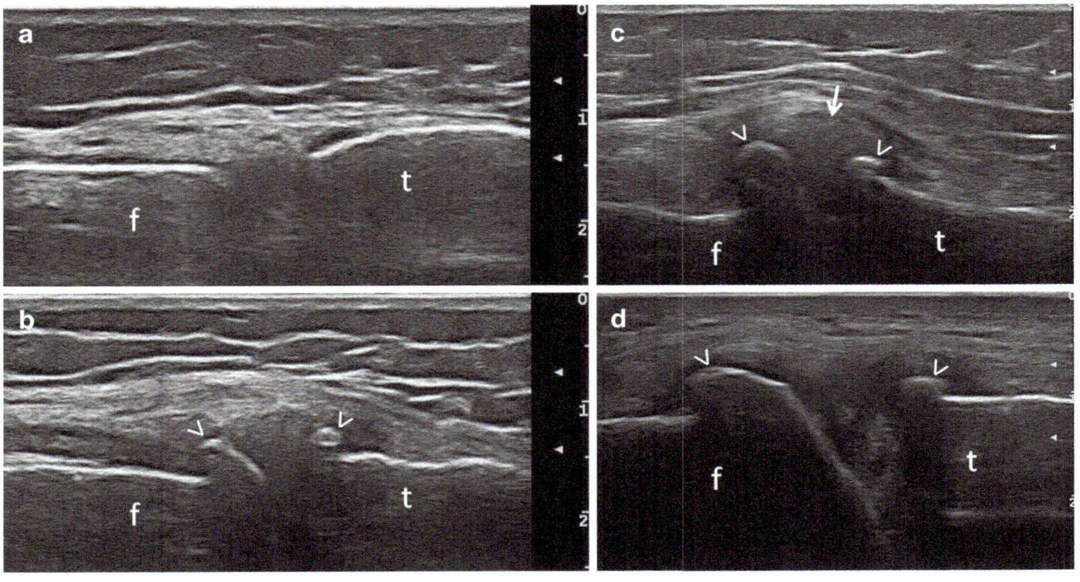

Fig. 7.7 Healthy subject (**a**) and osteoarthritis (**b–d**). Knee. Medial longitudinal scan showing the normal appearance of the femoral and tibial bone profiles and medial meniscus (**a**), osteophytes of different size (**b–d**), and medial meniscal protrusion (**c**). *arrow* medial meniscal protrusion; *arrowheads* osteophytes; *f* femur; *t* tibia

with the acoustic window for the US assessment of the medial meniscus being wider than the one for the lateral meniscus.

There is evidence supporting the use of US to detect medial meniscal extrusion (Fig. 7.7c), a typical OA lesion positively correlated with medial joint space narrowing documented by conventional radiography.

7.5 Osteophytes

Osteophytes are pathological bony prominences at the margins of the articular surface of the bone. From a prognostic point of view, the size of osteophytes correlates with the duration and severity of OA.

Using US, osteophytes appear as abnormal step-up prominences of the bone which may exhibit acoustic shadowing (Fig. 7.7b–d).

Compared to conventional radiography, US has proven to be a sensitive imaging technique to detect osteophytes, especially at small joints of the hand (Figs. 7.8 and 7.9).

Moreover, there is evidence documenting the US ability to reveal the presence of osteophytes at the medial femoral condyle of the knee joint in a relevant proportion of patients with no radiographic findings indicative of osteophytes.

The main advantage of the US over conventional radiography is the possibility to perform a multiplanar study which allows the visualization of areas of the joint margin where osteophytes may result hidden to the radiographic examination.

Some US grading systems have been developed to score osteophytes and some studies have found a significant correlation between the radiographic and US assessments of femoral osteophyte size at knee level, both on the medial and lateral joint aspects.

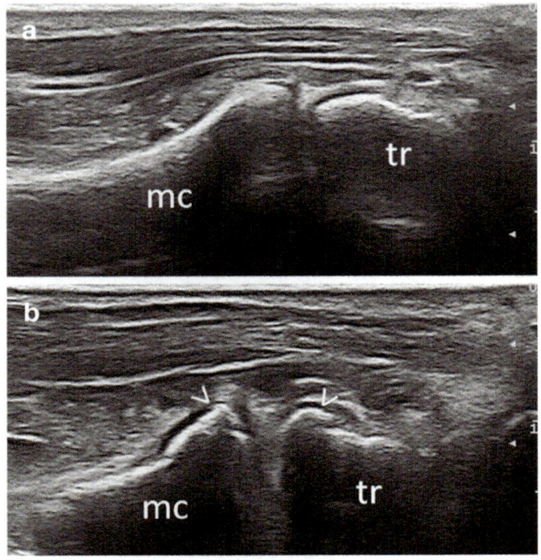

Fig. 7.8 Healthy subject (**a**) and osteoarthritis (**b**). Trapeziometacarpal joint. Longitudinal scan through the thenar eminence shows normal appearance of the bony cortex (**a**) and osteophytes (**b**). *mc* base of the first metacarpal bone; *tr* trapezius

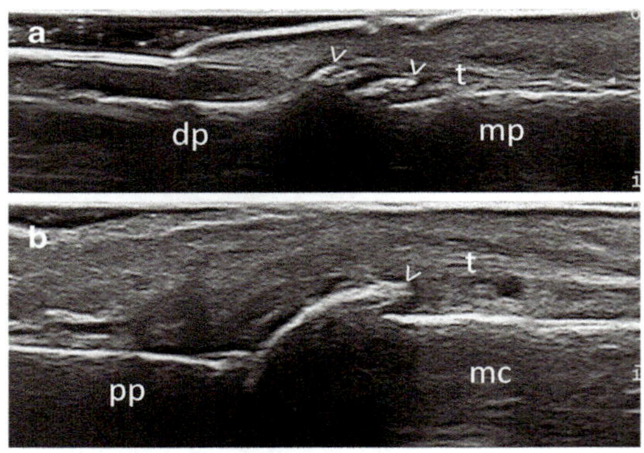

Fig. 7.9 Osteoarthritis. Hand. Longitudinal dorsal scan of distal interphalangeal joint (**a**) and metacarpophalangeal joint (**b**) showing osteophytes (arrowheads). *dp* distal phalanx; *mp* middle phalanx; *pp* proximal phalanx; *mc* metacarpal bone; *t* finger extensor tendon

Further Readings

Altman RD, Gold GE. Atlas of individual radiographic features in osteoarthritis, revised. Osteoarthr Cartil. 2007;15 Suppl A:A1–56.

Amin S, LaValley MP, Guermazi A, Grigoryan M, Hunter DJ, Clancy M, Niu J, Gale DR, Felson DT. The relationship between cartilage loss on magnetic resonance imaging and radiographic progression in men and women with knee osteoarthritis. Arthritis Rheum. 2005;52:3152–9.

Bruyn GA, Naredo E, Damjanov N, et al. An OMERACT reliability exercise of inflammatory and structural abnormalities in patients with knee osteoarthritis using ultrasound assessment. Ann Rheum Dis. 2016;75:842–6.

Bruyn GA, Iagnocco A, Naredo E, et al. OMERACT definitions for ultrasonographic pathologies and elementary lesions of rheumatic disorders 15 years on. J Rheumatol. 2019;46:1388–93.

Buck RJ, Wyman BT, Le Graverand MP, Hudelmaier M, Wirth W, Eckstein F, investigators A. Osteoarthritis may not be a one-way-road of cartilage loss - comparison of spatial patterns of cartilage change between osteoarthritic and healthy knees. Osteoarthr Cartil. 2010;18:329–35.

Conaghan PG, D'Agostino MA, Le Bars M, et al. Clinical and ultrasonographic predictors of joint replacement for knee osteoarthritis: results from a large, 3-year, prospective EULAR study. Ann Rheum Dis. 2010;69:644–7.

D'Agostino MA, Iagnocco A, Aegerter P, et al. Does subclinical inflammation contribute to impairment of function of knee joints in aged individuals? High prevalence of ultrasound inflammatory findings. Rheumatology (Oxford). 2015;54:1622–9.

Dawson J, Linsell L, Zondervan K, Rose P, Randall T, Carr A, Fitzpatrick R. Epidemiology of hip and knee pain and its impact on overall health status in older adults. Rheumatology (Oxford). 2004;43:497–504.

Guermazi A, Hayashi D, Eckstein F, Hunter DJ, Duryea J, Roemer FW. Imaging of osteoarthritis. Rheum Dis Clin N Am. 2013;39:67–105.

Hunter DJ, Zhang YQ, Tu X, Lavalley M, Niu JB, Amin S, Guermazi A, Genant H, Gale D, Felson DT. Change in joint space width: hyaline articular cartilage loss or alteration in meniscus? Arthritis Rheum. 2006;54:2488–95.

Kawaguchi K, Enokida M, Otsuki R, Teshima R. Ultrasonographic evaluation of medial radial displacement of the medial meniscus in knee osteoarthritis. Arthritis Rheum. 2012;64:173–80.

Kellgren JH, Lawrence JS. Radiological assessment of osteo-arthrosis. Ann Rheum Dis. 1957;16:494–502.

Koski JM, Kamel A, Waris P, et al. Atlas-based knee osteophyte assessment with ultrasonography and radiography: relationship to arthroscopic degeneration of articular cartilage. Scand J Rheumatol. 2016;45:158–64.

Iagnocco A, Naredo E. Ultrasound of the osteoarthritic joint. Clin Exp Rheumatol. 2017;35:527–34.

Martino F, Ettorre GC, Patella V, et al. Articular cartilage echography as a criterion of the evolution of osteoarthritis of the knee. Int J Clin Pharmacol Res. 1993;13:35–42.

Mathiessen A, Haugen IK, Slatkowsky-Christensen B, Bøyesen P, Kvien TK, Hammer HB. Ultrasonographic assessment of osteophytes in 127 patients with hand osteoarthritis: Exploring reliability and associations with MRI, radiographs and clinical joint findings. Ann Rheum Dis. 2013;72:51–6.

Mathiessen A, Slatkowsky-Christensen B, Kvien TK, Haugen IK, Berner HH. Ultrasound-detected osteophytes predict the development of radiographic and clinical features of hand osteoarthritis in the same finger joints 5 years later. RMD Open. 2017;3:e000505.

Möller I, Bong D, Naredo E, Filippucci E, Carrasco I, Moragues C, et al. Ultrasound in the study and monitoring of osteoarthritis. Osteoarthr Cartil. 2008;16:S4.

Naredo E, Cabero F, Palop MJ, Collado P, Cruz A, Crespo M. Ultrasonographic findings in knee osteoarthritis: a comparative study with clinical and radiographic assessment. Osteoarthr Cartil. 2005;13:568–74.

Okano T, Filippucci E, Di Carlo M, Draghessi A, Carotti M, Salaffi F, Wright G, Grassi W. Ultrasonographic evaluation of joint damage in knee osteoarthritis: feature-specific comparisons with conventional radiography. Rheumatology (Oxford). 2016;55:2040–9.

Østergaard M, Pedersen SJ, Døhn UM. Imaging in rheumatoid arthritis - status and recent advances for magnetic resonance imaging, ultrasonography, computed tomography and conventional radiography. Best Pract Res Clin Rheumatol. 2008;22:1019–44.

Podlipská J, Guermazi A, Lehenkari P, Niinimäki J, Roemer FW, Arokoski JP, et al. Comparison of diagnostic performance of semi-quantitative knee ultrasound and knee radiography with MRI: Oulu Knee osteoarthritis study. Sci Rep. 2016;6:22365.

Pradsgaard D, Fiirgaard B, Spannow AH, Heuck C, Herlin T. Cartilage thickness of the knee joint in juvenile idiopathic arthritis: comparative assessment by ultrasonography and magnetic resonance imaging. J Rheumatol. 2015;42:534–40.

Reichmann WM, Maillefert JF, Hunter DJ, Katz JN, Conaghan PG, Losina E. Responsiveness to change and reliability of measurement of radiographic joint space width in osteoarthritis of the knee: a systematic review. Osteoarthr Cartil. 2011;19:550–6.

Riecke BF, Christensen R, Torp-Pedersen S, Boesen M, Gudbergsen H, Bliddal H. An ultrasound score for knee osteoarthritis: a cross-sectional validation study. Osteoarthr Cartil. 2014;22:1675–91.

Roemer FW, Eckstein F, Hayashi D, Guermazi A. The role of imaging in osteoarthritis. Best Pract Res Clin Rheumatol. 2014;28:31–60.

Saarakkala S, Waris P, Waris V, Tarkiainen I, Karvanen E, Aarnio J, et al. Diagnostic performance of knee ultrasonography for detecting degenerative changes of articular cartilage. Osteoarthr Cartil. 2012;20:376–81.

Stammberger T, Eckstein F, Englmeier KH, Reiser M. Determination of 3D cartilage thickness data from MR imaging: computational method and reproducibility in the living. Magn Reson Med. 1999;41:529–36.

Takase K, Ohno S, Takeno M, et al. Simultaneous evaluation of long-lasting knee synovitis in patients undergoing arthroplasty by power Doppler ultrasonography and contrast-enhanced MRI in comparison with histopathology. Clin Exp Rheumatol. 2012;30:85–92.

Wakefield RJ, Balint PV, Szkudlarek M, et al. Musculoskeletal ultrasound including definitions for ultrasonographic pathology. J Rheumatol. 2005;32:2485–24.

Wang Y, Wluka AE, Jones G, Ding C, Cicuttini FM. Use magnetic resonance imaging to assess articular cartilage. Ther Adv Musculoskelet Dis. 2012;4:77–97.

8 Rheumatoid Arthritis

Marina Carotti, Emilio Filippucci, Fausto Salaffi, and Fabio Martino

Contents

8.1 Introduction

Rheumatoid arthritis (RA) is the archetypal inflammatory arthritis. It primarily targets the synovium of peripheral joints. RA can be defined as an inflammatory autoimmune disease, characterized by chronic synovitis mainly involving the small joints of the hands and feet. In the absence of appropriate treatment, RA leads to irreversible anatomical damage, disability and premature death.

In North America and Europe, the prevalence of RA is estimated to be 0.5–1.0% and annual incidence is approximately 0.02–0.05%, with the age of onset highest in the fifth decade of life. Epidemiologic studies suggest genetic and environmental contributions in the aetiology of RA. This multifactorial hypothesis is confirmed by the presence of multiple risk factors for RA. Females have a higher risk of disease by 2–3 times and smoking is also associated with an increased risk of seropositive RA by 1.5 times.

RA patients have an increased risk of cardiovascular disease morbidity and mortality. Overall, patients with RA have a 3–10 years reduction of life expectancy, depending on both their age at disease onset and RA severity.

M. Carotti
Clinica di Radiologia, Dipartimento di Scienze Radiologiche – Azienda Ospedali Riuniti di Ancona Universita' Politecnica delle Marche, Ancona, Italy

E. Filippucci · F. Salaffi
Clinica Reumatologica, Dipartimento di Scienze Cliniche e Molecolari, Università Politecnica delle Marche, Jesi (Ancona), Italy

F. Martino (✉)
Radiology, Sant'Agata Diagnostic Center, Bari, Italy

F. Martino et al. (eds.), *Musculoskeletal Ultrasound in Orthopedic and Rheumatic disease in Adults*,
https://doi.org/10.1007/978-3-030-91202-4_8

Joint pain and swelling are two of the hallmark manifestations of RA, usually characterized by a symmetric distribution usually involving wrist, metacarpophalangeal (MCP), proximal interphalangeal (PIP) and metatarsophalangeal (MTP) joints. Larger joints (e.g. elbow and knee) may be involved during the disease course. Synovial inflammation is typically related to morning stiffness lasting more than half an hour and may be associated with a relevant impairment of daily living activities.

RA should be suspected in a patient who presents with inflammatory polyarthritis. The initial evaluation of such patients requires a careful history and physical examination, along with selected laboratory testing to identify features that are characteristic of RA or that suggest an alternative diagnosis. Symptoms of arthritis should be present for more than 6 weeks to increase the specificity of the diagnosis. In fact, symptoms that have been present for a shorter time may be due to an acute viral polyarthritis rather than to RA. Laboratory tests may support the diagnosis. Rheumatoid factor (RF) and anti-cyclic citrullinated peptide (ACPA) antibody positivity increases overall diagnostic accuracy. Despite this, both tests are negative on presentation in up to 50% of patients and remain negative during follow-up in 20% of patients with RA. According to serological status, RA patients can be classified as seropositive or seronegative. This distinction has a prognostic value in terms of disease severity, and clinical responsiveness to some medications.

In 2010, the ACR and the European League Against Rheumatism (EULAR) developed the latest classification criteria for RA. These criteria required the presence of synovitis in at least one joint and the absence of an alternative diagnosis that offered a more suitable explanation for the synovitis.

Traditionally, conventional radiography (CR) has been the imaging technique most used in the assessment of RA and it remains widely used both in daily practice and in clinical trials. CR allows to assess multiple joints simultaneously in a reasonable amount of time and without important radiation exposure. Juxta-articular osteoporosis is a feature usually detected in the early stages of the disease. Bone erosions are the hallmark of the structural damage in RA. Erosive process usually appears in the "bare areas" of the joint, where the intra-articular bone surface is not covered by the hyaline cartilage and is exposed to the hyperplastic synovial tissue. In later stages, concentric joint space narrowing (JSN) could occur. Subchondral radiolucent areas are common in RA and usually are the consequence of the extension of synovial proliferation into the trabecular bone. In end stages of the disease, irreversible joint deformities can be observed. However, the main limitations of CR are the lack of sensitivity in detecting RA joint structural changes especially in early disease phases and the inability to assess directly soft tissues (such as synovium, tendons) and cartilage.

The use of magnetic resonance imaging (MRI) and ultrasound (US) has undoubtedly enhanced the understanding of the pathological processes at both articular and periarticular levels. MRI allows the detection of all relevant changes of RA (i.e. synovitis, tenosynovitis, bone marrow oedema, bone erosions and cartilage damage). MRI allows the identification of bone marrow oedema, which represents a strong predictor of subsequent radiographic progression in early RA.

US permits an accurate and real-time analysis of articular and periarticular structures. Moreover, US is increasingly used to guide interventional procedures in rheumatological daily practice. However, US cannot assess osteitis and its accuracy depends on the equipment used and the correctness of the procedure.

US provides additional benefits over the physical examination in the early identification of inflammation and may increase the performance of the 2010 ACR/EULAR criteria in the early diagnosis of RA especially in subjects negative for ACPA and RF.

Colour Doppler and power Doppler modalities are able to detect even small changes of the synovial vascularization, estimating the inflammatory activity at joint level. Power Doppler mode is theoretically more sensitive than colour Doppler one in the assessment of small-vessel flow, because of its higher sensitivity for low-volume, low-velocity blood flow at the microvascular level. It has been shown that both synovial vascularization and power Doppler signal increase in active joint inflammation and decrease after an appropriate treatment. In addition to a dichotomous scoring method (presence or absence of pathological synovial vascularization), several semiquantitative scoring systems have been proposed to evaluate the synovial blood flow. In 2017, the OMERACT/EULAR ultrasound taskforce described a four-grade scoring system of power Doppler (grade 0: no Doppler signal, grade 1: up to three single Doppler spots or up to one confluent spots and two single spots or up to two confluent spots, grade 2: more than grade 1 but less than 50% of Doppler signals in the total greyscale background, grade 3: more than 50% of Doppler signals in the total greyscale background) to be applied in MCP, PIP, MTP joints, wrist and knee.

Moreover, US evaluation of synovitis has been shown to have internal and external validity allowing the US assessment of treatment response. Finally, US has been used to guide therapy decisions such as biologics discontinuation, showing that power Doppler was a predictor of biologics tapering failure.

US in patients with RA allows the detection of a wide range of morphostructural abnormalities. The main pathological findings detectable by US at joint and tendon level can be divided into two major categories, those revealing inflammation and those indicative of anatomic damage.

Inflammatory changes in RA include joint space/tendon sheath widening, synovial effusion and synovial hypertrophy. The most relevant structural changes are bone erosions, cartilage damage and tendon tears.

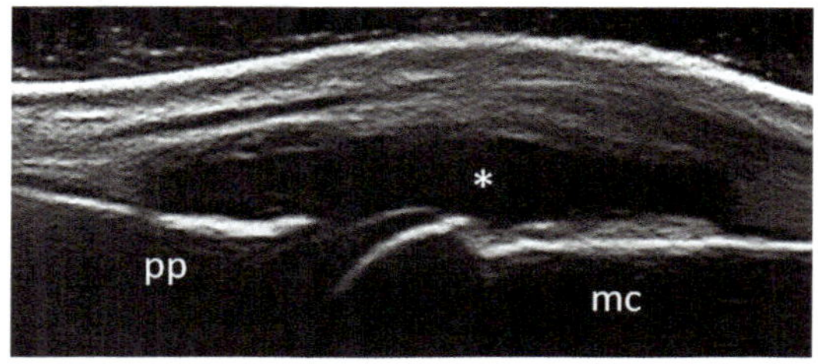

Fig. 8.1 Rheumatoid arthritis. Metacarpophalangeal joint on longitudinal dorsal scan showing a representative example of exudative synovitis. Note the anechoic joint cavity widening. *mc* metacarpal bone; *pp* proximal phalanx; *synovial fluid

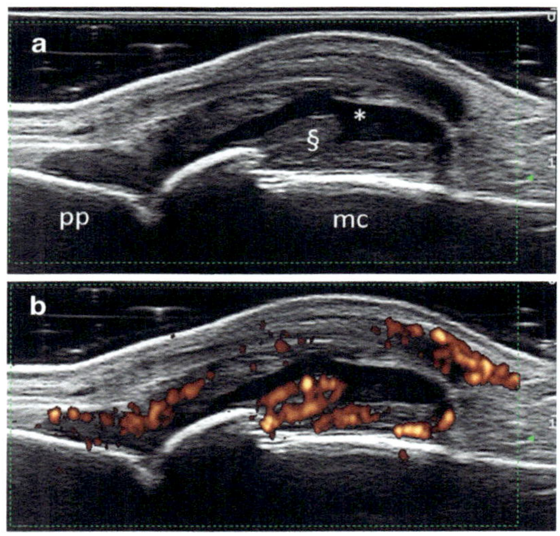

Fig. 8.2 Rheumatoid arthritis. Metacarpophalangeal joint on longitudinal dorsal scan showing a representative example of proliferative synovitis using B-mode (**a**) and power mode (**b**). Note the marked joint widening due to an abnormal amount of synovial fluid and areas of synovial hypertrophy showing intense power Doppler signal. *mc* metacarpal bone; *pp* proximal phalanx; §synovial hypertrophy; *synovial fluid

8.2 Synovitis

Joint cavity widening is the key finding indicative of synovitis and may depend on a variable amount of synovial fluid and synovial proliferation. Synovial effusion appears as an anechoic or a hypoechoic (relative to subdermal fat, but sometimes isoechoic or hyperechoic) material which is easily displaceable and compressible by pressure exerted using the examining probe and does not exhibit power Doppler signal (Fig. 8.1). Synovial effusion is virtually the first step of the inflammatory process detectable by US. Even a minimal intra-articular effusion can be detected by US. However, due to the lack of specificity of this finding, very recently, the Outcome Measures in Rheumatology (OMERACT) US Task Force stated that synovial effusion alone is not enough to be indicative of synovitis in RA.

On the other hand, synovial proliferation is a hypoechoic (relative to subdermal fat, but sometimes isoechoic or hyperechoic) not displaceable

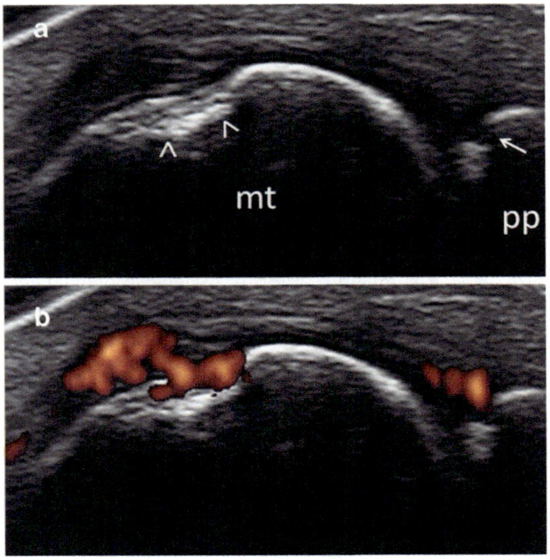

Fig. 8.3 Rheumatoid arthritis. Fifth toe. Metatarsophalangeal joint on longitudinal lateral scan showing pre-erosive changes at the bare area of the metatarsal head (arrowheads) and bone erosion at the base of the proximal phalanx (arrow) using B-mode (**a**) and power Doppler mode (**b**). Note the distribution of the power Doppler signal at the areas of bony damage. *mt* metatarsal bone; *pp* proximal phalanx

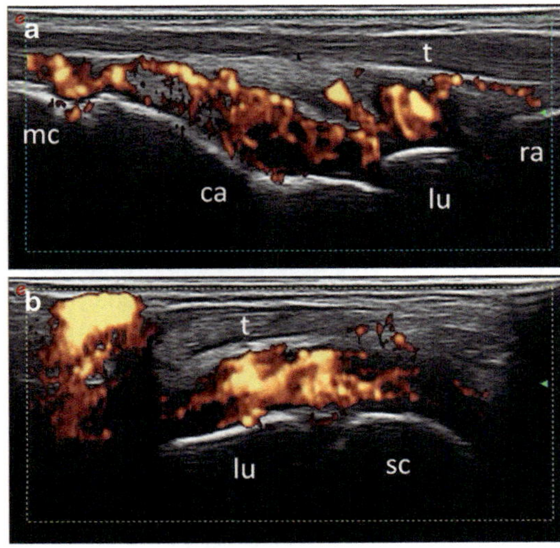

Fig. 8.4 Rheumatoid arthritis. Wrist on longitudinal (**a**) and transverse (**b**) dorsal scans showing "active" synovitis. Radio-carpal, intercarpal and carpo-metacarpal joints present evident joint cavity widening with intense intra-articular power Doppler signal (score 3 of OMERACT/EULAR ultrasound taskforce). *mc* base of the third metacarpal bone; *ca* capitate bone; *lu* lunate bone; *ra* radius; *sc* scaphoid bone; *t* common extensor tendons of the fingers

and poorly compressible intra-articular tissue which may exhibit power Doppler signal (Fig. 8.2).

Synovial effusion can be easily distinguished from the "dark-grey" hypoechogenicity of synovial proliferation, which can appear as a homogenous or irregular (villous, polypoid or bushy appearance) thickening of the synovial membrane. Currently, synovial hypertrophy is the mandatory US abnormality for the definition of synovitis even in the absence of power Doppler signal.

The presence of a highly vascularized synovial proliferation has been identified as a strong predictor of the subsequent development of structural damage both at joint and tendon level (Fig. 8.3) and it has been linked with the amount of inflammatory changes in histological specimens. Despite synovial hypertrophy, power Doppler signal may be considered the best US biomarker of inflammation in RA because its identification is independent of disease duration (Fig. 8.4).

8.3 Bone Erosions

Bone erosion is one of the hallmarks of RA. The presence of a bone erosion is a predictor of poor outcome. According to its presence RA is classified into two different prognostic categories: erosive and non-erosive disease.

Over the last two decades, several studies confirmed that US allows an accurate and detailed analysis of the bony changes induced by the inflammatory process. US has been shown to be more sensitive than CR for the detection of bone erosions because of a higher spatial resolution and the multiplanar assessment of the bone surface. A disadvantage of US is its relative inaccessibility to certain sites due to the lack of an acoustic window (e.g. lateral sides of III and IV metacarpal heads). When US was compared with micro-CT scan a large proportion of bone lesions detected by US were identified by micro-CT. In general, the sensitivity for detecting erosions is higher than 85% when the US examination is confined to well-accessible joint regions such as II and V MCP joints and V MTP joint.

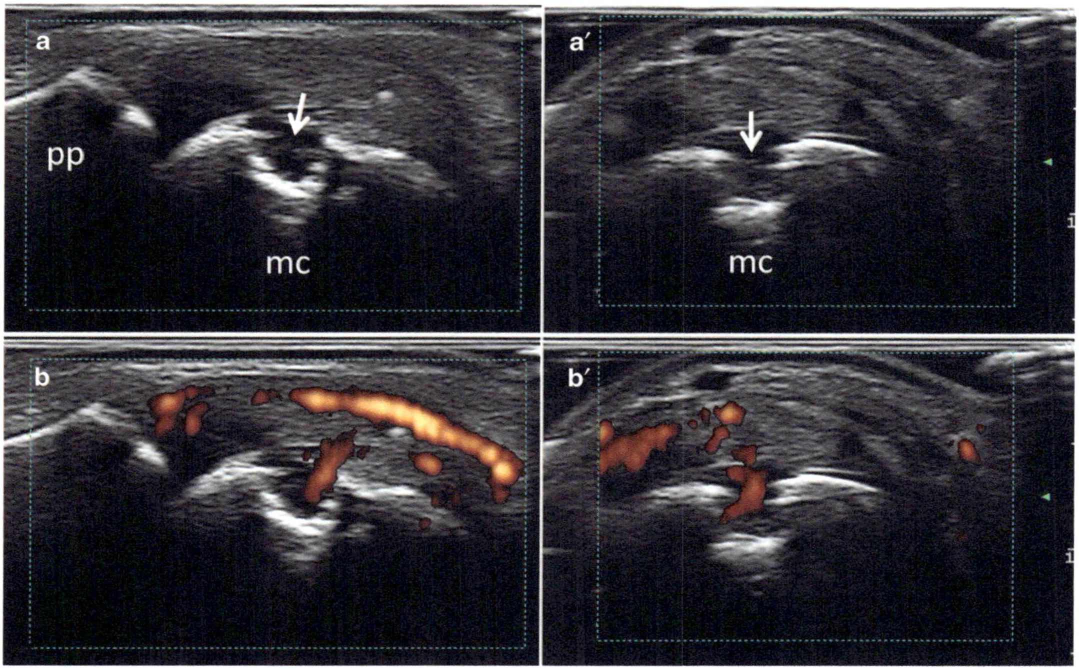

Fig. 8.5 Rheumatoid arthritis. Second finger dominant hand. Metacarpophalangeal joint on longitudinal (**a, b**) and transverse (**a′**, **b′**) lateral scans showing bone erosion at the bare area of the metacarpal head (arrows) using B-mode (**a**–**a′**) and power Doppler mode (**b**–**b′**). Note the presence of power Doppler signal inside the erosive crater indicative of "hot" erosion. *mc* metacarpal bone; *pp* proximal phalanx

Bone erosions are defined as an intra-articular discontinuity of the bone surface that is visible in at least two perpendicular planes (Fig. 8.5).

While assessing bone defects, particular attention should be paid especially when these abnormalities are smaller than 1 mm in size. In fact, it is essential to distinguish true bone erosions from other causes of cortical bone irregularities including physiologic small vascular bone channels, and wider smooth depression at the metaphysis, bone microfracture, multiple osteophytes in osteoarthritis and bone proliferation in psoriatic arthritis. US depicts the walls and the floor of the erosive crater that is generally filled by rheumatoid pannus. Erosion borders usually appear as irregular and jagged. At the level of the MCP joints, US can identify bone erosions more frequently than CR in early RA (Fig. 8.6).

Several studies showed the US bone erosions are "true erosions" using computed tomography as the gold standard. The lateral aspect of the II and V metacarpal heads, of the V metatarsal head and of the ulnar styloid should be included in a dedicated scanning protocol aiming at revealing bone erosions. Humeral head and first metatarsal head should not be assessed, being relatively high the prevalence of US abnormalities totally fulfilling the definition of bone erosions in healthy subjects.

Greyscale assessment should always be completed with power Doppler evaluation to distinguish between "hot" and "cold" bone erosions (Figs. 8.5 and 8.6).

8.4 Cartilage Damage

Cartilage thinning is one of the most relevant factors in the development of irreversible loss of the joint function and long-term disability in RA patients. In fact, as showed by CR studies, cartilage damage appears to be more clearly associated

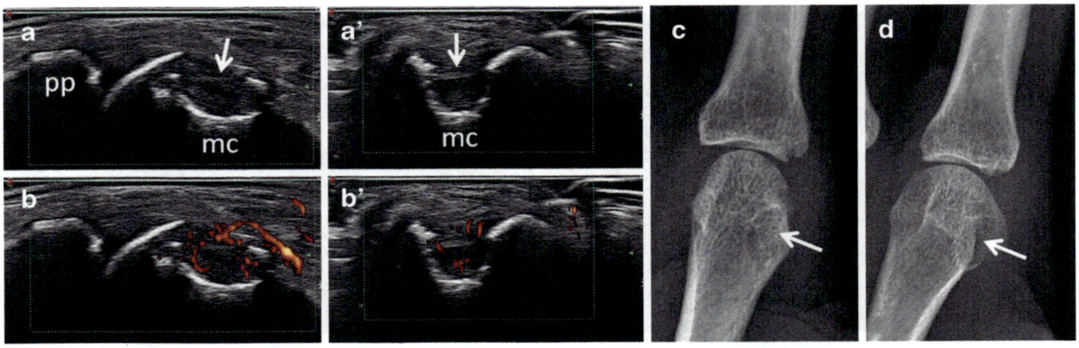

Fig. 8.6 Rheumatoid arthritis. Second finger dominant hand. Metacarpophalangeal joint on longitudinal (**a**, **b**) and transverse (**a′**–**b′**) lateral scans showing a large "hot" bone erosion at the bare area of the metacarpal head (arrows) using B-mode (**a**–**a′**) and power Doppler mode (**b**–**b′**). (**c** and **d**) Conventional radiography using frontal (**c**) and oblique (**d**) views. *mc* metacarpal bone; *pp* proximal phalanx

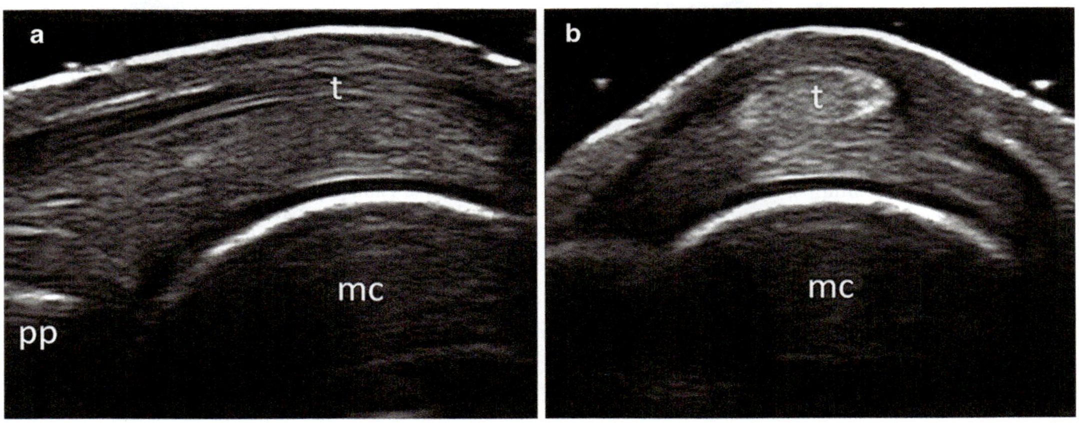

Fig. 8.7 Healthy subject. Metacarpophalangeal joint on longitudinal (**a**) and transverse (**b**) dorsal scans with joint in flexed position to enhance the visualization of the metacarpal head hyaline cartilage appearing as a subtle anechoic layer with sharp continuous hyperechoic margins. *mc* metacarpal bone; *pp* proximal phalanx; *t* finger extensor tendon

with irreversible physical disability than bony damage.

US is not routinely performed to assess the hyaline cartilage of both small and large joints in RA. In fact, there is only limited US evidence about the burden of cartilage damage in RA and its natural history. Moreover, in most of the US studies aiming at assessing hyaline cartilage involvement in RA, the MCP joints were investigated. The hyaline cartilage of metacarpal heads should be explored with the subject seated with hands placed on the examination table and MCP joints in maximal flexion (more than 60°). This position increases the extent of the metacarpal head hyaline cartilage detectable by US on the dorsal aspect. Normal appearance of hyaline cartilage is characterized by homogenous anechoic band delimited by two hyperechoic sharp, regular and continuous interfaces, when it is perpendicularly insonated by the US beam (Fig. 8.7). The

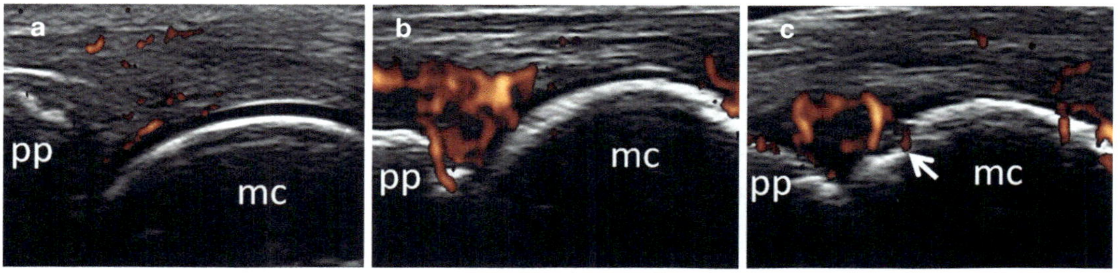

Fig. 8.8 Rheumatoid arthritis. Metacarpophalangeal joint on longitudinal dorsal scan with joint in flexed position to enhance the visualization of the metacarpal head hyaline cartilage, showing initial (**a**), established (**b**) and long-standing cartilage damage. (**a**) The early stages of the cartilage involvement are characterized by the loss of the sharpness of the chondrosynovial margin. (**b**) More advanced stages of the cartilage damage which show partial and complete thinning of the cartilage layer. (**c**) Cartilage is completely reabsorbed and a subchondral bone erosion is refilled by an inflamed pannus (arrow). *mc* metacarpal bone; *pp* proximal phalanx

loss of the sharpness of the chondrosynovial margin is the initial US abnormality of cartilage involvement. In advanced stages, partial or complete thinning of the cartilage layer and subchondral bone erosion can occur (Fig. 8.8).

8.5 Tenosynovitis

In RA, tenosynovitis is a well-known, but underestimated, component of the disease. In addition, tenosynovitis is often misinterpreted as joint inflammation by physical examination.

Although US is particularly useful in the evaluation of tendon involvement in RA, to date, only few studies have been performed to investigate its role in the assessment of tendon inflammatory changes in RA patients. The tendons most frequently involved in RA are the flexor tendons of the II, III and IV fingers; posterior tibialis tendon and extensor carpi ulnaris tendon. The US assessment of tendon pathology has been shown to have a prognostic factor. In fact, the presence of an extensor carpi ulnaris tendon tenosynovitis has been linked to the development of ulnar styloid bone erosions in early RA, and tibial posterior tenosynovitis to flatfoot deformity in RA.

Tendon sheath widening is the hallmark of tenosynovitis in RA. Tenosynovitis can be defined on greyscale US imaging as an abnormal anechoic and/or hypoechoic (relative to tendon fibres) tendon sheath widening, which can be related to both the presence of tenosynovial abnormal fluid and hypertrophy.

Tendon sheath effusion can be defined as an abnormal anechoic or hypoechoic (relative to tendon fibres) material within the synovial sheath, either localized or surrounding the tendon that is displaceable and seen in two perpendicular planes. Tenosynovial hypertrophy appears as the presence of abnormal hypoechoic (relative to tendon fibres) tissue within the synovial sheath that is not displaceable and poorly compressible and seen in two perpendicular planes.

In greyscale US, transverse view allows for a more sensitive detection of abnormal synovial fluid at tendon sheath level, revealing small collections on the sides of the tendon.

While using power Doppler mode, particular attention must be paid to avoid misinterpretation of power Doppler signal due to normal feeding vessels. Tenosynovitis is characterized by the detection of peritendinous power Doppler signal within a widened synovial sheath; such a finding

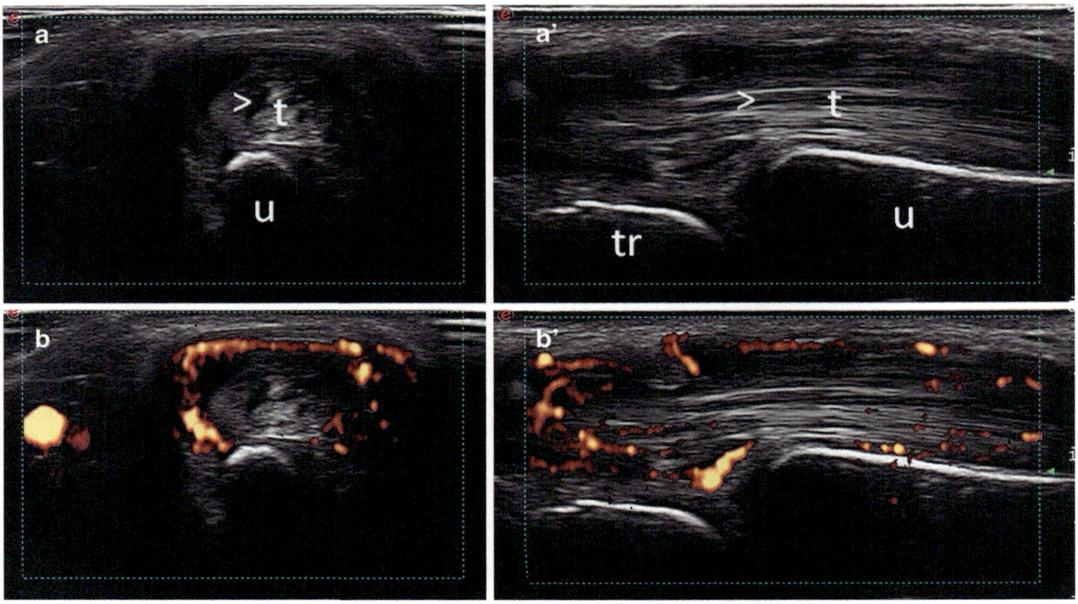

Fig. 8.9 Rheumatoid arthritis. Extensor carpi ulnaris tendon on transverse (**a**, **b**) and longitudinal (**a′**, **b′**) scans showing "active" tenosynovitis and partial tendon tear (arrowheads) using B-mode (**a**–**a'**) and power Doppler mode (**b**–**b′**). t=extensor ulnaris carpi tendon; tr=triquetrum; u = ulna

should be documented on at least two perpendicular planes (Fig. 8.9).

Several US patterns of tendon sheath widening can be identified. Tenosynovitis can be furtherly characterized by the extent of the widening and the presence of synovial proliferation. The amount of synovial fluid within a tendon sheath may be considerably different, ranging from minimal diffuse widening to important focal enlargement. No direct relationship between the extent of tenosynovitis and clinical symptoms has been reported. The profile of a widened tendon sheath can be regular or extremely nonhomogeneous with saccular or aneurysmal appearance, especially in chronic tenosynovitis.

8.6 Tendon Damage

The range of tendon tears in RA is wide and includes loss of "fibrillar" echotexture and partial and complete tendon rupture. Physical examination provides only limited information on the presence and extent of a partial tendon tear.

Analysis of tendon echotexture is one of the fundamental roles of US assessment. In the early phases of persistent tenosynovitis the initial abnormality is the loss of the fibrillar echotexture.

This finding can precede a partial rupture of tendon (Fig. 8.10) and the subsequent evolution into a complete tendon tear. Tendon damage should always be assessed by dynamic examination (to exclude anisotropy artefacts). To avoid

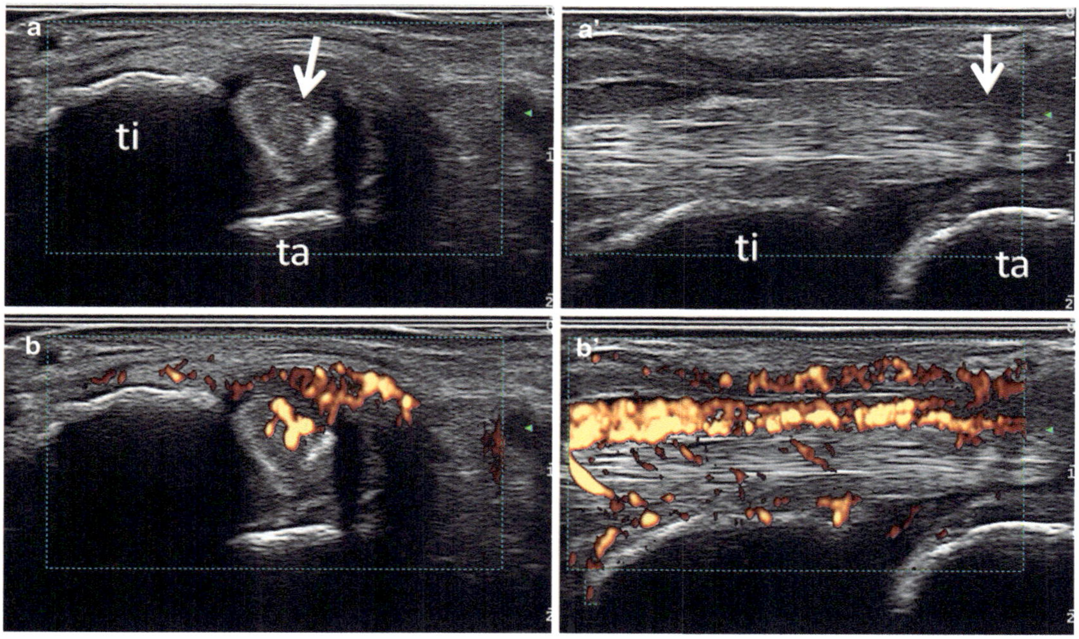

Fig. 8.10 Rheumatoid arthritis. Tibialis posterior tendon on transverse (**a**, **b**) and longitudinal (**a′**–**b′**) scans showing "active" tenosynovitis and partial tendon tear (arrows) using B-mode (**a**–**a′**) and power Doppler mode (**b**–**b′**). Note the loss of the fibrillar echotexture and the presence of intra-tendinous power Doppler signal. *ti* tibia; *ta* talus

anisotropy artefacts, the suspicion of a tendon tear on a single scanning plane must be verified changing the US beam direction. Complete tendon tear is characterized by the depiction of both the complete loss of fibrillar structure and the gap between the retracted tendon edges, frequently refilled by fluid or synovial proliferation.

Further Readings

Bruyn GAW, Hanova P, Iagnocco A, D'Agostino MA, Möller I, Terslev L, et al. Ultrasound definition of tendon damage in patients with rheumatoid arthritis. Results of a OMERACT consensus-based ultrasound score focussing on the diagnostic reliability. Ann Rheum Dis. 2014;73:1929–34.

Cipolletta E, Hurnakova J, Di Matteo A, et al. Prevalence and distribution of cartilage and bone damage at metacarpal head in healthy subjects. Clin Exp Rheumatol. 2021;39(6):1394–401.

Cipolletta E, Mandl P, Di Matteo A, et al. Sonographic assessment of cartilage damage at the metacarpal head in rheumatoid arthritis: qualitative versus quantitative methods. Rheumatology (Oxford). 2022;61(3):1018–25. https://doi.org/10.1093/rheumatology/keab472.

Cipolletta E, Filippucci E, Di Matteo A, et al. The reliability of ultrasound in the assessment of hyaline cartilage in rheumatoid arthritis and healthy metacarpal heads [published online ahead of print, 2020 Oct 30]. Ultraschall Med. 2020. https://doi.org/10.1055/a-1285-4602.

D'Agostino MA, Terslev L, Wakefield R, Østergaard M, Balint P, Naredo E, et al. Novel algorithms for the pragmatic use of ultrasound in the management of patients with rheumatoid arthritis: From diagnosis to remission. Ann Rheum Dis. 2016;75:1902–8.

Døhn UM, Ejbjerg BJ, Court-Payen M, Hasselquist M, Narvestad E, Szkudlarek M, et al. Are bone erosions detected by magnetic resonance imaging and ultrasonography true erosions? A comparison with computed tomography in rheumatoid arthritis metacarpophalangeal joints. Arthritis Res Ther. 2006;8:R110. https://doi.org/10.1186/ar1995.

Filippou G, Sakellariou G, Scirè CA, Carrara G, Rumi F, Bellis E, et al. The predictive role of ultrasound-detected tenosynovitis and joint synovitis for flare in patients with rheumatoid arthritis in stable remission. Results of an Italian multicentre study of the Italian Society for Rheumatology Group for Ultrasound: The STARTER study. Ann Rheum Dis. 2018;77:1283–9.

Filippucci E, Iagnocco A, Meenagh G, Riente L, Delle Sedie A, Bombardieri S, et al. Ultrasound imaging for the rheumatologist VII. Ultrasound imaging in rheumatoid arthritis. Clin Exp Rheumatol. 2007;25:5–10.

Filippucci E, Cipolletta E, Mashadi Mirza R, Carotti M, Giovagnoni A, Salaffi F, et al. Ultrasound imaging in rheumatoid arthritis. Radiol Med. 2019;124:1087–100.

Finzel S, Ohrndorf S, Englbrecht M, Stach C, Messerschmidt J, Schett G, et al. A detailed comparative study of high-resolution ultrasound and micro-computed tomography for detection of arthritic bone erosions. Arthritis Rheum. 2011;63:1231–6.

Han J, Geng Y, Deng X, Zhang Z. Subclinical synovitis assessed by ultrasound predicts flare and progressive bone erosion in rheumatoid arthritis patients with clinical remission: A systematic review and meta-analysis. J Rheumatol. 2016;43:2010–8.

Koski JM, Saarakkala S, Helle M, Hakulinen U, Heikkinen JO, Hermunen H. Power Doppler ultrasonography and synovitis: Correlating ultrasound imaging with histopathological findings and evaluating the performance of ultrasound equipments. Ann Rheum Dis. 2006;65:1590–5.

Jindal S, Kaushik R, Raghuvanshi S, Kaushik RM, Kakkar R. Gray scale and power doppler ultrasonographic findings in the assessment of disease activity and their correlation with disease activity parameters in rheumatoid arthritis. Curr Rheumatol Rev. 2017;14:153–62.

Mandl P, Studenic P, Filippucci E, Bachta A, Backhaus M, Bong D, et al. Development of semiquantitative ultrasound scoring system to assess cartilage in rheumatoid arthritis. Rheumatology (United Kingdom). 2019;58:1802–11.

Naredo E, D'Agostino MA, Wakefield RJ, Möller I, Balint PV, Filippucci E, et al. Reliability of a consensus-based ultrasound score for tenosynovitis in rheumatoid arthritis. Ann Rheum Dis. 2013;72:1328–34.

Szkudlarek M, Klarlund M, Narvestad E, Court-Payen M, Strandberg C, Jensen KE, et al. Ultrasonography of the metacarpophalangeal and proximal interphalangeal joints in rheumatoid arthritis: a comparison with magnetic resonance imaging, conventional radiography and clinical examination. Arthritis Res Ther. 2006;8:R52. https://doi.org/10.1186/ar1904.

Szkudlarek M, Terslev L, Wakefield RJ, Backhaus M, Balint PV, Bruyn GAW, et al. Summary findings of a systematic literature review of the ultrasound assessment of bone erosions in rheumatoid arthritis. J Rheumatol. 2016;43:12–21.

Tămaş M-M, Filippucci E, Becciolini A, Gutierrez M, Di Geso L, Bonfiglioli K, et al. Bone erosions in rheumatoid arthritis: ultrasound findings in the early stage of the disease. Rheumatology (Oxford). 2014;53:1100–7.

Terslev L, Østergaard M, Sexton J, Hammer HB. Is synovial hypertrophy without Doppler activity sensitive to change? Post-hoc analysis from a rheumatoid arthritis ultrasound study 11 Medical and Health Sciences 1103 Clinical Sciences. Arthritis Res Ther. 2018;20 https://doi.org/10.1186/s13075-018-1709-6.

Vreju FA, Filippucci E, Gutierrez M, Di Geso L, Ciapetti A, Ciurea ME, et al. Subclinical ultrasound synovitis in a particular joint is associated with ultrasound evidence of bone erosions in that same joint in rheumatoid patients in clinical remission. Clin Exp Rheumatol. 2016;34:673–8.

Zayat AS, Ellegaard K, Conaghan PG, Terslev L, Hensor EMA, Freeston JE, et al. The specificity of ultrasound-detected bone erosions for rheumatoid arthritis. Ann Rheum Dis. 2015;74:897–903.

Seronegative Spondyloarthritis 9

Edoardo Cipolletta, Marco Di Carlo, Emilio Filippucci, and Fabio Martino

Contents

9.1 Introduction

Seronegative spondyloarthritides represent a group of heterogeneous inflammatory joint diseases characterized by shared epidemiology, pathogenesis, and clinical manifestations. The typical musculoskeletal manifestations are peripheral and axial joint involvement, enthesitis, and dactylitis. Uveitis, psoriasis, and inflammatory bowel diseases are characteristic extra-articular features of spondyloarthritides.

Spondyloarthritides can be classified as follows:

- Ankylosing spondylitis
- Psoriatic arthritis
- Reactive arthritis
- Enteropathic arthritis (spondyloarthritis related to inflammatory bowel diseases)
- Undifferentiated spondyloarthritis

The prevalence of spondyloarthritides ranges between 0.2% and 2%. Males in the second and third decades are the most affected by spondyloarthritides.

HLA-B27 antigen is closely related to the development of spondyloarthritides; however, its prevalence varies considerably in the different subsets of spondyloarthritides (up to 95% of

E. Cipolletta · M. Di Carlo · E. Filippucci
Clinica Reumatologica,
Dipartimento di Scienze Cliniche e Molecolari,
Università Politecnica delle Marche,
Jesi (Ancona),
Italy

F. Martino (✉)
Radiology, Sant'Agata Diagnostic Center,
Bari, Italy

F. Martino et al. (eds.), *Musculoskeletal Ultrasound in Orthopedic and Rheumatic disease in Adults*,
https://doi.org/10.1007/978-3-030-91202-4_9

ankylosing spondylitis patients are HLA-B27 positive in comparison with the 40% of psoriatic arthritis patients).

Moreover, bacterial infections have been recognized as trigger factors of spondyloarthritides. Chlamydia, Mycoplasma, and several Enterobacteriaceae species are able to trigger a reactive arthritis in susceptible individuals, through a molecular mimicry mechanism.

The two main spondyloarthritides are the ankylosing spondylitis as the archetypal inflammatory disease that primarily targets axial skeleton (sacroiliac joints and spine), and psoriatic arthritis as the one that primarily targets peripheral joints.

Psoriatic arthritis may be defined as an inflammatory joint disease associated with psoriasis and is usually negative for rheumatoid factor; it affects up to 30% of patients with psoriasis. Wright and Moll described five clinical patterns of joint involvement in psoriatic arthritis:

- Asymmetric oligoarthritis
- Symmetric polyarthritis
- Predominant distal interphalangeal (DIP) joint involvement
- Predominant spondyloarthritis
- Destructive (mutilans) arthritis

More recently, an international study [The Classification of Psoriatic Arthritis (CASPAR)] reported that polyarticular joint involvement was the most common (63%) followed by the oligoarticular pattern.

Characteristic features of psoriatic arthritis include dactylitis and enthesitis. Dactylitis clinically presents as a sausage-shaped swelling of the digit. It may be found in one-third of patients with psoriatic arthritis at first presentation, and in up to 50% during the disease course. Dactylitis affects the right more than left side, involves feet more than hands, and often affects multiple digits at the same time. Acute dactylitis usually presents as a tender, warm, and often erythematous digit while chronic dactylitis as a swollen and often asymptomatic digit. Ultrasound (US) and magnetic resonance imaging (MRI) studies have shown that dactylitis corresponds to a multitissue inflammation of tendons, subcutaneous tissues, and joints.

Enthesitis is an inflammation at tendon and ligament insertion into a bony structure. The most commonly involved entheses are the distal insertion of Achilles tendon, the calcaneus insertion of plantar fascia, both the proximal and distal insertions of patellar tendon, the distal insertion of the quadriceps tendon, the triceps insertion into the olecranon process, and the common extensor tendon insertion into the lateral epicondyle of the elbow.

According to the European League Against Rheumatism (EULAR), conventional radiography and MRI are the only recommended imaging techniques in the diagnosis of the axial involvement in spondyloarthritides. Thus, the role of US in the assessment of sacroiliac and spine involvement in ankylosing spondylitis and other types of axial spondyloarthritis is currently limited to research purposes. In patients with peripheral involvement, US may be used to detect the presence of enthesitis, since US has shown to be more sensitive than clinical examination in the identification of the entheseal abnormalities. Furthermore, as in rheumatoid arthritis, US might be used to detect peripheral arthritis, tenosynovitis, and bursitis, in doubtful cases.

The EULAR recommendations support the use of US to monitor disease activity, since US may provide additional information on top of clinical and laboratory data. However, the decision on when to repeat US depends on the clinical circumstances and, until now, a standardized protocol has not been proposed. The evaluation of structural damage in peripheral spondyloarthritis is predominantly the prerogative of conventional radiography.

The radiographic picture of psoriatic arthritis is quite variable, but it is often distinctive. Peripheral joint involvement is common, and the hand and wrist are most often involved. Joint involvement is usually asymmetric; in contrast to rheumatoid arthritis, the distal interphalangeal joints may be more frequently involved; juxta-articular osteoporosis is frequently absent whereas there is a propensity for bone proliferation. This may be in the form of periostitis of the shafts of the phalanges or in the form of irregular bony spurs at joints or entheses. Bone damage can present the simultaneous coexistence of bone erosions and of new bone formation resulting in a particularly characteristic "whiskering" appearance. In advanced disease, "pencil-in-cup" deformity may be observed as severe marginal erosion of the metacarpal or phalanx head producing the appearance of a pencil, and deep central erosion of phalangeal base, of a cup.

9.2 General Concepts

Psoriatic arthritis and in general seronegative spondyloarthritides are characterized by multiple targets. Therefore, US assessment can be focused on joints, tendons with and without synovial sheaths, entheses, skin, and nails. Basic sonographic changes of joint and tendons with synovial sheaths can be similar to those of RA (e.g., synovial effusion and synovial proliferation). However, in psoriatic arthritis synovial hypertrophy is usually more vascularized than in rheumatoid arthritis.

US is more sensitive than clinical examination for the detection of synovitis, tenosynovitis, and enthesitis in patients with seronegative spondyloarthritides. Although several US findings have been proposed as highly specific features of spondyloarthritides (i.e., peritendinous extensor tendon inflammation and enthesitis), to date, no studies have evaluated the role of US in distinguishing spondyloarthritides (i.e., psoriatic arthritis) from other arthritides in early undifferentiated arthritis. Only a few studies aimed at evaluating the role of US in the prediction of psoriatic arthritis development in patients with psoriasis. There is some evidence supporting that subclinical enthesitis and nail bed vascular changes may be predictors of psoriatic arthritis development.

9.3 Joint Involvement

Every single US finding in seronegative spondyloarthritides is nonspecific as it may occur also in patients with other inflammatory conditions such as rheumatoid arthritis. Synovial effusion and synovial hypertrophy are common features of articular involvement in seronegative spondyloarthritides (Figs. 9.1, 9.2, 9.3, and 9.4). US can be used to assess all the elementary findings of joint involvement: synovitis, bone erosions, and cartilage damage. The dynamic examination may be helpful in the differentiation between synovial effusion (compressible by the probe pressure) and synovial proliferation (only poorly compressible by probe pressure). Although not fully validated, in recent years, several US findings have been proposed to differentiate hand involvement in rheumatoid arthritis and psoriatic arthritis. Peritendinitis, entheseal involvement (i.e., extensor tendon enthesitis at proximal interphalangeal joint and collateral ligament enthesitis) (Fig. 9.4), periarticular soft tissue edema, and palmar plate inflammation are more indicative of psoriatic arthritis than rheumatoid arthritis.

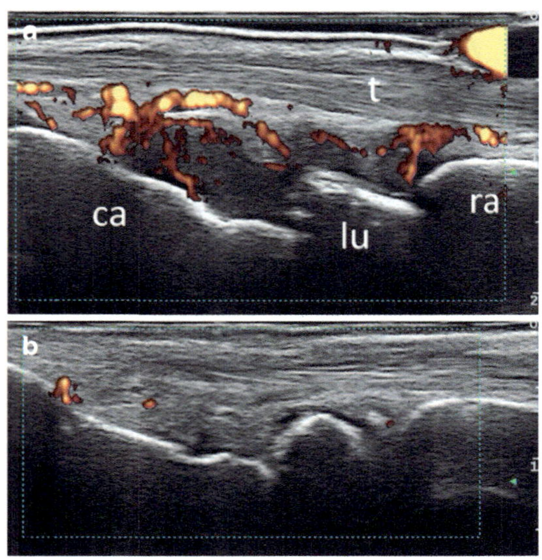

Fig. 9.1 Psoriatic arthritis. Wrist. Right (**a**)–left (**b**) comparison. Longitudinal dorsal scan showing "active" synovitis of radio-carpal and intercarpal joints. *ca* capitate bone; *lu* lunate bone; *ra* radius

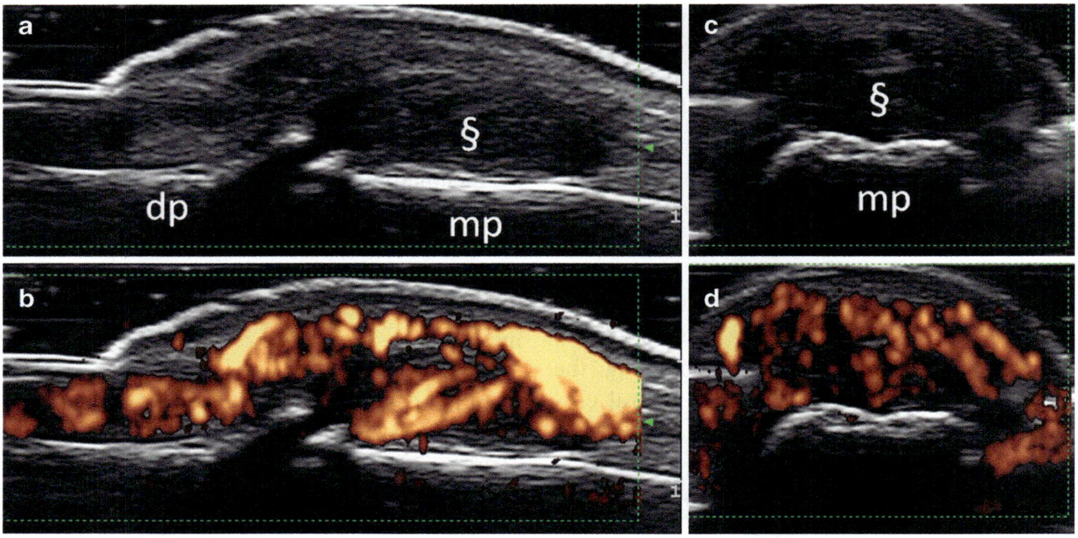

Fig. 9.2 Psoriatic arthritis. Distal interphalangeal joint on longitudinal (**a**, **b**) and transverse (**c**, **d**) dorsal scans showing a representative example of proliferative synovitis with intense intra-articular power Doppler signal. Note the hyperemia of the surrounding periarticular soft tissues (i.e., distal insertion of the finger extensor tendon into the basis of the distal phalanx and nail bed). *dp* distal phalanx; *mp* middle phalanx; §synovial hypertrophy

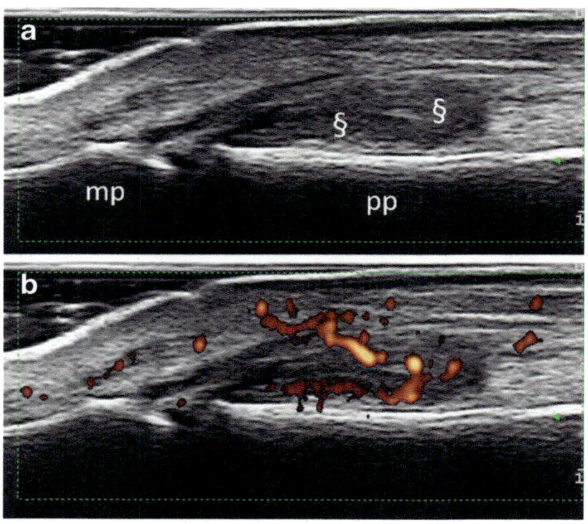

Fig. 9.3 Psoriatic arthritis. Proximal interphalangeal joint. Longitudinal dorsal scan showing proliferative synovitis with evident intra-articular power Doppler signal. (**a**) gray scale mode, (**b**) power Doppler mode. mp=middle phalanx; pp=proximal phalanx; § = synovial hypertrophy

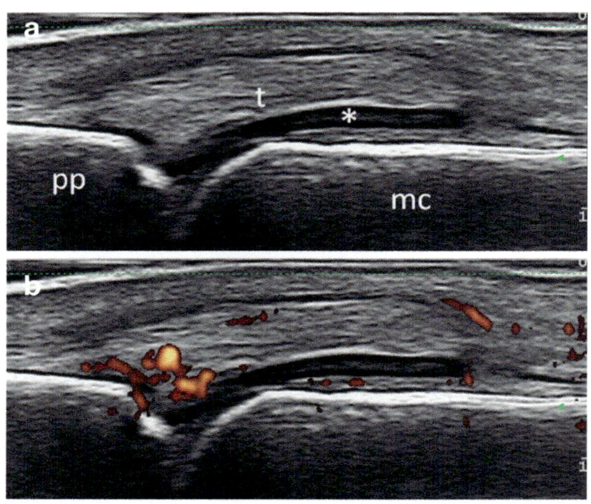

Fig. 9.4 Psoriatic arthritis. Longitudinal dorsal scan showing exudative synovitis of the second metacarpophalangeal joint and "active" enthesitis of the insertion of the finger extensor tendon into the base of the proximal phalanx. (**a**) gray scale mode, (**b**) power Doppler mode. *pp* proximal phalanx; *mc* metacarpal bone; *t* finger extensor tendon; *synovial fluid

9.4 Dactylitis

The "sausage" digit, which is a common finding in psoriatic arthritis, is characterized by a variable combination of the following US features: tenosynovitis of flexor digitorum tendons (Fig. 9.5), synovitis of metacarpophalangeal and interphalangeal joints, and diffuse edema of the soft tissues.

9.5 Enthesitis

US can identify a wide range of abnormalities at the entheseal level. Bone erosions (Fig. 9.6), calcification, and enthesophytes (Figs. 9.7 and 9.8) are regarded as elements indicative of "structural changes," whereas power Doppler signal (Fig. 9.9), hypoechogenicity, and entheseal thickening as inflammatory changes. Recently, the Outcome Measures in Rheumatology US Working Group defined each elementary findings as reported in Table 9.1.

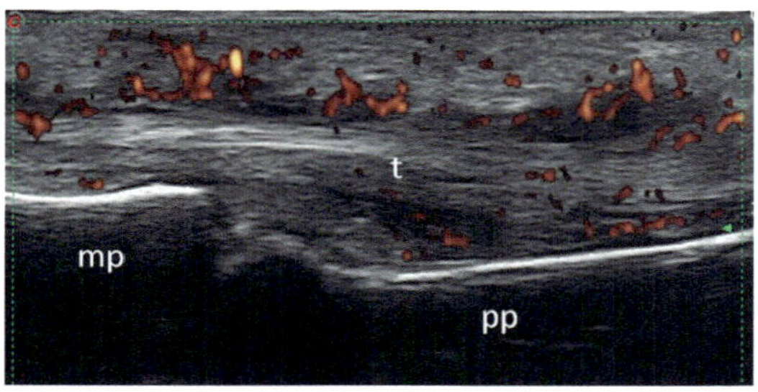

Fig. 9.5 Psoriatic arthritis. Dactylitis. Longitudinal volar scan showing finger flexor tendon tenosynovitis. Note the hypoechoic widening of the synovial tendon sheath with evident abnormal power Doppler signal at synovial tissue level. *mp* middle phalanx; *pp* proximal phalanx; *t* finger flexor tendons

The same group of experts performed a reliability exercise on those definitions. The accepted US elementary findings of entheseal involvement are reported in Table 9.2.

Due to the poor reliability of calcification and enthesophyte definitions, the OMERACT US Working Group decided to merge the two definitions with an improvement in the reliability.

The final OMERACT definition of US enthesitis is "a hypoechoic and/or thickened insertion of the tendon close to the bone (within 2 mm from the bony cortex) which exhibits Doppler signal if active and which may show erosions and enthesophytes/calcifications as a sign of structural damage."

However, several issues should be still clarified. Defining enthesitis as being within 2 mm of the bony cortex remains an area of active debate. In fact, the Group for Research and Assessment of Psoriasis and Psoriatic Arthritis US Working Group supports the concept that the enthesis could also extend beyond the cutoff of 2 mm. Thus, the OMERACT US Working Group definition may not fully capture the entire spectrum of entheseal abnormalities.

US has shown to be more sensitive than clinical examination in the detection of entheseal involvement in seronegative spondyloarthritides. Although most studies explored the entheses of the lower limbs, there is an increasing evidence

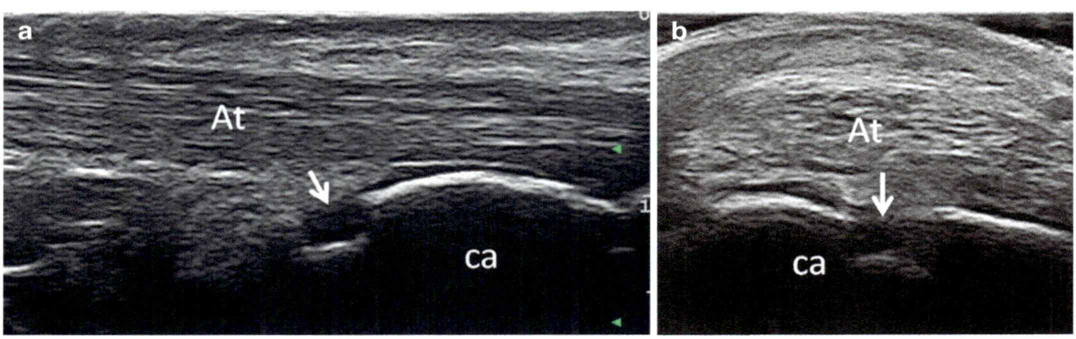

Fig. 9.6 Psoriatic arthritis. Longitudinal (**a**) and transverse (**b**) scans showing Achilles tendon (At) and a bone erosion (arrows) of the calcaneal bone (ca)

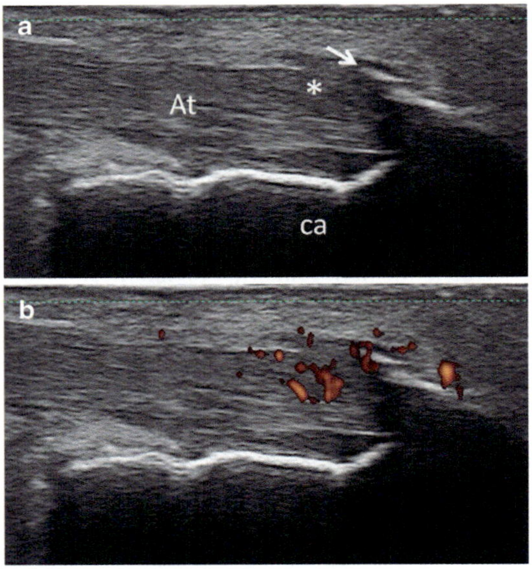

Fig. 9.7 Psoriatic arthritis. Achilles tendon insertion into the calcaneal bone. Longitudinal scan showing "active" enthesitis with evident enthesophytes (arrow). (**a**) gray scale mode, (**b**) power Doppler mode. *At* Achilles tendon; *ca* calcaneal bone

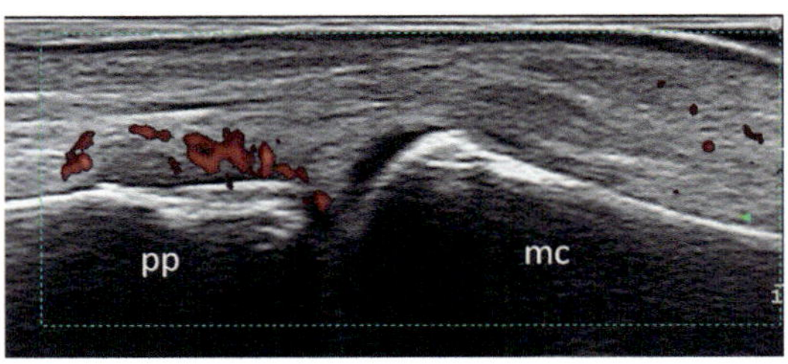

Fig. 9.8 Psoriatic arthritis. First metacarpophalangeal joint. Longitudinal dorsal scan showing "active" enthesitis of the insertion of the finger extensor tendon into the base of the proximal phalanx. *pp* proximal phalanx; *mc* metacarpal bone

of US ability to evaluate enthesitis of the upper limbs and, in particular, of small joints of the hands.

In the early stages, the enthesis may reveal mainly inflammatory changes such as entheseal thickening, hypoechogenicity due to intratendinous edema, with or without associated bursitis, and different amounts of Doppler signal. In later stages, structural changes may be related to

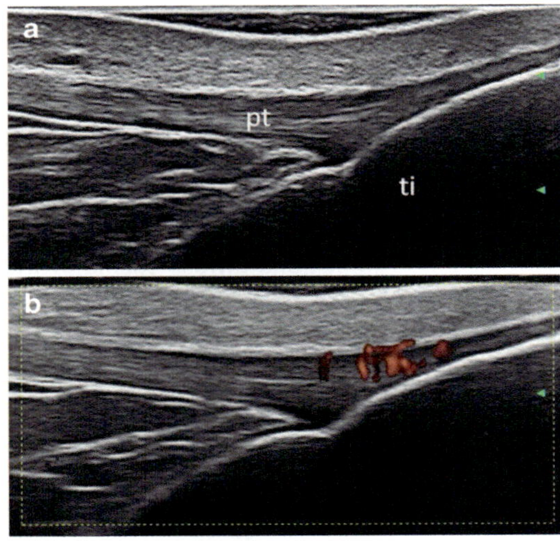

Fig. 9.9 Psoriatic arthritis. Distal patellar tendon insertion into the anterior tibial tuberosity. Longitudinal scan showing "active" enthesitis. (**a**) gray scale mode, (**b**) power Doppler mode. *pt* patellar tendon; *ti* anterior tibial tuberosity

the presence of enthesophytes, calcifications, and/or bone erosions.

9.6 Tendon Involvement

Tenosynovitis is relatively common in psoriatic arthritis. US appearance of tenosynovitis is similar to that described in rheumatoid arthritis. Hands, wrists, and ankles are the most frequently involved anatomical areas. At ankle level, posterior tibialis and peroneal tendons are frequently involved in PsA patients (Fig. 9.10). At hand level, particular attention should be paid in distinguishing flexor digitorum tendon tenosynovitis and finger tendon pulley inflammation. Dynamic maneuvers could help in distinguishing fluid and pulleys.

Among tendons without synovial sheath, Achilles tendon, plantar fascia, and patellar tendon are the most frequently involved. US findings indicative of tendinitis include tendon thickening, usually leading to a fusiform appearance, hypoechogenicity due to edema, and focal derangement of tendon echotexture with a vari-

Table 9.1 OMERACT definitions of US elementary pathologic findings at entheseal level

Findings indicative of structural changes	
Bone irregularity	Bone profile changes not including definite enthesophytes nor bone erosions.
Calcification	Hyperechoic foci, with or without acoustic shadow, detected at the enthesis (<2 mm from the cortical bone).
Enthesophyte	Enthesophyte was defined as a step-up of bony prominence, seen in two perpendicular planes at the end of the bone contour of the enthesis.
Bone erosion	Cortical break with a step-down contour defect, seen in two perpendicular planes, at the insertion of the enthesis.
Inflammatory findings	
Hypoechogenicity at the enthesis	Lack of the homogeneous fibrillar pattern in the enthesis (<2 mm from the cortical bone) with loss of the tightly packed echogenic lines after correcting for anisotropy.
Entheseal thickening	Increased thickness of the tendon insertion into the bone (<2 mm from the cortical bone) as compared with the body of tendon, with or without blurring of the tendon margins.
Doppler signal at enthesis	Doppler signal seen at bone insertion (<2 mm from the cortical bone), different from reflecting surface artifact or nutrition vessel signal, with or without cortical irregularities, erosions, or enthesophytes.
Doppler signal outside the enthesis	Doppler signal far from the enthesis (i.e., >2 mm from the cortical bone, within the body of tendon) and clearly different from nutrition vessel signals.
Bursitis	An enlargement (i.e., increase in diameter of the bursa), with well-defined, anechoic or hypoechoic area inside, with or without Doppler signal.

Table 9.2 Accepted US elementary findings for OMERACT US definition of enthesitis

Inflammatory findings	Findings indicative of structural changes
Doppler signal at the enthesis	Calcification/enthesophyte at the enthesis
Hypoechogenicity at the enthesis	Bone erosion at the enthesis
Thickened enthesis	

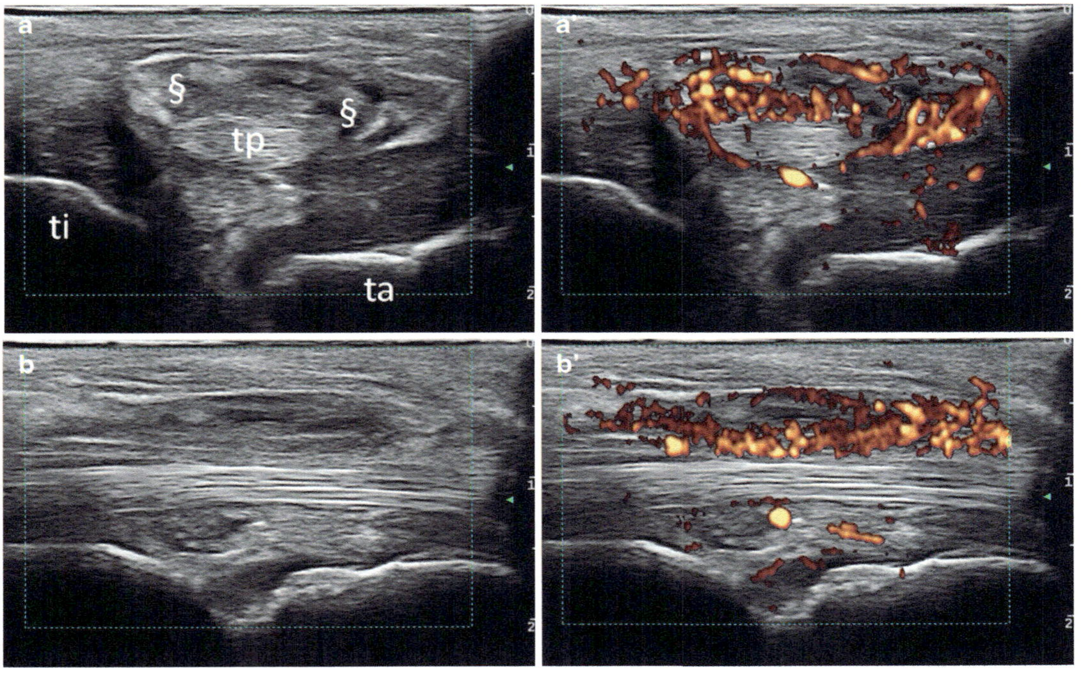

Fig. 9.10 Psoriatic arthritis. Ankle. Tibialis posterior tendon. Transverse (**a–a′**) and longitudinal (**b–b′**) scans showing "active" tenosynovitis (§) . *ti* tibia; *ta* talus; *tp* tibialis posterior tendon

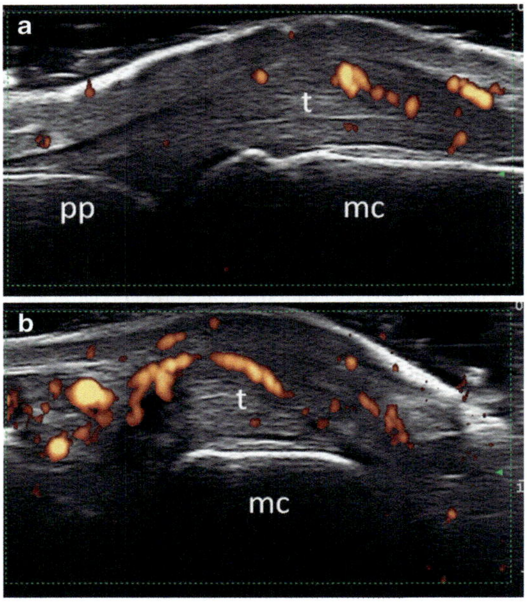

Fig. 9.11 Psoriatic arthritis. Peritendinous inflammation at second finger metacarpophalangeal joint level. Longitudinal (**a**) and transverse (**b**) dorsal scans showing power Doppler signal surrounding the finger extensor tendon. *pp* proximal phalanx; *mc* metacarpal bone; t=finger extensor tendon

able amount of intra-tendinous Doppler signal. Moreover, a peritendinous inflammation may appear as a hypoechoic swelling of the soft tissue surrounding the tendon with or without the presence of power Doppler signal (i.e., peritendinous involvement of finger extensor tendon at metacarpophalangeal joint) (Fig. 9.11).

Further Readings

Aydin SZ, Bas E, Basci O, Filippucci E, Wakefield RJ, Çelikel Ç, et al. Validation of ultrasound imaging for Achilles entheseal fibrocartilage in bovines and description of changes in humans with spondyloarthritis. Ann Rheum Dis. 2010;69:2165–8. https://doi.org/10.1136/ard.2009.127175.

Aydin SZ, Castillo-Gallego C, Ash ZR, Marzo-Ortega H, Wakefield R, McGonagle D. Vascularity of nail bed by ultrasound to discriminate psoriasis, psoriatic arthritis and healthy controls. Clin Exp Rheumatol. n.d.;35:872.

Aydin SZ, Karadag O, Filippucci E, Atagunduz P, Akdogan A, Kalyoncu U, Grassi W, Direskeneli H. Monitoring Achilles enthesitis in ankylosing spondylitis during TNF-alpha antagonist therapy: an ultrasound study. Rheumatology (Oxford). 2010;49(3):578–82. https://doi.org/10.1093/rheumatology/kep410. Epub 2009 Dec 29

Balint PV, Kane D, Wilson H, McInnes IB, Sturrock RD. Ultrasonography of entheseal insertions in the lower limb in spondyloarthropathy. Ann Rheum Dis. 2002;61:905–10. https://doi.org/10.1136/ard.61.10.905.

Balint PV, Terslev L, Aegerter P, Bruyn GAW, Chary-Valckenaere I, Gandjbakhch F, et al. Reliability of a consensus-based ultrasound definition and scoring for enthesitis in spondyloarthritis and psoriatic arthritis: An OMERACT US initiative. Ann Rheum Dis. 2018;77:1730–5. https://doi.org/10.1136/annrheumdis-2018-213609.

Delle Sedie A, Riente L, Filippucci E, Scirè CA, Iagnocco A, Gutierrez M, et al. Ultrasound imaging for the rheumatologist XXVI. Sonographic assessment of the knee in patients with psoriatic arthritis. Clin Exp Rheumatol. n.d.;28:147–52.

Delle Sedie A, Riente L, Filippucci E, Scirè CA, Iagnocco A, Meenagh G, et al. Ultrasound imaging for the rheumatologist. XXXII. Sonographic assessment of the foot in patients with psoriatic arthritis. Clin Exp Rheumatol. n.d.;29:217–22.

Filippucci E, Aydin SZ, Karadag O, Salaffi F, Gutierrez M, Direskeneli H, Grassi W. Reliability of high-resolution ultrasonography in the assessment of Achilles tendon enthesopathy in seronegative spondyloarthropathies. Ann Rheum Dis. 2009;68(12):1850–5. https://doi.org/10.1136/ard.2008.096511. Epub 2009 Apr 8

Filippucci E, Smerilli G Di Matteo A, Cipolletta E, Destro Castaniti GM, et al. Reliability assessment of the definition of ultrasound enthesitis in SpA: results of a large, multicentre, international web-based study [published online ahead of print, 2022 Mar 16]. Rheumatology (Oxford). 2022;keac162. https://doi.org/10.1093/rheumatology/keac162.

Filippucci E, Smerilli G, Di Matteo A, Grassi W. Ultrasound definition of enthesitis in spondyloarthritis and psoriatic arthritis: arrival or starting point?. Ann Rheum Dis. 2021;80(11):1373–5. https://doi.org/10.1136/annrheumdis-2021-220478.

Girolimetto N, Macchioni P, Tinazzi I, Costa L, Peluso R, Tasso M, et al. Predominant ultrasonographic extracapsular changes in symptomatic psoriatic dactylitis: results from a multicenter cross-sectional study comparing symptomatic and asymptomatic hand dactylitis. Clin Rheumatol. 2019; https://doi.org/10.1007/s10067-019-04683-2.

Gutierrez M, Filippucci E, De Angelis R, Filosa G, Kane D, Grassi W. A sonographic spectrum of psoriatic arthritis: "the five targets.". Clin Rheumatol. 2010;29:133–42. https://doi.org/10.1007/s10067-009-1292-y.

Gutierrez M, Filippucci E, De Angelis R, Salaffi F, Filosa G, Ruta S, et al. Subclinical entheseal involvement in patients with psoriasis: an ultrasound study. Semin Arthritis Rheum. 2011;40:407–12. https://doi.org/10.1016/j.semarthrit.2010.05.009.

Gutierrez M, Filippucci E, Salaffi F, Di Geso L, Grassi W. Differential diagnosis between rheumatoid arthritis and psoriatic arthritis: the value of ultrasound findings at metacarpophalangeal joints level. Ann Rheum Dis. 2011;70:1111–4. https://doi.org/10.1136/ard.2010.147272.

Mandl P, Navarro-Compán V, Terslev L, Aegerter P, Van Der Heijde D, D'Agostino MA, et al. EULAR recommendations for the use of imaging in the diagnosis and management of spondyloarthritis in clinical practice. Ann Rheum Dis. 2015;74:1327–39. https://doi.org/10.1136/annrheumdis-2014-206971.

Martínez-Vidal MP, Fernández-Carballido C. Is the SCORE chart underestimating the real cardiovascular (CV) risk of patients with psoriatic arthritis? Prevalence of subclinical CV disease detected by carotid ultrasound. Joint Bone Spine. 2018;85:327–32. https://doi.org/10.1016/j.jbspin.2017.07.002.

Tinazzi I, McGonagle D, Aydin SZ, Chessa D, Marchetta A, Macchioni P. "Deep Koebner" phenomenon of the flexor tendon-associated accessory pulleys as a novel factor in tenosynovitis and dactylitis in psoriatic arthritis. Ann Rheum Dis. 2018;77:922–5. https://doi.org/10.1136/annrheumdis-2017-212681.

Tinazzi I, McGonagle D, Macchioni P, Aydin SZ. Power Doppler enhancement of accessory pulleys confirming disease localization in psoriatic dactylitis. Rheumatology. 2020; https://doi.org/10.1093/rheumatology/kez549.

Tinazzi I, McGonagle D, Zabotti A, Chessa D, Marchetta A, Macchioni P. Comprehensive evaluation of finger flexor tendon entheseal soft tissue and bone changes by ultrasound can differentiate psoriatic arthritis and rheumatoid arthritis. Clin Exp Rheumatol. n.d.;36:785–90.

Tom S, Zhong Y, Cook R, Aydin SZ, Kaeley G, Eder L. Development of a preliminary ultrasonographic enthesitis score in psoriatic arthritis – GRAPPA ultrasound working group. J Rheumatol. 2019;46:384–90. https://doi.org/10.3899/jrheum.171465.

Zabotti A, Piga M, Canzoni M, Sakellariou G, Iagnocco A, Scirè CA, et al. Ultrasonography in psoriatic arthritis: Which sites should we scan? Ann Rheum Dis. 2018;77 https://doi.org/10.1136/annrheumdis-2018-213025.

Zabotti A, Salvin S, Quartuccio L, De Vita S. Differentiation between early rheumatoid and early psoriatic arthritis by the ultrasonographic study of the synovio-entheseal complex of the small joints of the hands. Clin Exp Rheumatol. 2016;34:459–65.

Crystal-Related Arthropathies

10

Marina Carotti, Emilio Filippucci, Fausto Salaffi, and Fabio Martino

Contents

10.1 Introduction

Crystal-related arthropathies are diseases characterized by crystal deposition at articular and periarticular level. There are three main types of crystals: monosodium urate (MSU) crystals, responsible for the gout; calcium pyrophosphate (CPP) crystals, responsible for calcium pyrophosphate deposition disease (CPPD); and basic calcium phosphate crystals.

In recent years, several articles have shown that ultrasound (US) is an accurate imaging technique to detect crystal deposits, and in experienced hands, US may change the standard diagnostic approach in patients with suspicion of crystal-related arthropathies.

Either the MSU or the CCP crystal deposits are characterized by a high reflectivity of the US beam, independently of the angle of insonation. The US appearance of crystal deposits is heterogeneous in size (from millimetric spots to large aggregates), shape (rounded or poorly defined), and echostructure (homogeneous or heterogeneous). Although CPP crystals can sometimes be undistinguishable from those of MSU, the identification of US pat-

M. Carotti
Clinica di Radiologia, Dipartimento di Scienze Radiologiche – Azienda Ospedali Riuniti di Ancona Universita' Politecnica delle Marche, Ancona, Italy

E. Filippucci · F. Salaffi
Clinica Reumatologica, Dipartimento di Scienze Cliniche e Molecolari, Università Politecnica delle Marche, Jesi (Ancona), Italy

F. Martino (✉)
Radiology, Sant'Agata Diagnostic Center, Bari, Italy

F. Martino et al. (eds.), *Musculoskeletal Ultrasound in Orthopedic and Rheumatic disease in Adults*, https://doi.org/10.1007/978-3-030-91202-4_10

terns defined by the topographic distribution of crystal deposits at different tissues has been shown to be accurate in distinguishing MSU from CPP crystal deposits. In fact, the value of each US finding depends mainly on its characteristics and its topographic distribution in the different tissues (e.g., hyperechoic spots within the hyaline cartilage are indicative of CPPD, whereas an enhancement of the chondrosynovial interface is indicative of gout).

These differences account for a large spectrum of US features and this wide heterogeneity generates many different scenarios not only in different patients but also in the same subject. Such a high variety has prompted the development of a standardization for the definition of each single US finding as reported later in this chapter.

The diagnostic potential of US in the diagnosis of crystal-related arthropathies depends on the high- resolution power (<0.1 mm) at superficial tissues (targets not deeper than 1 cm), the possibility to carry out a multisite and multitissue examination, and the capability of real-time imaging providing a safe guidance for the aspiration of even minimal synovial fluid collections in order to obtain a definite diagnosis.

Unlike polarized light microscopy, US assessment does not need the presence of synovial fluid or tophi to identify crystal deposits. Thus, US can be performed during intercritical phases to obtain information useful to reach a definite diagnosis.

10.2 Gout

Gout occurs when body tissues become supersaturated with urate, leading to the formation of MSU crystals in and around joints. The traditional clinical features of gout include acute painful synovitis, tophaceous deposits, chronic joint damage, renal stones, and chronic kidney disease. Gout leads to impaired quality of life and it is associated with a variety of cardiovascular and metabolic comorbidities.

Gout is mainly diagnosed by identification of the pathognomonic MSU crystals by synovial fluid analysis or by clinical evidence of tophi.

The assessment of joint damage in gout traditionally relied on conventional radiography (CR). However, CR has been shown to be frequently normal especially in the early disease. Early radiological findings are limited at soft tissue level and mainly restricted to asymmetric swelling in the joints with tophaceous deposits. In later phases of the disease, gout may determine intra-articular and extra-articular bone erosions. Typically, bone erosions in gout are well-defined, "punched-out," periarticular erosions with overhanging edges, often located next to a tophus. Joint involvement is usually asymmetric and joint space is relatively preserved until late stage. Thus, the CR findings suggestive of gout are absence of juxta-articular osteoporosis and of joint space narrowing, sharply marginated erosions with sclerotic borders and overhanging edges, and asymmetric distribution of the joint. Despite highly characteristic of gout these CR findings are indicative of structural damage and CR may underestimate the extent of MSU crystal deposition.

10.2.1 Ultrasound Findings at Joint Level

US findings in gout include joint effusion, synovitis, bone erosions, and MSU deposits at joint and periarticular soft tissue level.

Acute gouty arthritis is typically characterized by a joint space widening due to the presence of variable amount of synovial fluid. In some patients a "snowstorm" appearance can be seen, when hyperechoic spots can be identified floating in the synovial fluid (Fig. 10.1).

Synovitis in gout appears as a heterogeneous, but predominantly hyperechoic intra-articular tissues because of MSU deposits. The presence of hyper-reflective spots of MSU deposits may be helpful to further differentiate gout from other inflammatory arthritis such as rheumatoid arthritis.

Bone erosions are seen in long-standing gouty arthropathy. Bone erosions are defined as an intra- and/or extra-articular discontinuity of the bone surface, visible in at least two perpendicular planes. Bone erosions are usually located next to tophi, due to the osteoclastogenic activity of MSU deposits. The overhanging edges of bone erosions and the presence of hyperechoic deposits filling the bone cavity are characteristic features of gout. Moreover, bone erosions in gout

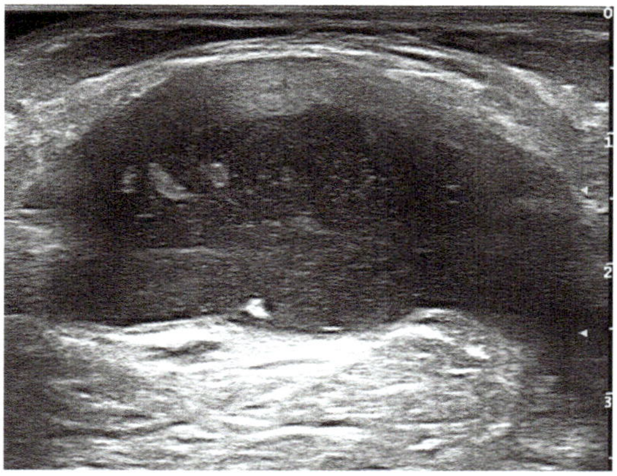

Fig. 10.1 Gout. Popliteal cyst. Snowstorm appearance of the synovial fluid, characterized by multiple hyperechoic spots with different shape and size. The probe compression during real-time examination shows their floating in the synovial fluid

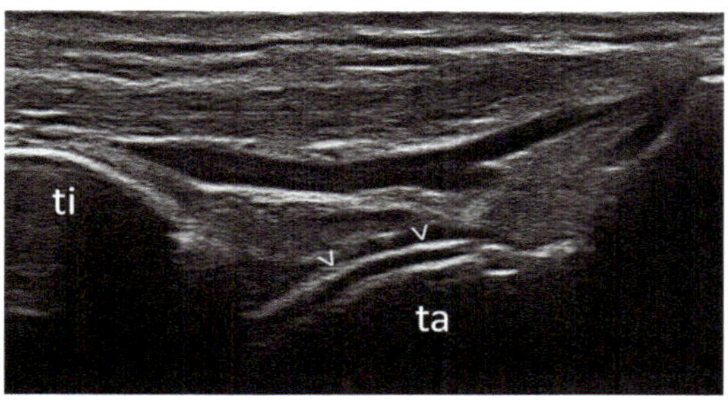

Fig. 10.2 Gout. Tibiotalar joint on longitudinal anterior scan showing double-contour sign due to urate deposits on the surface of the talar hyaline cartilage. Note the enhancement of the chondrosynovial interface (arrowheads). *ti* tibia; *ta* talus

can be either intra- or extra-articular and tend to be deep and destructive.

According to OMERACT definitions MSU deposits can be defined as:

- **Double-contour sign**: "Abnormal hyperechoic band over the superficial profile of the joint hyaline cartilage, independent of the angle of insonation and which may be either irregular or regular, continuous or intermittent and can be distinguished from the cartilage interface sign" (Fig. 10.2). The deposits are found on the outer layer of the hyaline cartilage and appear as an irregular enhancement of the cartilage surface. Although this is a specific sign for the diagnosis of gout (i.e., more than 90%), it is not very sensitive (i.e., between 60% and 80%). The reported sensitivity of the double-contour sign is highly variable mainly according to the number of scanned anatomic sites, the width of the cartilage surface explorable by US, and the disease duration. Special care should be paid avoiding to misinterpret the normal cartilage interface as double-contour sign. Normal cartilage surface is hyperechoic only when it is insonated perpendicularly or in the presence of overlying fluid.

  Double-contour sign does not disappear where the cartilage curves away from the horizontal plane, and where the US beam is not perpendicular to the cartilage. For example, the presence of synovial effusion in the first metatarsophalangeal joint can enhance the visualization of the outer margin of the hyaline cartilage. In such cases, the dislocation of the synovial fluid applying a gentle probe compression can help in the correct interpretation of this finding. Finally, the double-contour sign should be differentiated from intracartilaginous hyperechoic spots, seen in CPPD.
- **Tophi**: [independent of location (e.g., extra-articular/intra-articular/intra-tendinous)]: "A circumscribed, inhomogeneous, hyperechoic, and/or hypoechoic aggregation (which may or may not generate posterior acoustic shadow) which may be surrounded by a subtle 'anechoic halo'" (Fig. 10.3). Tophaceous deposits may show a different degree of reflectivity according

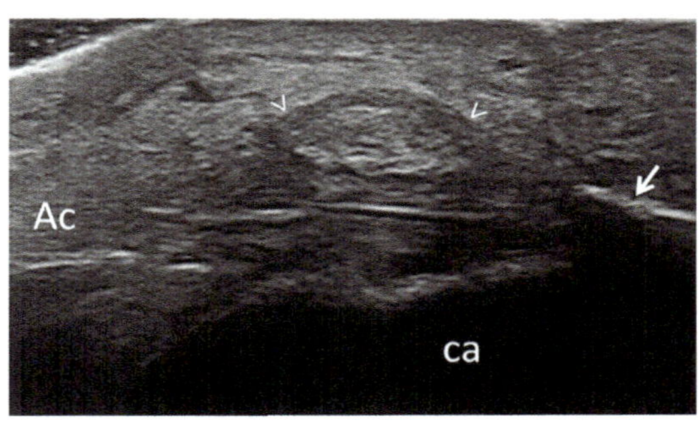

Fig. 10.3 Tophaceous gout. Achilles tendon insertion into the calcaneal bone on longitudinal scan showing a peri-tendinous tophus appearing as an oval shaped area. The arrow indicates a retrocalcaneal spur. *Ac* Achilles tendon; *ca* calcaneal bone

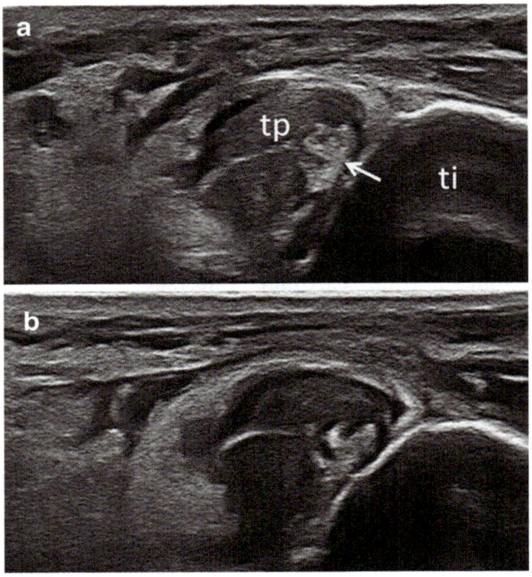

Fig. 10.4 Gout. (**a**) Tibialis posterior tendon on transverse scan at tibial malleolus level. The arrow indicates an intra-tendinous urate deposit. (**b**) Note the reduction of the tendon echogenicity induced by the change of the probe inclination; conversely the crystal deposit did not decrease its echogenicity. *tp* tibialis posterior tendon; *ti* tibia

to the density of the deposits. These vary from soft tophi, with an inhomogeneous echogenicity and polymorphic appearance, to hard tophi characterized by dense and compact aggregates of MSU crystals that generate a hyperechoic band and a posterior acoustic shadow.

- **Aggregates** [independent of location (intra-articular/intra-tendinous)]: "Heterogeneous hyperechoic foci that maintain their high degree of reflectivity even when the gain setting is minimized or the insonation angle is changed and which occasionally may generate posterior acoustic shadow" (Fig. 10.4). Aggregates are the least defined form of MSU deposits. The appearance of aggregates can vary considerably ranging from the smallest form of aggregates, the "isolated shining dots," described as submillimeter homogenous hyperechoic punctiform spots, to dense microdotted deposits inside the joint cavity with or without small or large hyperechoic spots.

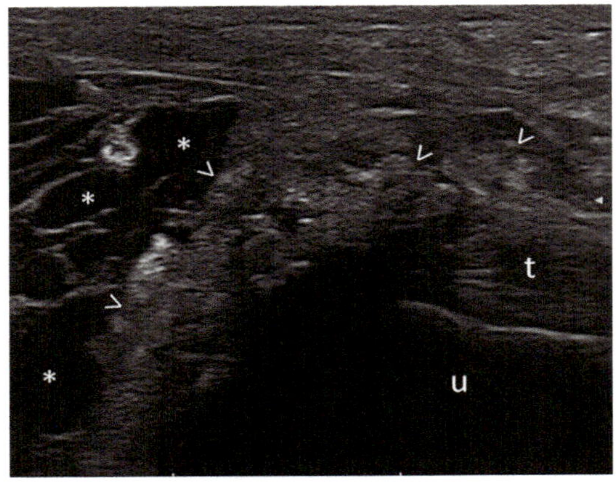

Fig. 10.5 Olecranon bursitis in patient with tophaceous gout. The longitudinal view shows bursal enlargement due to anechoic synovial fluid (*) in-between echogenic branches of synovial hypertrophy. Tophus is made of inhomogeneous echogenic aggregate deposits with rounded edges (arrowheads). *u* ulna, olecranon process; *t* triceps tendon

10.2.2 Ultrasound Findings at Tendon, Bursa, and Subcutaneous Level

US is able to clearly depict tophaceous deposits in bursae, tendons, and subcutaneous tissues. The olecranon bursa is the commonly involved site in gout. US features of an acute gouty bursitis are substantially similar to those of acute arthritis. The high sensitivity of US in the detection of even a minimal amount of synovial fluid allows easy identification of inflammation even in case of small bursae (i.e., retrocalcaneal bursa and olecranon bursa) (Fig. 10.5) or deep ones (i.e., iliopsoas bursa).

Deposition of MSU crystals may also involve both sliding and supporting tendons. MSU deposits can be found both at intra- and peri-tendinous level. Knowledge of the most frequently involved tendons can also be helpful in the diagnosis of gout. The Achilles and peroneal tendons are common sites of involvement at ankle level, whereas the popliteus and the patellar tendons are common locations at knee level. Moreover, the triceps tendon has been indicated as frequently involved tendon in the upper limb.

The identification of MSU crystals within tendons is easy because in the background of the typical fibrillar echotexture of the tendon, they appear as inhomogeneous spots or bands deranging the tendon echostructure. Extensive and/or multiple crystal clouds have a variable and inhomogeneous echotexture with aggregates of different reflectivity, mainly related to crystal density. Tendon deposits maintain their high degree of reflectivity, even when the gain value is reduced and the tendon is not perpendicularly insonated. Finally, the main findings indicating acute gouty tendinopathy include hypoechoic thickening and intra-tendinous Doppler signal which may be found in between and outside the MSU deposits.

10.2.3 Scanning Protocol

Even if US allows for rapid, safe, and easy multisite and multitissue evaluation, in daily practice the sonographic examination should be guided by patient history and physical examination.

Nevertheless, US can reveal the presence of crystal deposits in asymptomatic sites without previous involvement. Thus, in gouty patients, the first MTP joint, the elbow, the patellar, and the Achilles tendons could be considered sites to scan even if not clinically involved. Recently a dedicated US protocol was developed. The assessment of radio-carpal joint, patellar tendon, and triceps tendon for the presence of hyperechoic aggregates, and of the articular cartilage of the first metatarsophalangeal, tibiotalar, and knee joints for double-contour sign, showed the best balance between sensitivity and specificity (84.6% and 83.3%) in patients with gout.

MSU crystal deposits were documented also in subjects with asymptomatic hyperuricemia. In asymptomatic hyperuricemia, scanning of the first metatarsophalangeal joint and knee femoral condyles for double contour and the first metatarsophalangeal joint for tophus has the highest discriminative power in comparison with normouricemic subjects.

A correct position of the joint to be examined is essential to ensure the best exposure of the cartilaginous structure. For instance, the maximal flexion of the knee joint allows the perpendicular insonation of the femoral trochlea hyaline cartilage using suprapatellar axial views.

10.2.4 Disease Monitoring

With appropriate and effective treatment, primarily involving urate-lowering drugs, MSU deposits may reduce in size and completely resolve. Thus, the efficacy of urate-lowering therapy can be monitored by US by the disappearance of MSU crystal deposits. However, to date, despite the great potential of US, there are only few studies supporting the ability of US to monitor changes induced by urate-lowering therapy. Still unresolved issues are the lack of standardization of monitoring parameters (i.e., tophus largest diameter or volume), the identification of the best MSU deposit to be followed up (double-contour sign or tophus), and the different speed of dissolution process at different anatomical areas.

10.3 Pyrophosphate Arthropathy

Calcium pyrophosphate deposition disease (CPPD) is characterized by the deposition of calcium pyrophosphate (CPP) crystals in and around the joints. Although the main target of CPPD is the cartilaginous structure, both fibrocartilage and hyaline cartilage, CPP crystal deposits may occur also at tendon, joint capsule, and ligament level. CPPD occurs mainly in the elderly, although a mono-oligo articular form of young-onset CPPD (<55 years old) may happen at sites of prior joint injury and osteoarthritis (OA), whereas a polyarticular form may be due to genetic or metabolic disorders. CPPD is frequently asymptomatic and it is usually an incidental finding of chondrocalcinosis on imaging studies. In a minority of patients, CPPD can cause an acute CPP-crystal arthritis or a chronic CPP-crystal inflammatory arthritis or may be associated with a form of OA with chondrocalcinosis. CPPD can occur in any synovial or fibrocartilaginous joint; however, knee, wrist, symphysis pubis, hip, and shoulder are the most frequent targets.

The "definite" diagnosis of CPPD is based on the identification of CPP crystals in the synovial fluid. However, during intercritical phases, a "probable" diagnosis of CPPD is generally established on the typical CR findings displaying cartilage calcification and structural changes typical of OA.

Although CR is traditionally considered as the reference imaging modality in daily practice, other imaging techniques such as US and computed tomography (CT) can be used to identify CPP crystal deposits. Of these, US is more commonly used because it is inexpensive, safe, and well accepted by patients, but it requires experienced operators. On the other hand, CT may be particularly useful in demonstrating axial CPPD, such as in the crowned dens syndrome.

In recent years, a growing body of evidence has shown that US is more sensitive than CR in the detection of CPP crystal deposits at knee and wrist level.

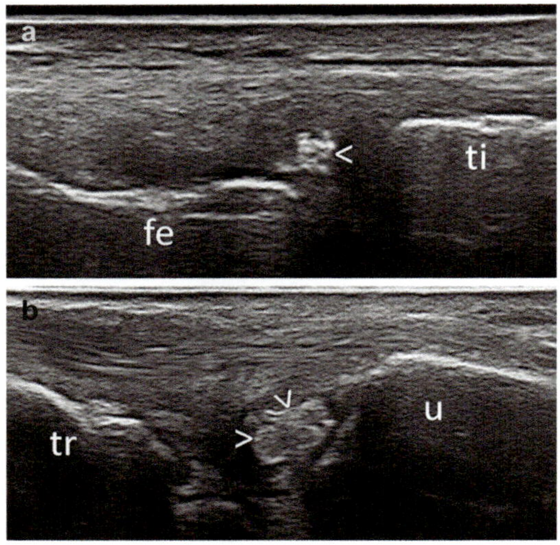

Fig. 10.6 Calcium pyrophosphate deposition disease. (**a**) Knee. Medial longitudinal scan showing meniscal calcification (arrowhead). (**b**) Wrist. longitudinal scan on the ulnar side showing calcification of the triangular fibrocartilage complex (arrowheads). *fe* medial femoral condyle; *ti* medial tibia; *tr* triquetral bone; *u* ulna

10.3.1 Ultrasound Findings at Joint Level

CPP crystals appear as hyperechoic dots which may be isolated or aggregated, typically without acoustic shadowing and usually located within the cartilaginous structures. According to OMERACT definitions CPP crystal deposits can be defined as follows:

- **Fibrocartilaginous calcifications**: deposits of variable shape, hyperechoic (similar to the bone cortex echogenicity), localized within the fibrocartilage structure, that remain fixed and move together with the fibrocartilage during dynamic assessment (i.e., joint movement and probe compression) (Fig. 10.6).
- **Hyaline cartilage calcifications**: deposits of variable size and shape, hyperechoic (similar to the bone cortex echogenicity) that do not create posterior shadowing, localized within the hyaline cartilage and that remain fixed and move together with the hyaline cartilage during the joint movement (Fig. 10.7).
- **Synovial fluid calcifications**: deposits of variable size (from punctuate to large), hyperechoic (similar to the bone cortex echogenicity), that generally do not create posterior shadowing, localized within the synovial fluid and mobile according to joint movement and probe pressure.

In healthy subjects, the hyaline cartilage appears as an anechoic layer having two sharp, continuous, and regular hyperechoic margins (of note the outer chondrosynovial interface is detectable only where the US beam is perpendicular to the cartilage surface), whereas the fibrocartilage shows a mild and homogeneous punctate echogenicity. Fibrocartilaginous calcifications detectable on US in CPPD can show widely variable appearance, depending on the size, distribution, and density of crystal aggregates, ranging from isolated hyperechoic dots to large and heterogeneous aggregates.

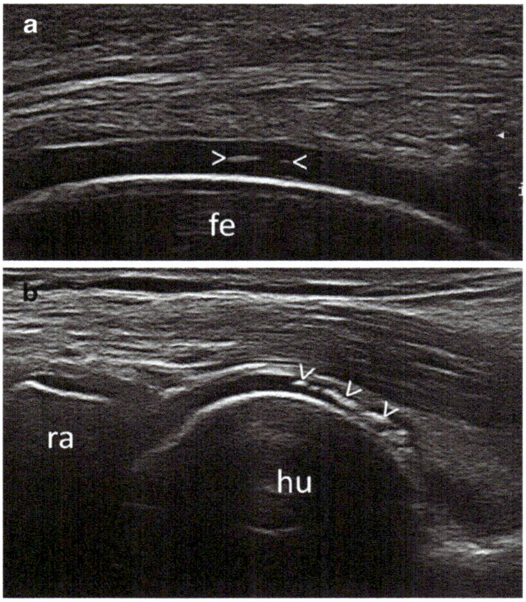

Fig. 10.7 Calcium pyrophosphate deposition disease. (**a**) Medial femoral condyle of the knee on longitudinal parapatellar scan (**a**) and longitudinal anterior radial scan of the elbow (**b**) showing hyperechoic deposits (arrowheads) not generating acoustic shadowing within the hyaline cartilage layer. *fe* medial femoral condyle; *ra* radius; *hu* humerus

In the hyaline cartilage, the intracartilaginous distribution of the crystal deposits differs from that of the MSU deposits, which are on the cartilage surface.

Fibrocartilage is the most frequent anatomical target of CPPD disease. Meniscal calcification was reported as highly prevalent in patients with CPPD disease, being identified in more than 75% of cases.

Although a multisite scanning protocol in CPPD patients was not already described, the hyaline cartilage of femoral condyles, humeral head, humeral trochlea and capitellum, the talus and the metacarpal heads and the fibrocartilage of menisci, triangular fibrocartilage complex and acromioclavicular joint could be considered sites to scan even if not clinically involved.

CPP crystal deposits are usually easy to detect, by their characteristic appearance. However, they must be distinguished from other "shining dots" such as the MSU aggregates, osteoarthritic debris and proteinaceous material floating within the synovial fluid, and intra-articular air bubbles. Characteristically the CPP crystal deposits maintain their hyperechogenicity despite changing the insonation angle and reducing the gain level (Fig. 10.8).

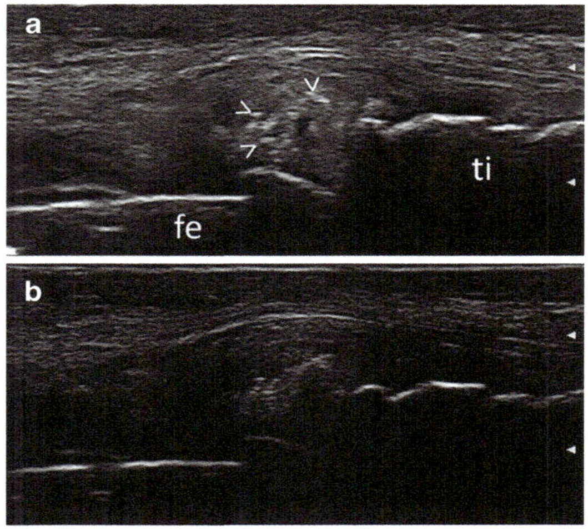

Fig. 10.8 Calcium pyrophosphate deposition disease. (**a**) Medial aspect of the knee on longitudinal scan showing meniscal calcifications (arrowheads). (**b**) Same view after reducing the gain value; note the disappearance of the meniscus while calcifications are still detectable. *fe* medial femoral condyle; *ti* tibia

The dynamic assessment can help in discriminating the exact position of the deposits. It is particularly useful in the assessment of the knee menisci to distinguish whether the crystals are on the condylar hyaline cartilage or within the meniscal fibrocartilage and in the evaluation of hyaline cartilage to differentiate between cartilaginous calcification and capsular calcification.

10.3.2 Ultrasound Findings at Tendon and Periarticular Level

Calcifications in tendons are also typical imaging features of CPPD. CPP crystal deposits appear as hyperechoic bands and spots, generally, without posterior acoustic shadow and often distributed along the major axis of the tendon. According to OMERACT definition, tendon calcifications are multiple hyperechoic (in relation to the tendon echogenicity) and linear deposits (parallel to the tendon fibrillar structure and not in continuity with the bone profile) that generally will not create posterior shadowing, localized within the tendon, and that remain fixed and move together with the tendon during movement and probe compression (Fig. 10.9). Achilles tendon and plantar fascia are frequently involved in patients with CPPD. The identification of crystals is easy when they are located within tissues showing anisotropy, such as the tendons. In these cases, changing the probe inclination allows the enhancement of the crystals, which maintain their brightness while the surrounding tendon fibers reduce their echogenicity.

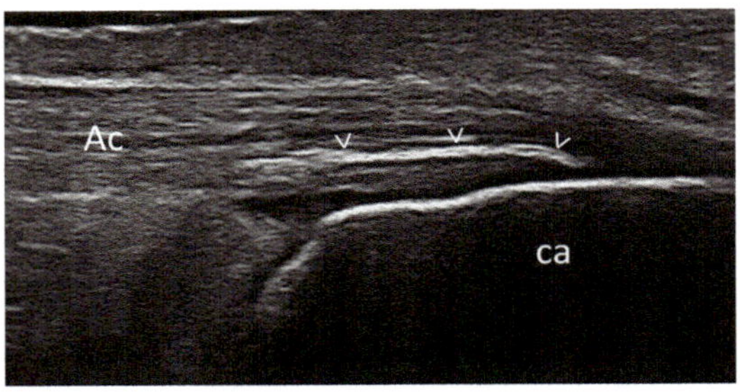

Fig. 10.9 Calcium pyrophosphate deposition disease. Achilles tendon insertion into the calcaneal bone on longitudinal scan showing an intra-tendinous linear deposit appearing as a hyperechoic band (arrowheads) not attached to the bone and without posterior acoustic shadowing. *Ac* Achilles tendon; *ca* calcaneal bone

10.4 Basic Calcium Phosphate Crystal Deposition Disease

Basic calcium phosphate (BCP) crystal-related musculoskeletal pathology can be divided into two main conditions, osteoarthritis secondary to intra-articular BCP crystals and calcific periarthritis due to BCP crystal deposition in tendons, bursae, and other soft tissues around joints.

The term "hydroxyapatite" is often used as a synonymous of "basic calcium phosphate," with carbonated hydroxyapatite being the most prevalent mineral type in BCP crystal-related arthropathy.

Calcific periarthritis is the main BCP-related condition. Calcium deposits are easily detected by US because of their high reflectivity. Differently to calcium pyrophosphate (CPP) crystals, BCP crystals usually generate a posterior acoustic shadow (Fig. 10.10a). However, as in other crystal-related arthropathies, BCP crystal deposits may have different degrees of compaction of the crystalline aggregates. Moreover, their size, shape, and location can vary significantly. Shoulder results the most frequently affected anatomic site and ultrasound (US) examination allows for an accurate assessment of inflammatory and structural changes at shoulder level.

Among inflammatory findings, tenosynovitis of the long head of the biceps tendon, subacromial-

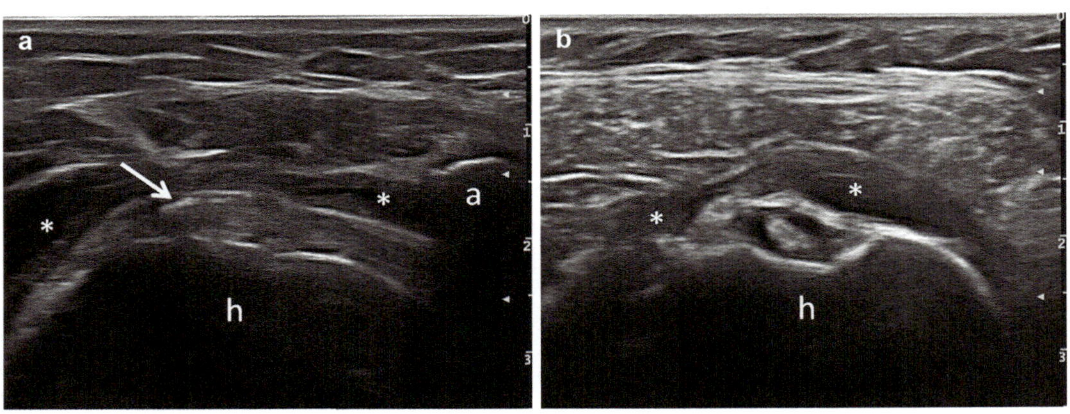

Fig. 10.10 (**a**) Calcific tendinopathy of the supraspinatus tendon and subdeltoid bursitis (*). (**b**) Transverse view at the bicipital groove shows subdeltoid bursitis and tenosynovitis of the long head of the biceps tendon. *h* humerus; *a* acromion

subdeltoid bursitis, and rotator cuff tendonitis are the most frequent (Fig. 10.10b). In tenosynovitis of the long head of the biceps tendon, the most characteristic US finding is distension of the tendon sheath. Subacromial-deltoid bursitis appears as an anechoic or hyperechoic, generally conspicuous, fluid collection that separates the bursal walls.

In lesions of the rotator cuff, US allows the identification of a wide range of structural changes: partial or complete tendon tear, supra- and/or infraspinatus tendon thinning, and BCP crystal deposits. Single or multiple calcifications can often be observed also in clinically asymptomatic patients.

All patients with acute "painful shoulder" must be examined using a comprehensive and standardized scanning protocol, given the possibility that there may be more than one pathologic condition within the same patient.

Finally, apart from reliably assessing calcific tendonitis, US allows for a real-time guidance of needle percutaneous treatment.

Further Readings

Barskova VG, Kudaeva FM, Bozhieva LA, Smirnov AV, Volkov AV, Nasonov EL. Comparison of three imaging techniques in diagnosis of chondrocalcinosis of the knees in calcium pyrophosphate deposition disease. Rheumatology. 2013;52:1090–4.

Chianca V, Albano D, Messina C, Midiri F, Mauri G, Aliprandi A, Catapano M, Pescatori LC, Monaco CG, Gitto S, Pisani Mainini A, Corazza A, Rapisarda S, Pozzi G, Barile A, Masciocchi C, Sconfienza LM. Rotator cuff calcific tendinopathy: from diagnosis to treatment. Acta Biomed. 2018;89(1-S):186–96.

Chowalloor PV, Keen HI. A systematic review of ultrasonography in gout and asymptomatic hyperuricaemia. Ann Rheum Dis. 2013;72:638–45.

Cipolletta E, Di Matteo A, Smerilli G, et al. Ultrasound findings of calcium pyrophosphate deposition disease at metacarpophalangeal joints [published online ahead of print, 2022 Feb 1]. Rheumatology (Oxford). 2022;keac063. https://doi.org/10.1093/rheumatology/keac063.

Cipolletta E, Di Battista J, Di Carlo M, et al. Sonographic estimation of monosodium urate burden predicts the fulfillment of the 2016 remission criteria for gout: a 12-month study. Arthritis Res Ther. 2021;23(1):185. Published 2021 Jul 9. https://doi.org/10.1186/s13075-021-02568-x.

Cipolletta E, Filippou G, Scirè CA, et al. The diagnostic value of conventional radiography and musculoskeletal ultrasonography in calcium pyrophosphate deposition disease: a systematic literature review and meta-analysis. Osteoarthritis Cartilage. 2021;29(5):619–32. https://doi.org/10.1016/j.joca.2021.01.007.

Cipolletta E, Smerilli G, Mashadi Mirza R, et al. Sonographic assessment of calcium pyrophosphate deposition disease at wrist. A focus on the dorsal scapholunate ligament. Joint Bone Spine. 2020;87(6):611–7. https://doi.org/10.1016/j.jbspin.2020.04.012.

Delle Sedie A, Riente L, Iagnocco A, Filippucci E, Meenagh G, Grassi W, et al. Imaging Ultrasound imaging for the rheumatologist X. Ultrasound imaging in crystal-related arthropathies. Clin Exp Rheumatol. 2007;25:513–7.

Di Matteo A, Filippucci E, Salaffi F, Carotti M, Carboni D, Di Donato E, et al. Diagnostic accuracy of musculoskeletal ultrasound and conventional radiography in the assessment of the wrist triangular fibrocartilage complex in patients with definite diagnosis of calcium pyrophosphate dihydrate deposition disease. Clin Exp Rheumatol. 2017;35:647–52.

Di Matteo A, Filippucci E, Cipolletta E, Ausili M, Martire V, Di Carlo M, et al. The popliteal groove region: a new target for the detection of monosodium urate crystal deposits in patients with gout. An ultrasound study. Joint Bone Spine. 2018; https://doi.org/10.1016/j.jbspin.2018.06.008.

Di Matteo A, Filippucci E, Cipolletta E, Musca A, Carotti M, Mashadi Mirza R, et al. Hip involvement in patients with calcium pyrophosphate deposition disease: potential and limits of musculoskeletal ultrasound. Arthritis Care Res (Hoboken). 2018; https://doi.org/10.1002/acr.23814.

Ellabban AS, Kamel SR, Omar HAA, El-Sherif AM, Abdel-Magied RA. Ultrasonographic findings of Achilles tendon and plantar fascia in patients with calcium pyrophosphate deposition disease. Clin Rheumatol. 2012;31:697–704.

Filippou G, Scanu A, Adinolfi A, et al. Criterion validity of ultrasound in the identification of calcium pyrophosphate crystal deposits at the knee: an OMERACT ultrasound study. Ann Rheum Dis. 2021;80(2):261–7. https://doi.org/10.1136/annrheumdis-2020-217998.

Filippou G, Filippucci E, Tardella M, Bertoldi I, Di Carlo M, Adinolfi A, et al. Extent and distribution of CPP deposits in patients affected by calcium pyrophosphate dihydrate deposition disease: an ultrasonographic study. Ann Rheum Dis. 2013;72:1836–9.

Filippou G, Adinolfi A, Cimmino MA, Scirè CA, Carta S, Lorenzini S, et al. Diagnostic accuracy of ultrasound, conventional radiography and synovial fluid analysis in the diagnosis of calcium pyrophosphate dihydrate crystal deposition disease. Clin Exp Rheumatol. 2016;34:254–60.

Filippou G, Scirè CA, Damjanov N, Adinolfi A, Carrara G, Picerno V, et al. Definition and reliability assessment of elementary ultrasonographic findings in calcium pyrophosphate deposition disease: a study by the OMERACT calcium pyrophosphate deposition disease ultrasound subtask force. J Rheumatol. 2017;44:1744–9.

Filippou G, Scirè CA, Adinolfi A, Damjanov NS, Carrara G, Bruyn GAW, et al. Identification of calcium pyrophosphate deposition disease (CPPD) by ultrasound: reliability of the OMERACT definitions in an extended set of joints—an international multiobserver study by the OMERACT Calcium Pyrophosphate Deposition Disease Ultrasound Su. Ann Rheum Dis. 2018;77:1194–9.

Filippucci E, Gutierrez M, Georgescu D, Salaffi F, Grassi W. Hyaline cartilage involvement in patients with gout and calcium pyrophosphate deposition disease. An ultrasound study. Osteoarthr Cartil. 2009;17:178–81.

Filippucci E, Scirè CA, Delle Sedie A, Iagnocco A, Riente L, Meenagh G, et al. Ultrasound imaging for the rheumatologist. XXV Sonographic assessment of the knee in patients with gout and calcium pyrophosphate deposition disease. Clin Exp Rheumatol. 2010;28:2–5.

Filippucci E, Di Geso L, Grassi W. Tips and tricks to recognize microcrystalline arthritis. Rheumatology. 2012;51:vii18–21.

Filippucci E, Delle Sedie A, Riente L, Di Geso L, Carli L, Ceccarelli F, Sakellariou G, Iagnocco A, Grassi W. Ultrasound imaging for the rheumatologist. XLVII. Ultrasound of the shoulder in patients with gout and calcium pyrophosphate deposition disease. Clin Exp Rheumatol. 2013;31(5):659–64.

Filippucci E, Di Geso L, Girolimetti R, Grassi W. Ultrasound in crystal-related arthritis. Clin Exp Rheumatol. 2014;32:S42–7.

Forien M, Combier A, Gardette A, Palazzo E, Dieudé P, Ottaviani S. Comparison of ultrasonography and radiography of the wrist for diagnosis of calcium pyrophosphate deposition. Joint Bone Spine. 2018;85:615–8.

Frediani B, Filippou G, Falsetti P, Lorenzini S, Baldi F, Acciai C, et al. Diagnosis of calcium pyrophosphate dihydrate crystal deposition disease: ultrasonographic criteria proposed. Ann Rheum Dis. 2005;64:638–40.

Grassi W, Meenagh G, Pascual E, Filippucci E. "Crystal Clear"—sonographic assessment of gout and calcium pyrophosphate deposition disease. Semin Arthritis Rheum. 2006;36:197–202.

Grassi W, Okano T, Di Geso L, Filippucci E. Imaging in rheumatoid arthritis: options, uses and optimization. Expert Rev. Clin Immunol. 2015;11:1131–46.

Gutierrez M, Di Geso L, Salaffi F, Carotti M, Girolimetti R, De Angelis R, et al. Ultrasound detection of cartilage calcification at knee level in calcium pyrophosphate deposition disease. Arthritis Care Res (Hoboken). 2014;66:69–73.

Lee KA, Lee SH, Kim HR. Diagnostic value of ultrasound in calcium pyrophosphate deposition disease of the knee joint. Osteoarthr Cartil. 2019;27:781–7.

Löffler C, Sattler H, Löffler U, et al. Size matters: observations regarding the sonographic double contour sign in different joint sizes in acute gouty arthritis. Z Rheumatol. 2018;77(9):815–23.

Louwerens JKG, Sierevelt IN, Kramer ET, Boonstra R, van den Bekerom MPJ, van Royen BJ, Eygendaal D, van Noort A. Comparing ultrasound-guided needling combined with a subacromial corticosteroid injection versus high-energy extracorporeal shockwave therapy for calcific tendinitis of the rotator cuff. A randomized controlled trial. Arthroscopy. 2020;36(7):1823–1833.e1.

Naredo E, Uson J, Jiménez-Palop M, Martínez A, Vicente E, Brito E, et al. Ultrasound-detected musculoskeletal urate crystal deposition: which joints and what findings should be assessed for diagnosing gout? Ann Rheum Dis. 2014;73:1522–8.

Ogdie A, Taylor WJ, Neogi T, Fransen J, Jansen TL, Schumacher HR, et al. Performance of ultrasound in the diagnosis of gout in a multicenter study: comparison with monosodium urate monohydrate crystal analysis as the gold standard. Arthritis Rheumatol. 2017;69:429–38.

Ottaviani S, Juge P-A, Aubrun A, Palazzo E, Dieude P. Sensitivity and reproducibility of ultrasonography in calcium pyrophosphate crystal deposition in knee cartilage: a cross-sectional study. J Rheumatol. 2015;42:1511–3.

Pascual E, Sivera F. Time required for disappearance of urate crystals from synovial fluid after successful hypouricaemic treatment relates to the duration of gout. Ann Rheum Dis. 2007;66:1056–8.

Peiteado D, De Miguel E, Villalba A, Ordóñez MC, Castillo C, Martín-Mola E, et al. Value of a short four-joint ultrasound test for gout diagnosis: a pilot study. Clin Exp Rheumatol. 2012;30:830–7.

Perez-Ruiz F, Calabozo M, Pijoan JI, Herrero-Beites AM, Ruibal A. Effect of urate-lowering therapy on the velocity of size reduction of tophi in chronic gout. Arthritis Rheum. 2002;47:356–60.

Perez-Ruiz F, Martin I, Canteli B. Ultrasonographic measurement of tophi as an outcome measure for chronic gout. J Rheumatol. 2007;34:1888–93.

Pineda C, Amezcua-Guerra LM, Solano C, Rodriguez-Henriquez P, Hernandez-Diaz C, Vargas A, et al. Joint and tendon subclinical involvement suggestive of gouty arthritis in asymptomatic hyperuricemia: an ultrasound controlled study. Arthritis Res Ther. 2011;13:R4.

Roddy E, Menon A, Hall A, Datta P, Packham J. Polyarticular sonographic assessment of gout: a hospital-based cross-sectional study. Joint Bone Spine. 2013;80:295–300.

Rosenthal AK. Basic calcium phosphate crystal-associated musculoskeletal syndromes: an update. Curr Opin Rheumatol. 2018;30(2):168–72.

Ruta S, Catay E, Marin J, Rosa J, García-Monaco R, Soriano ER. Knee effusion: ultrasound as a useful tool for the detection of calcium pyrophosphate crystals. Clin Rheumatol. 2016;35:1087–91.

Stewart S, Dalbeth N, Vandal AC, Allen B, Miranda R, Rome K. Ultrasound features of the first metatarsophalangeal joint in gout and asymptomatic hyperuricemia: comparison with normouricemic individuals. Arthritis Care Res. 2017;69:875–83.

Terslev L, Gutierrez M, Christensen R, Balint PV, Bruyn GA, Delle Sedie A, et al. Assessing elementary lesions in gout by ultrasound: Results of an OMERACT patient-based agreement and reliability exercise. J Rheumatol. 2015;42:2149–54.

Thiele RG, Schlesinger N. Ultrasonography shows disappearance of monosodium urate crystal deposition on hyaline cartilage after sustained normouricemia is achieved. Rheumatol Int. 2010;30:495–503.

Ventura-Ríos L, Sánchez-Bringas G, Pineda C, Hernández-Díaz C, Reginato A, Alva M, et al. Tendon involvement in patients with gout: an ultrasound study of prevalence. Clin Rheumatol. 2016;35:2039–44.

Wright SA, Filippucci E, McVeigh C, Grey A, McCarron M, Grassi W, et al. High-resolution ultrasonography of the first metatarsal phalangeal joint in gout: a controlled study. Ann Rheum Dis. 2007;66:859–64.

Zhang T, Duan Y, Chen J, Chen X. Efficacy of ultrasound-guided percutaneous lavage for rotator cuff calcific tendinopathy: a systematic review and meta-analysis. Medicine (Baltimore). 2019;98(21):e15552.

Zufferey P, Pascal Z, Valcov R, Fabreguet I, Dumusc A, Omoumi P, et al. A prospective evaluation of ultrasound as a diagnostic tool in acute microcrystalline arthritis. Arthritis Res Ther. 2015;17:188.

Connective Tissue Disorders

11

Marina Carotti, Emilio Filippucci, Fausto Salaffi, and Fabio Martino

Contents

11.1 Systemic Lupus Erythematosus

Joint involvement was long regarded as a minor clinical feature in systemic lupus erythematosus (SLE), although almost all patients refer musculoskeletal symptoms (i.e., arthralgias, which are usually transient and migratory) during the disease course. In a minority of patients, the presence of an arthritis may be documented (Fig. 11.1).

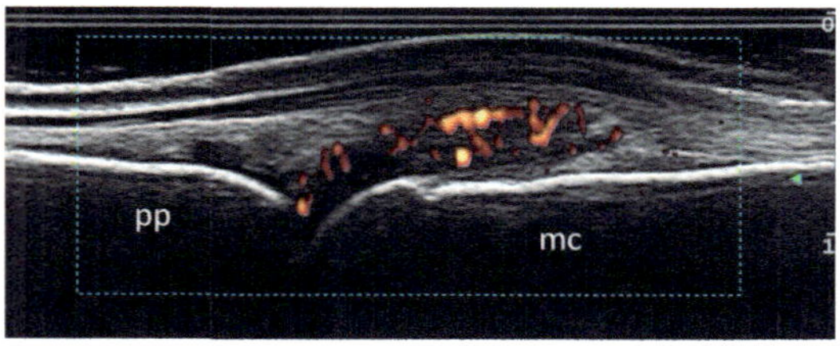

Fig. 11.1 Systemic lupus erythematosus. Dorsal longitudinal scan of a metacarpophalangeal joint showing "active" synovitis. *mc* metacarpal bone; *pp* proximal phalanx

Together with the joint disorders, the spectrum of musculoskeletal disease in SLE also includes tenosynovitis, tendon rupture, tendonitis, osteonecrosis, myositis, and fibromyalgia. Three main forms of SLE arthropathy based on the evidence and degree of deformities and the presence/absence of erosive damage were traditionally described: nondeforming and nonerosive arthritis, Jaccoud's arthropathy, and Rhupus syndrome.

Despite being promising, the use of ultrasound (US) in the assessment of musculoskeletal manifestations in patients with SLE is still limited. A wide heterogeneity of US pathologic findings in the joints and tendons of patients with SLE was

M. Carotti
Clinica di Radiologia, Dipartimento di Scienze Radiologiche – Azienda Ospedali Riuniti di Ancona Universita' Politecnica delle Marche, Ancona, Italy

E. Filippucci · F. Salaffi
Clinica Reumatologica, Dipartimento di Scienze Cliniche e Molecolari, Università Politecnica delle Marche, Jesi (Ancona), Italy

F. Martino (✉)
Radiology, Sant'Agata Diagnostic Center, Bari, Italy

F. Martino et al. (eds.), *Musculoskeletal Ultrasound in Orthopedic and Rheumatic disease in Adults*, https://doi.org/10.1007/978-3-030-91202-4_11

reported. Synovial effusion, synovial hypertrophy, "mixed" synovitis (coexistence of synovial effusion and synovial hypertrophy), joint dislocation, abnormal power Doppler signal, bone erosion, and cartilage damage were all reported in SLE.

Cartilage damage and bone erosions are more frequently detected in Rhupus syndrome, while joint dislocation is more common in Jaccoud's arthropathy. Besides the synovial targets, US also revealed inflammatory changes in non-synovial areas, such as tendons with no synovial sheath (peritendinous extensor tendon inflammation) and their entheses (patellar tendon insertion into the anterior tibial tuberosity).

11.2 Systemic Sclerosis

Very-high-frequency ultrasound (>20 MHz) offers a potential for quantitative assessment of skin thickness and skin echogenicity in patients with systemic sclerosis. The degree of skin involvement is a very important outcome measure in patients with systemic sclerosis. Although US is a promising technique there have been relatively few studies examining the use of dermal ultrasound in patients with systemic sclerosis. A significant correlation between US findings and Rodnan Skin Score was reported.

US findings in systemic sclerosis include soft tissue calcification and narrowing of the distance between phalangeal apex and skin surface at the distal phalanx.

In the musculoskeletal system, US was found more sensitive than clinical examination in the detection of synovitis and tenosynovitis at hand and foot level, and US synovitis of the hand was found to be associated with higher hand disability.

Finally, color and power Doppler techniques may play a valuable role in the assessment of blood perfusion, especially of the hand and foot extremities, and elastography has been described as effective in the assessment of affected tissue stiffness.

11.3 Salivary Gland Ultrasonography in Sjögren's Syndrome

Sjögren's syndrome is a systemic autoimmune disease primarily characterized by a focal chronic inflammation of glandular parenchyma, with chronic and persistent involvement of major salivary gland remaining a key element of the disease. In the last decade, advances in ultrasound technology and practice have resulted in a noninvasive method to investigate the major salivary gland in different diseases, including Sjögren's syndrome. Several studies published over the past 20 years reported a sensitivity of 80% and a specificity of more than 90% for the diagnosis of Sjögren's syndrome. Salivary gland ultrasonography is also of high value for the identification of patients prone to systemic disease complications, high disease activity, and lymphoma development. The useful combination of US gray scale and color/power Doppler technique provides more valuable details regarding the presence and the degree of soft tissue blood perfusion and may be valuable in narrowing the differential diagnosis.

The main echostructural abnormalities detectable on ultrasound are represented by the parenchymal inhomogeneity, hypoanechoic or hyperechoic areas (due to multiple cysts or calcifications, respectively), increased or reduced size, irregularity of the margins, and presence of peri-intraglandular lymph nodes (Fig. 11.2). As underlined by several authors, the most relevant sonographic sign in primary Sjögren's syndrome is the bilateral parenchymal inhomogeneity which is considered to be the most relevant anatomical structural change in these patients, with good agreement between salivary gland scintigraphy, sialography, and minor labial salivary gland biopsy. Ultrasound abnormalities are strongly correlated to the histological changes and the proposed ultrasound scoring system correlates well with sialographic gradings.

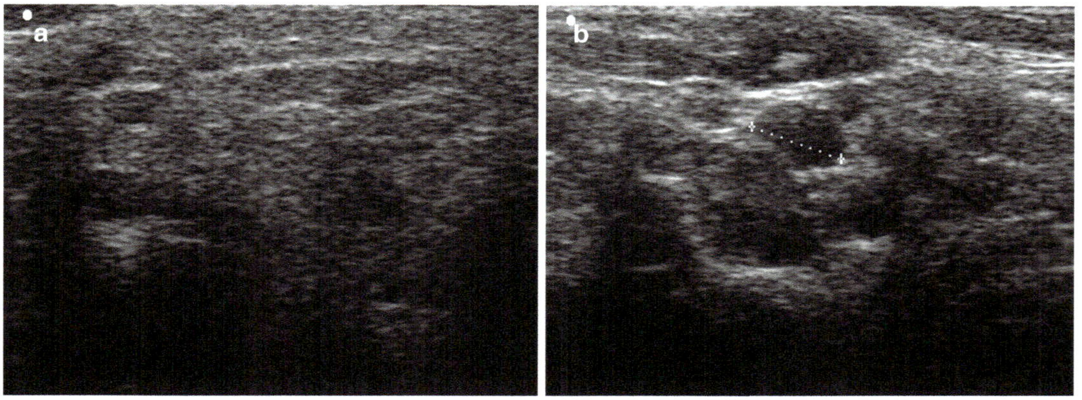

Fig. 11.2 (**a**) US longitudinal scan of parotid gland in a pSS patient. The parenchyma is completely heterogeneous with hypoechogenic areas and echogenic bands due to replacement of connective fibrous tissue. The borders of the glands are not well defined. (**b**) The parenchyma shows irregular contour, multiple large confluent hypoechogenic areas (with a maximal diameter >6 mm as indicated by calipers), and multiple cysts with echogenic bands, resulting in severe damage to the glandular architecture, decreased glandular volume, and posterior glandular border not well visible

At present, there are several different scoring systems suggested in the literature for the ultrasound assessment of major salivary glands in patients with Sjögren's syndrome. An echographic score, ranging from 0 to 16, was obtained from the sum of the scores (0–4) for each parotid and submandibular gland. The following ultrasound parameters were recorded: parenchymal homogeneity, echogenicity, size of the glands, and posterior glandular border. Each of these parameters was scored according to the previously described scoring system (Table 11.1). A sonographic pattern was considered abnormal if both parotids or both submandibular glands exhibited a minimum score of 1. According to this ultrasound scoring system grade 2 corresponds to a clear parenchymal inhomogeneity, characterized by multiple scattered hypoechogenic areas of variable size (<2 mm) and not uniformly distributed. Setting the cutoff ultrasound score >6 resulted in the best ratio of sensitivity (75.3%) to specificity (83.5%), with a likelihood ratio of 4.58.

Vitali C et al. suggested to include ultrasound as a complementary diagnostic tool in the American–European Consensus Group classifi-

Table 11.1 Ultrasound grading score proposed by Salaffi F et al.

Grade 0	Normal glands
Grade 1	Regular contour, small hypoechoic spots/areas, without echogenic bands, regular or increased glandular volume (mean values 20 + 3 mm for the parotids and 13 + 2 mm for the submandibular glands), and ill-defined posterior glandular border (definite echogenic border with respect to the neighboring structures)
Grade 2	Regular contour, evident multiple scattered hypoechogenic areas usually of variable size (<2 mm) and not uniformly distributed, without echogenic bands, regular or increased glandular volume, and ill-defined posterior glandular border
Grade 3	Irregular contour, multiple large circumscribed or confluent hypoechogenic areas (2–6 mm) and/or multiple cysts, with echogenic bands, regular or decreased glandular volume, and no visible posterior glandular border
Grade 4	Irregular contour, multiple large circumscribed or confluent hypoechogenic areas (>6 mm), and/or multiple cysts or multiple calcifications, with echogenic bands, resulting in severe damage to the glandular architecture, decreased glandular volume, and posterior glandular border not visible.

cation criteria for primary Sjögren's syndrome. Ultrasound contributes significantly to the performance of the criteria, because it is more widely available and cheaper than both sialography, which is an invasive and obsolete imaging procedure for major salivary gland investigation, and salivary scintigraphy, which has low specificity and limited availability and involves radiation exposure. However, for early detection of Sjögren's syndrome, however, and probably for follow-up monitoring within clinical trials and of lymphoma development, more advanced and elaborate scoring systems, including color/power Doppler assessments of vascularity, will be necessary.

11.4 Lung Ultrasound in Patients with Connective Tissue Disease

Interstitial lung disease (ILD) is a frequent manifestation of lung involvement in patients with systemic autoimmune disease. ILD mortality is increased in patients with rheumatoid arthritis (RA) and systemic lupus erythematosus, and in diffuse and limited systemic sclerosis lung involvement is the leading cause of death. Therefore, patients with CTD-ILD require aggressive and personalized treatment.

The role of pulmonary ultrasound in the evaluation of a variety of lung conditions has been widely reported in the literature. Recently, lung ultrasound validity in the evaluation of CTD-ILD has been investigated using high-resolution computed tomography (HRCT) as the contemporary "gold standard." In fact, HRCT provides a detailed morphological representation of even minimal lung involvement, even in patients without any alteration of lung volumes and the diffusion capacity of carbon monoxide. However, HRCT carries the risk of radiation exposure. Sonographic signs (Fig. 11.3) such as B-lines and pleural irregularities are suitable screening tools for the presence of ILD. B-lines consist of artifacts appearing as hyperechoic comet tails generated by the reflection of the US beam from thickened subpleural interlobar septa. B-lines are

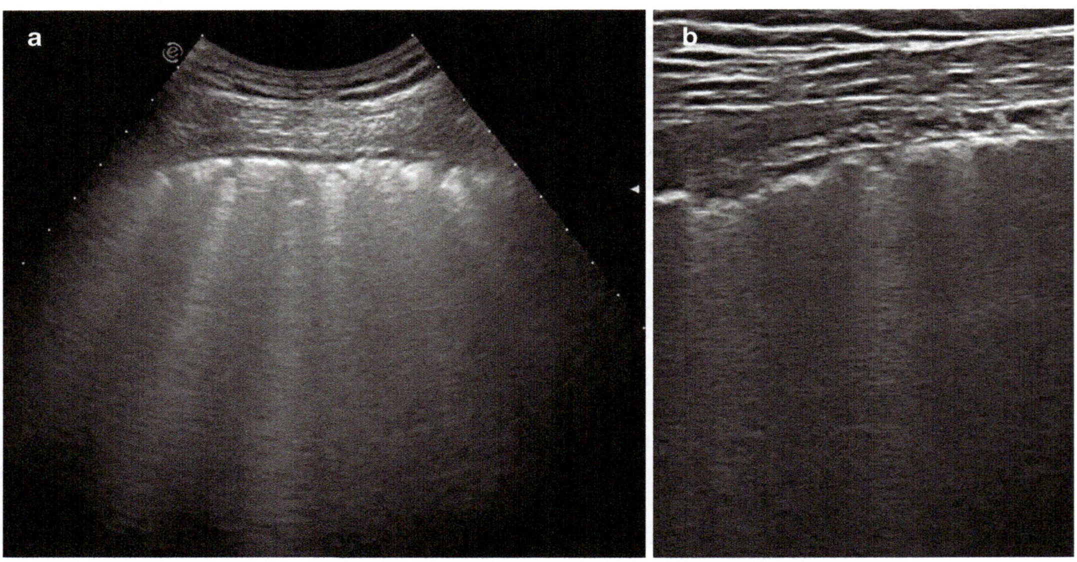

Fig. 11.3 Ultrasound (US) evaluation of a patient with interstitial lung disease and systemic sclerosis, showing pleural irregularities and B-lines at the level of the eighth intercostal space on the right subscapular line. (**a**) US scanning performed with a 2–7 MHz broadband convex transducer; (**b**) US scanning performed with a 4–13 MHz broadband linear transducer

a reliable instrument for assessing diffuse parenchymal lung disease, because their presence and number correlate with the HRCT extension of ILD, although the mechanisms for generating B-lines are not yet clear. A recent meta-analysis of published studies and a review of the literature revealed that lung ultrasound has high diagnostic accuracy, correlates well with HRCT results, and could be considered as the first lung imaging technique in subjects with suspected CTD-ILD. Therefore, in order to validate the use of lung ultrasound as a management tool for ILD in patients with rheumatic diseases, an OMERACT-LUS Sub-Task Force provided an overview of the potential role of lung ultrasound in the evaluation of ILD in patients with systemic sclerosis based on a review of the systemic literature. Current evidence and validation status are discussed, supporting their clinical relevance and usefulness in daily clinical practice. Lung ultrasound passed the filter of face, content validity, and feasibility. However, there is no evidence to support the criterion validity, reliability, and sensitivity to change.

Further Readings

Cannaò PM, Vinci V, Caviggioli F, Klinger M, Orlandi D, Sardanelli F, Serafini G, Sconfienza LM. Technical feasibility of real-time elastography to assess the perioral region in patients affected by systemic sclerosis. J Ultrasound. 2014;17(4):265–9.

Carotti M, Ciapetti A, Jousse-Joulin S, Salaffi F. Ultrasonography of the salivary glands: the role of grey-scale and colour/power Doppler. Clin Exp Rheumatol. 2014;32(1 Suppl 80):S61–7.

Carotti M, Salaffi F, Di Carlo M, Barile A, Giovagnoni A. Diagnostic value of major salivary gland ultrasonography in primary Sjögren's syndrome: the role of grey-scale and colour/power Doppler sonography. Gland Surg. 2019;8(Suppl 3):S159–67.

Di Geso L, Filippucci E, Girolimetti R, Tardella M, Gutierrez M, De Angelis R, Salaffi F, Grassi W. Reliability of ultrasound measurements of dermal thickness at digits in systemic sclerosis: role of elastosonography. Clin Exp Rheumatol. 2011;29(6):926–32.

Di Matteo A, Isidori M, Corradini D, Cipolletta E, McShane A, De Angelis R, Filippucci E, Grassi W. Ultrasound in the assessment of musculoskeletal involvement in systemic lupus erythematosus: state of the art and perspectives. Lupus. 2019;28(5):583–90.

Ferro F, Delle Sedie A. The use of ultrasound for assessing interstitial lung involvement in connective tissue diseases. Clin Exp Rheumatol. 2018;36 Suppl 114(5):165–70.

Gabba A, Piga M, Vacca A, Porru G, Garau P, Cauli A, Mathieu A. Joint and tendon involvement in systemic lupus erythematosus: an ultrasound study of hands and wrists in 108 patients. Rheumatology (Oxford). 2012;51(12):2278–85.

Gargani L, Doveri M, D'Errico L, Frassi F, Bazzichi ML, Delle Sedie A, Scali MC, Monti S, Mondillo S, Bombardieri S, Caramella D, Picano E. Ultrasound lung comets in systemic sclerosis: a chest sonography hallmark of pulmonary interstitial fibrosis. Rheumatology. 2009;48:1382–7.

Gutierrez M, Gomez-Quiroz LE, Clavijo-Cornejo D, Lozada CA, Lozada-Navarro AC, Labra RU, Fernandez-Torres J, Sanchez-Bringas G, Salaffi F, Bertolazzi C, Pineda C. Ultrasound in the interstitial pulmonary fibrosis. Can it facilitate a best routine assessment in rheumatic disorders? Clin Rheumatol. 2016;35(10):2387–95.

Gutierrez M, Soto-Fajardo C, Pineda C, Alfaro-Rodriguez A, Terslev L, Bruyn GA, Iagnocco A, Bertolazzi C, D'Agostino MA, Delle Sedie A. Ultrasound in the assessment of interstitial lung disease in systemic sclerosis. A systematic literature review by the OMERACT Ultrasound Group. J Rheumatol. 2019; https://doi.org/10.3899/jrheum.180940.

Han N, Tian X. Detection of subclinical synovial hypertrophy by musculoskeletal gray-scale/power Doppler ultrasonography in systemic lupus erythematosus patients: a cross-sectional study. Int J Rheum Dis. 2019;22(6):1058–69.

Hubac J, Gilson M, Gaudin P, Clay M, Imbert B, Carpentier P. Ultrasound prevalence of wrist, hand, ankle and foot synovitis and tenosynovitis in systemic sclerosis, and relationship with disease features and hand disability. Joint Bone Spine. 2020; https://doi.org/10.1016/j.jbspin.2020.01.011.

Jousse-Joulin S, Gatineau F, Baldini C, et al. Weight of salivary gland ultrasonography compared to other items of the 2016 ACR/EULAR classification criteria for Primary Sjögren's syndrome. J Intern Med. 2020;287(2):180–8.

Kaloudi O, Bandinelli F, Filippucci E, Conforti ML, Miniati I, Guiducci S, Porta F, Candelieri A, Conforti D, Grassiri G, Grassi W, Matucci-Cerinic M. High frequency ultrasound measurement of digital dermal thickness in systemic sclerosis. Ann Rheum Dis. 2010;69(6):1140–3.

Salaffi F, Argalia G, Carotti M, Giannini FB, Palombi C. Salivary gland ultrasonography in the evaluation of primary Sjogren's syndrome. Comparison with minor salivary gland biopsy. J Rheumatol. 2000;27:1229–36.

Salaffi F, Carotti M, Di Carlo M, Tardella M, Giovagnoni A. High-resolution computed tomography of the lung in patients with rheumatoid arthritis: Prevalence of interstitial lung disease involvement and determinants of abnormalities. Medicine (Baltimore). 2019;98(38):e17088.

Salaffi F, Carotti M, Iagnocco A, Luccioli F, Ramonda R, Sabatini E, De Nicola M, Maggi M, Priori R, Valesini G, Gerli R, Punzi L, Giuseppetti GM, Salvolini U, Grassi W. Ultrasonography of salivary glands in primary Sjögren's syndrome: a comparison with contrast sialography and scintigraphy. Rheumatology (Oxford). 2008;47(8):1244–9.

Salliot C, Denis A, Dernis E, et al. Ultrasonography and detection of subclinical joints and tendons involvements in Systemic Lupus erythematosus (SLE) patients: a cross-sectional multicenter study. Joint Bone Spine. 2018;85(6):741–5.

Santiago T, Santiago M, Ruaro B, Salvador MJ, Cutolo M, da Silva JAP. Ultrasonography for the assessment of skin in systemic sclerosis: a systematic review. Arthritis Care Res (Hoboken). 2019;71(4):563–74.

Schmidt WA, Krause A, Schicke B, Wernicke D. Color Doppler ultrasonography of hand and finger arteries to differentiate primary from secondary forms of Raynaud's phenomenon. J Rheumatol. 2008;35(8):1591–8. Epub 2008 Jul 15

Tani C, Carli L, Stagnaro C, Elefante E, Signorini V, Balestri F, Delle Sedie A, Mosca M. Imaging of joints in systemic lupus erythematosus. Clin Exp Rheumatol. 2018;36 Suppl 114(5):68–73.

Tardella M, Di Carlo M, Carotti M, Filippucci E, Grassi W, Salaffi F. Ultrasound B-lines in the evaluation of interstitial lung disease in patients with systemic sclerosis: cut-off point definition for the presence of significant pulmonary fibrosis. Medicine (Baltimore). 2018;97(18):e0566.

Vitali C, Carotti M, Salaffi F. Is it the time to adopt salivary gland ultrasonography as an alternative diagnostic tool for the classification of patients with Sjögren's syndrome? Comment on the article by Cornec et al. Arthritis Rheum. 2013;65:1950.

Metabolic Diseases

12

Marina Carotti, Emilio Filippucci, Fausto Salaffi, and Fabio Martino

Contents

12.1 Metabolic Diseases

Tendon involvement is a prominent feature in patients with metabolic syndrome. US has shown to be a useful imaging technique in establishing the diagnosis of heterozygous familial hypercholesterolemia in subjects with high levels of cholesterol and with no clinically evident xanthomata. The typical sonographic appearance of chronic tendinopathy is characterized by heterogeneous echotexture, loss of the normal fibrillar pattern, blurring of the tendon margins, and increased tendon size. In Achilles tendon, these abnormalities are usually located in the central third of tendon.

Detection of loss of the normal fibrillar structure and/or hypo-anechoic areas may be an important finding indicative of low mechanical tendon resistance. Lack of homogeneity of tendon structure may range from focal aspects of fibrillar interruption to diffuse blurring of the tendon texture.

Enthesophytes and/or calcification are frequent US pathological findings at the tendon insertions of patients with metabolic diseases (Fig. 12.1). Conversely, bone erosions and abnormal vascularization (i.e., intra-tendinous power Doppler signal) are more frequently detected at entheseal level in patients with seronegative spondyloarthropathy.

M. Carotti
Clinica di Radiologia, Dipartimento di Scienze Radiologiche – Azienda Ospedali Riuniti di Ancona Universita' Politecnica delle Marche, Ancona, Italy

E. Filippucci · F. Salaffi
Clinica Reumatologica, Dipartimento di Scienze Cliniche e Molecolari, Università Politecnica delle Marche, Jesi (Ancona), Italy

F. Martino (✉)
Radiology, Sant'Agata Diagnostic Center, Bari, Italy

F. Martino et al. (eds.), *Musculoskeletal Ultrasound in Orthopedic and Rheumatic disease in Adults*, https://doi.org/10.1007/978-3-030-91202-4_12

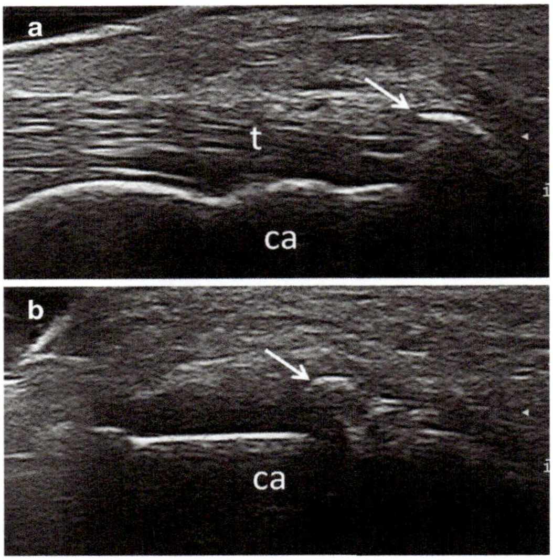

Fig. 12.1 Chronic enthesopathy of the Achilles tendon (**t**) insertion into the posterior calcaneal tuberosity. Longitudinal (**a**) and transverse (**b**) scans showing enthesophytes (**arrows**) generating an acoustic shadow. *ca* calcaneal bone

Further Readings

Bude RO, Nesbitt SD, Adler RS, Rubenfire M. Sonographic detection of xanthomas in normal-sized Achilles' tendons of individuals with heterozygous familial hypercholesterolemia. AJR. 1998;170:621–5.

Dagistan E, Canan A, Kizildag B, Barut AY. Multiple tendon xanthomas in patient with heterozygous familial hypercholesterolaemia: sonographic and MRI findings. BMJ Case Rep. 2013;2013:bcr2013200755.

Okur SC, Dogan YP, Mert M, Aksu O, Burnaz O, Caglar NS. Ultrasonographic evaluation of lower extremity entheseal sites in diabetic patients using Glasgow ultrasound enthesitis scoring system score. J Med Ultrasound. 2017;25(3):150–6.

Sakellariou G, Iagnocco A, Delle Sedie A, Riente L, Filippucci E, Montecucco C. Ultrasonographic evaluation of entheses in patients with spondyloarthritis: a systematic literature review. Clin Exp Rheumatol. 2014;32(6):969–78.

Terslev L, Naredo E, Iagnocco A, Balint PV, Wakefield RJ, Aegerter P, Aydin SZ, Bachta A, Hammer HB, Bruyn GA, Filippucci E, Gandjbakhch F, Mandl P, Pineda C, Schmidt WA, D'Agostino MA. Outcome measures in rheumatology ultrasound task force. defining enthesitis in spondyloarthritis by ultrasound: results of a Delphi process and of a reliability reading exercise. Arthritis Care Res (Hoboken). 2014;66(5):741–8.

Ursini F, Arturi F, D'Angelo S, Amara L, Nicolosi K, Russo E, Naty S, Bruno C, De Sarro G, Olivieri I, Grembiale RD. High prevalence of Achilles tendon enthesopathic changes in patients with type 2 diabetes without peripheral neuropathy. J Am Podiatr Med Assoc. 2017;107(2):99–105.

Synovial Osteochondromatosis

13

Alessandro Muda and Fabio Martino

Contents

13.1 Introduction

Synovial osteochondromatosis is a benign condition characterized by proliferation of synovial membrane, in which there is metaplasia of the synovial lining of a joint into cartilaginous or osteocartilaginous nodules. In more rare cases, an extra-articular form of the condition can be identified, in which lesions are found in bursal tissue and/or in tendon sheath.

There are two forms: primary (also referred to as Reichel syndrome) and secondary synovial chondromatosis. The primary form is uncommon, has unknown etiology, and is usually monoarticular, although rare cases of multiple joint involvements occur. Any joint may be affected, and the knee is the most commonly involved site (65%), followed by the hip (20%) and elbow. It preferentially occurs in between the third and fifth decades of life, with men affected two to four times more frequently than women. The secondary form is more common than primary and is believed to be due to or associated with joint abnormalities, such as mechanical or arthritic conditions that cause intra-articular chondral bodies.

Based on histopathology, synovial chondromatosis is classified into three stages: Stage 1 shows active chondroid metaplasia of synovium without intra-articular chondroid nodules. Stage 2 represents both intrasynovial chondroid metaplasia and intra-articular chondral nodules. Stage 3 documents the presence of intra-articular chondroid nodules, but no active synovial based disease. Later on, chondroid nodules spread and finally become calcified. Detachment of some calcified bodies embedded in the synovium gives rise to intra-articular loose bodies that are quite uniform in size and shape, which may eventually occupy the whole joint space. These nodules, nourished by synovial fluid, grow and most of them progressing to ossification. It should be pointed out that there is no correlation between these stages and duration of clinical symptoms or patient age.

A. Muda
Department of Radiology, IRCCS Policlinico San Martino-IST, Genova, Italy

F. Martino (✉)
Radiology, Sant'Agata Diagnostic Center, Bari, Italy

F. Martino et al. (eds.), *Musculoskeletal Ultrasound in Orthopedic and Rheumatic disease in Adults*, https://doi.org/10.1007/978-3-030-91202-4_13

At the beginning, the affected joints do not appear inflamed; however, joint effusion may be occasionally present. Symptoms are insidious and slowly progressive; they often include chronic joint pain, swelling, tenderness, and limitation of joint motility. The condition progresses slowly and can lead to secondary erosive and arthritic degenerative changes of joint bones. The disease may recur and malignant transformation has rarely been reported. Nevertheless, only few cases of true malignant transformation in chondrosarcomas have been described in literature.

13.2 Diagnostic Imaging

Conventional radiology usually represents the first-line imaging exam in the diagnostic suspicion of synovial osteochondrosis. In general, radiographic results are pathognomonic of synovial osteochondromatosis and vary in relation to the form (primary or secondary) and the evolutive stage of the diseases. Generally, the calcifications are ring-shaped; sometimes they have a calcified central focus and ring-shaped peripheral calcification, or a target sign with a radiolucent center and calcified periphery. In the case of secondary disease, signs of degenerative joint disease may be present. In case of suspected joint effusion sonography is usually the first-line examination technique and in such cases can detect also the presence of a mass-like process corresponding to chondroid nodule aggregate (Fig. 13.1).

The ultrasound appearance of synovial osteochondromatosis is characterized by numerous echogenic foci, representing the fronds of the growing process, and the synovium may be thickened; most of these are associated with distal acoustic shadowing, corresponding to the conglomeration of calcified chondroid islands. On ultrasound, the uncalcified component of the mass is hypoechoic and avascular. Calcifications are very commonly seen and when extensive will be the prominent feature visible on ultrasound.

Therefore, ultrasound can suggest the presence of synovial osteochondromatosis, but is not definitively diagnostic, and conventional radiography is usually required to confirm the suspected diagnosis. If loose bodies are present, they are visible as small echogenic lobules of cartilage, with possible posterior acoustic shadowing, free-floating in the effusion within the articular space. Extensive mineralization may hide lobular contours of chondral bodies.

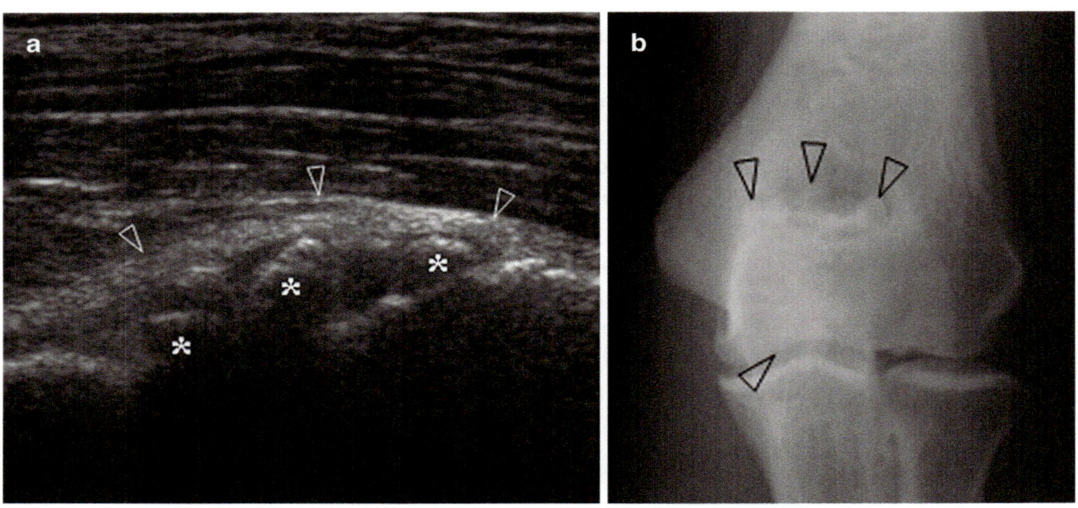

Fig. 13.1 Synovial osteochondromatosis of the elbow. (**a**) Longitudinal US scan of the volar aspect of the elbow showing bulge and thickening of the capsular profile (empty white arrowheads). Multiple echogenic foci with posterior acoustic shadowing (*) lining synovial profile are evident. (**b**) Frontal radiograph in same patient showing several rounded opacities (empty black arrowheads), corresponding to calcified chondroid islands

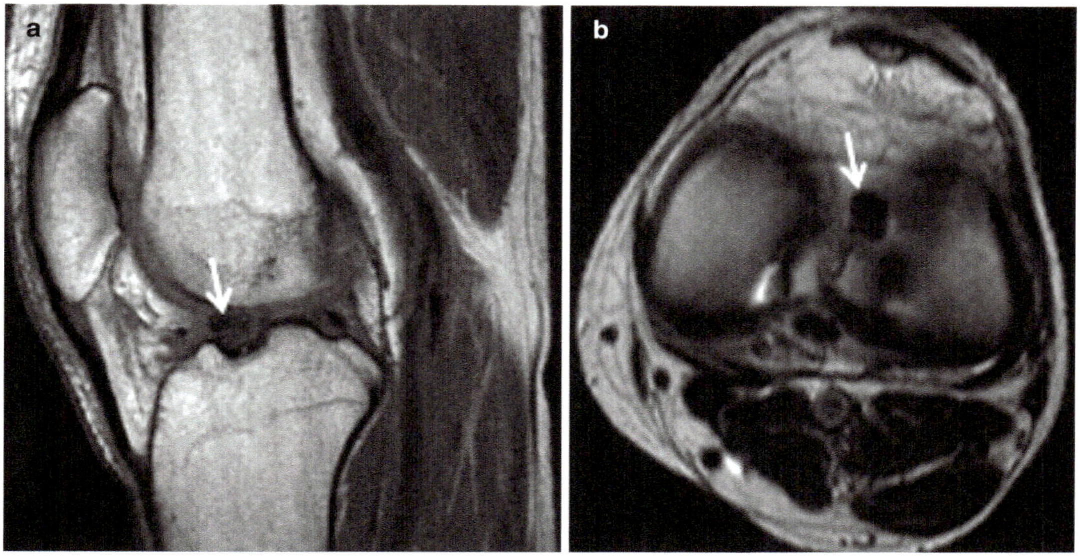

Fig. 13.2 MRI of the knee in patient with osteochondral nodule (arrows): (**a**) sagittal T1-weighted image; (**b**) axial T2-weighted image

Changing position during the examination can be helpful to reveal loose bodies and determine if they are indeed loose by assessing their possibility of free movement.

Color and power Doppler technique reveals no vascularity within the loose bodies and this feature may be useful to guide the examiner in the differential diagnosis.

MRI is sometimes required, particularly when the lesion is arising from a joint. MRI can be useful in identifying osteochondromatosis nodules, which if calcified have low signal in the T1 and T2 sequences weighted (Fig. 13.2).

Further Readings

Campeau NG, Lewis BD. Ultrasound appearance of synovial osteochondromatosis of the shoulder. Mayo Clin Proc. 1998;73:1079–81.

Fuerst M, Zustin J, Lohmann C, Rüther W. Synoviale chondromatose. Der Orthopäde. 2009;38(6):511–9.

Gille J, Krueger S, Aberle J, Boehm S, Ince A, Loehr JF. Synovial chondromatosis of the hip: a case report and clinicopathologic study. Acta Orthop Belg. 2004;70:182–8.

Kumar DS, Ethiraj D, Indiran V, Maduraimuthu P. Bilateral shoulder synovial chondromatosis: Multimodality imaging. Indian J Rheumatol. 2019;14:161–2.

Maghear L, Serban O, Papp I, Otel O, Manole S, Botan E, Fodor D. Multimodal ultrasonographic evaluation in a case with unossified primary synovial osteochondromatosis. Med Ultrasonogr. 2018;20(4):527–30.

Martino F, Silvestri E, Grassi W, Garlaschi G. Musculoskeletal sonography. New York: Springer; 2006.

McKenzie G, Raby N, Ritchie D. A pictorial review of primary synovial osteochondromatosis. EurRadiol. 2008;18:2662–9.

Murphey MD, Vidal JA, Fanburg-Smith JC, Gajewski DA. Imaging of synovial chondromatosis with radiologic-pathologic correlation. Radiographics. 2007;27(5):1465–88.

Roberts D, Miller TT, Erlanger SM. Sonographic appearance of primary synovial chondromatosis of the knee. J Ultrasound Med. 2004;23:707–9.

Terazaki CRT, Trippia CR, Trippia CH, Caboclo MFSF, Medaglia CRM. Synovial chondromatosis of the shoulder: imaging findings. Radiol Bras. 2014;47(1):38–42.

Pigmented Villonodular Synovitis

14

Alessandro Muda and Fabio Martino

Contents

14.1 Introduction

Pigmented villonodular synovitis (PVNS) is a slow-growing synovial proliferative disorder, which is locally invasive similar to a tumor and usually involves a single joint, tendon sheath, or bursa. It is a rare benign condition that primarily affects young adults. Patients are usually between the second and fourth decades of life, and both sexes are equally affected. Although the recurrence is high, malignant transformation is considered rare. The etiology is unknown but it is thought to be related to trauma, intra-articular hemorrhage, and recurrent inflammation; some cytogenetic abnormalities also seem to be implicated.

There are two forms of PVNS: (1) localized, that is, predominantly nodular, and (2) diffuse, that is, mostly villous.

Localized PVNS can be intra-articular, when it occurs in a restricted area of the joint, and grows inside the joint cavity as a nodular mass, or it can be extra-articular when it involves a bursa or a tendon sheath (termed "giant cell tumor of the tendon sheath"—GCTTS), which appears as nodular tenosynovitis nearly always related to the fingers or thumb. The localized (or nodular) intra-articular form is usually monoarticular and most commonly affects knee (up to 80% of cases), hip, and ankle. The localized PVNS (intra- or extra-articular form) usually responds well to treatment.

Diffuse PVNS is so called when the condition is more widespread and involves an entire joint. It is characterized by a diffused thickening of the synovium with coarse villi, finer fronds, and diffuse nodularity. It also tends to be more destructive and more difficult to treat.

The initial clinical presentation of intra-articular form is typically a monoarticular joint effusion with no history of trauma or inciting event. Aspiration of synovial fluid will lead to hemarthrosis in more than 60% of patients. They usually have mild discomfort and stiffness in the affected joint. Thereafter, painless or painful local swelling of chronic duration becomes the typical clinical pattern.

A. Muda
Department of Radiology, IRCCS Policlinico San Martino-IST, Genova, Italy

F. Martino (✉)
Radiology, Sant'Agata Diagnostic Center, Bari, Italy

F. Martino et al. (eds.), *Musculoskeletal Ultrasound in Orthopedic and Rheumatic disease in Adults*,
https://doi.org/10.1007/978-3-030-91202-4_14

Once the PVNS is confirmed by biopsy, the main and most effective treatment is complete surgical synovectomy. Since diffuse PVNS has a relatively high recurrence rate, radiation therapy or chemotherapy can be considered a treatment option.

Later on, the hypertrophic synovium and inflammation may damage the bone cortex producing erosions and cystic degeneration that can be evaluated by MRI, as well as by X-ray (Fig. 14.2) or sonography.

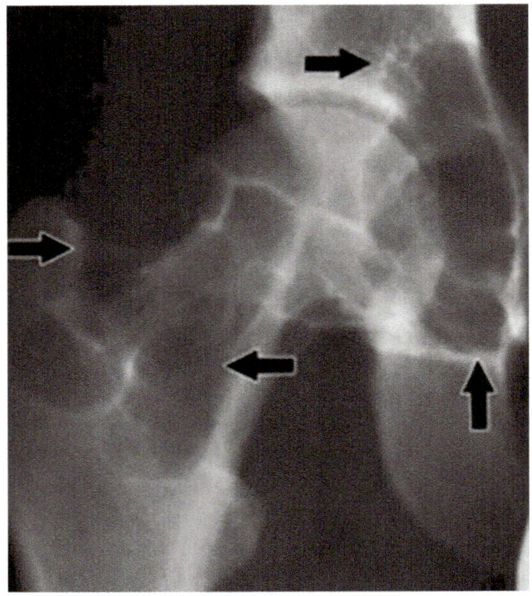

Fig. 14.2 Diffuse intra-articular PVNS of the hip with hip pain. Frontal X-ray shows extensive erosion of the femoral neck and acetabulum with sclerotic margins (arrows) and maintained hip joint space

14.2 Diagnostic Imaging

The histological composition of the PVNS is also relevant for diagnostic imaging. Indeed, histology reveals a state of chronic inflammation characterized by the presence of large amounts of mononuclear cells with hemosiderin deposits and multinucleated giant cells. Chronic inflammation increases the possibility of intra-articular bleeding, thereby providing more iron available for the PVNS tissue, which in turn probably constitutes an additional stimulus for mononuclear cells and fibroblasts, creating a vicious circle. So, the heavy deposition of hemosiderin inside the villous tissue and nodules enhances the diagnostic value of MRI, especially T2-weighted images, due to the "blooming" effect of hemosiderin deposits that return low signal intensity on all sequences. Therefore, MRI is considered the most appropriate investigation because it permits, in most cases, a wider identification of the full extent of the disease (Fig. 14.1).

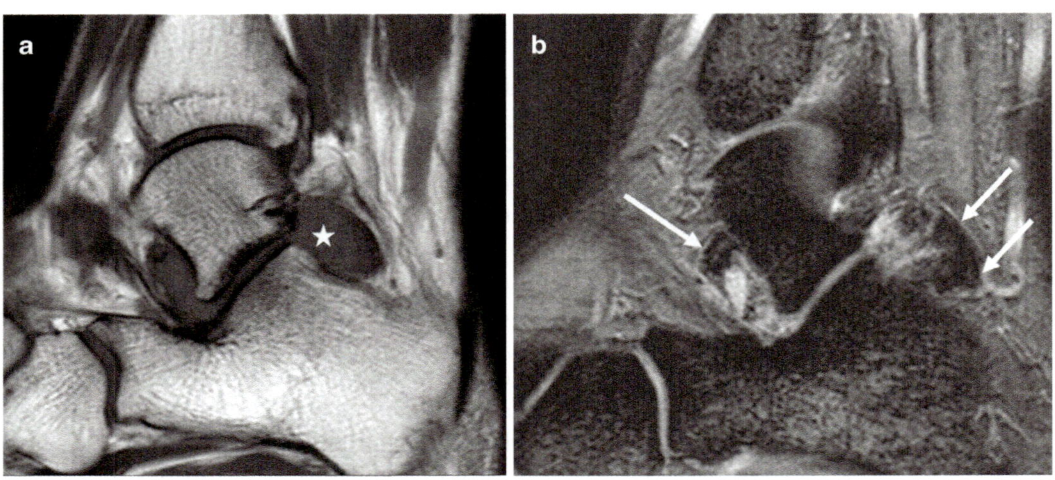

Fig. 14.1 (**a**) Sagittal T1-weighted image without gadolinium shows an intra-articular hypointense mass (white star) in the subtalar joint; (**b**) in sagittal gradient echo T2-weighted images, hemosiderin deposition appears more visible because of the blooming effect due to the magnetic susceptibility (white arrows)

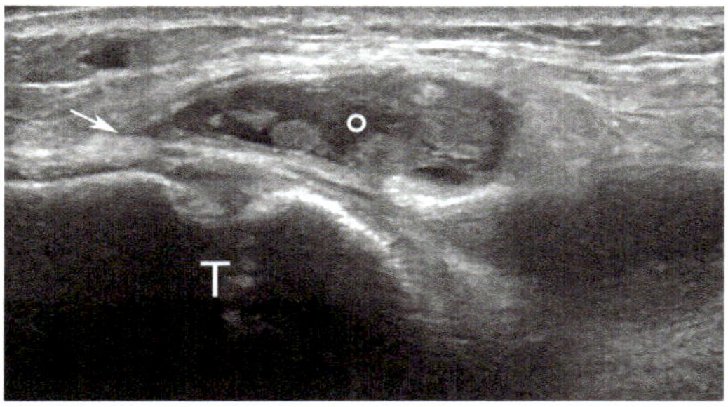

Fig. 14.3 Ultrasound examination of the medial side of the knee shows a cystic image (circles) with echoes inside emerging extra-articular from the pes anserine bursa (arrow). *T* tibia

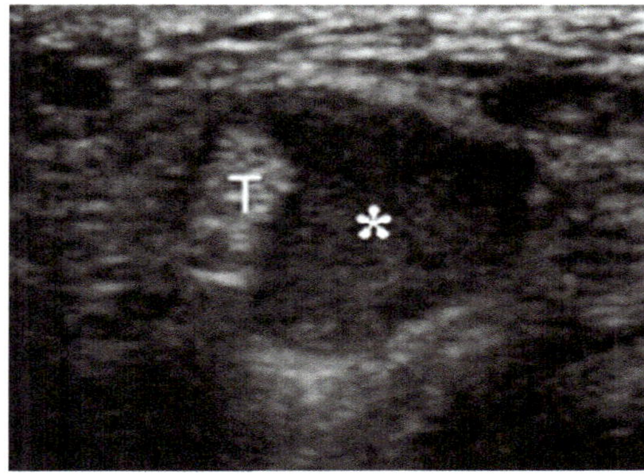

Fig. 14.4 Giant-cell tumor of the hand. Transverse US scan of the palmar surface of the finger demonstrates a solid, relatively homogeneous hypoechoic mass (*), filling the tendon sheath. Tendons (T) are peripherally dislocated

The ultrasound pattern in PVNS is nonspecific but it is helpful to understand if the mass is fluid or solid. It usually appears as hypoechoic hypertrophic synovium, with a widespread villous thickening or with a nodular aspect, corresponding to diffuse and localized type, respectively, with or without joint effusion (Fig. 14.3a, b).

Color and power Doppler ultrasound technique shows increased flow signals with a high degree of vessels in the mass. A pattern of increased flow may also be detected in the peripheral zone of the synovial capsule. Tenosynovial involvement by a giant-cell tumor most commonly appears as a single hypoechoic homogenous nodule, which tends to encircle and dislocate the affected tendon (Fig. 14.4).

Despite the fact that involvement of surrounding tissues is often extensive, when the tendon slides the mass does not move with it.

Ultrasound can detect blood-stained effusions both in the joint and in the tendon sheath, which might contain hemosiderin deposits in case of past bleedings.

Further Readings

Bianchi S, Mazzola CG, Martinoli C, Damiani S, Derchi LE. Quiz case of the month. Eur Radiol. 1998;8(7):1275.

Bianchi S, Martinoli C. Ultrasound of the musculoskeletal system. 1st ed. Berlin: Springer; 2007.

Bravo SM, Winalski CS, Weissman BN. Pigmented villonodular synovitis. Radiol Clin N Am. 1996;34:311–26.

Fałek A, Niemunis-Sawicka J, Wrona K, et al. Pigmented villonodular synovitis. Folia Med Cracov. 2018;58(4):93–104.

Martino F, Silvestri E, Grassi W, Garlaschi G. Musculoskeletal sonography. New York: Springer; 2006.

Murphey MD, Rhee JH, Lewis RB, Fanburg-Smith JC, Flemming DJ, Walker EA. Pigmented Villonodular synovitis: radiologic-pathologic correlation. Radiographics. 2008;28:1493–518.

Schvartzman P, Carrozza PV, Pascual T, Mazza L, Odesser M, San Román JL. Radiological features of pigmented villonodular synovitis and giant cell tumor of the tendon sheath. Rev Argent Radiol. 2015;79(1):4–11.

Yang PY, Wang CL, Wu CT, et al. Sonography of pigmented villonodular synovitis in the ankle joint. J Clin Ultrasound. 1998;26:166–70.

Shoulder Calcific Tendinopathy 15

Gianluigi Martino, Enzo Silvestri,
Davide Orlandi, Alessandro Muda,
and Fabio Martino

Contents

15.1 Introduction

Calcific tendinitis of the shoulder is a relatively common, painful disease, estimated to occur in 2.5–7.5% of adults. Although more common in the right shoulder, at least a 10–25% incidence of bilaterality has been reported.

G. Martino
Institute of Radiology, University of Bari, Bari, Italy

E. Silvestri
Radiology, Alliance Medical, Genova, Italy

D. Orlandi
Department of Radiology, Ospedale Evangelico Internazionale, Genova, Italy

A. Muda
Department of Radiology, IRCCS Policlinico San Martino-IST, Genova, Italy

F. Martino (✉)
Radiology, Sant'Agata Diagnostic Center, Bari, Italy

It predominantly affects individuals aged between 40 and 60 years, and 57–76.7% of patients are women. Calcific tendinitis is characterized by the presence of calcium salt deposits, primarily hydroxyapatite, in the substance of the rotator cuff tendons. Most calcification occurs in the supraspinatus tendon. Calcification is observed with decreasing frequency in the infraspinatus, teres minor, and subscapularis tendons. More than one tendon may be involved.

The calcific deposit usually is described as being approximately 1–2 cm proximal to the tendon insertion on the greater tuberosity. Calcifying tendinitis may be an incidental finding in 7.5–20% of asymptomatic adults, or it may be the cause of shoulder pain. Symptomatic patients usually present with impingement-type pain in the affected shoulder during overhead activity. Active and passive range of motion is painful and restricted. The pain may seem to be out of proportion to any objective physical findings. The patient may describe difficulty sleeping on the shoulder and trouble falling asleep. Symptoms may last for a

F. Martino et al. (eds.), *Musculoskeletal Ultrasound in Orthopedic and Rheumatic disease in Adults*,
https://doi.org/10.1007/978-3-030-91202-4_15

few weeks or a few months. The cause of calcifying tendinitis is not known. It is generally agreed that it is not caused by trauma, and it rarely is part of a systemic disease. The pathophysiology of calcifying tendinitis is controversial, and has been attributed to cell-mediated calcification and subsequent spontaneous phagocytic resorption.

Based on the pathogenesis of histic hypoxia, the hypoxic state produces a lack of irrigation of the "critical area" near the insertion of the tendon and induces calcified deposits. It is a self-limited process in which the calcifications tend to resolve after a period of worsening and intense pain. Therefore, many cases may resolve spontaneously and require no special treatment. Thus, it is a dynamic process (Fig. 15.1) that evolves through three distinct stages of the disease process: the **precalcific stage**, characterized by the asymptomatic change of the tenocytes into chondrocytes, and then fibrocartilage; the **calcific stage**, which is subdivided into three phases—*formation*, *resting*, and *resorption*; and the **postcalcific stage**, characterized by an attempt by the tendon to self-heal. The formation phase of calcific stage is characterized by deposition of amorphous calcium phosphate, and can be relatively painless. This phase is followed by the resting phase, which tends to be quiescent and may last for months to years. The resorptive phase of calcific stage tends to be painful, as calcium crystals are resorbed, inducing regional neoangiogenesis, beginning at the margin of the calcium deposit, and infiltration of phagocytes. The postcalcific stage, which can be painless, is characterized by the collagenization of the lesion by fibroblasts.

15.2 Imaging of Calcifying Tendinitis

The first-line imaging modalities are X-ray and ultrasound, as calcium deposits are readily identifiable on both. The evaluation of calcific tendinitis is based mainly on radiography. It is cost effective and useful, not only for determining the presence of calcium deposits but also for assessing their size, delineation, and density. Standard radiographic evaluation of the shoulder should include internal and external rotation anteroposterior views to help visualize calcific deposits and their relationship to

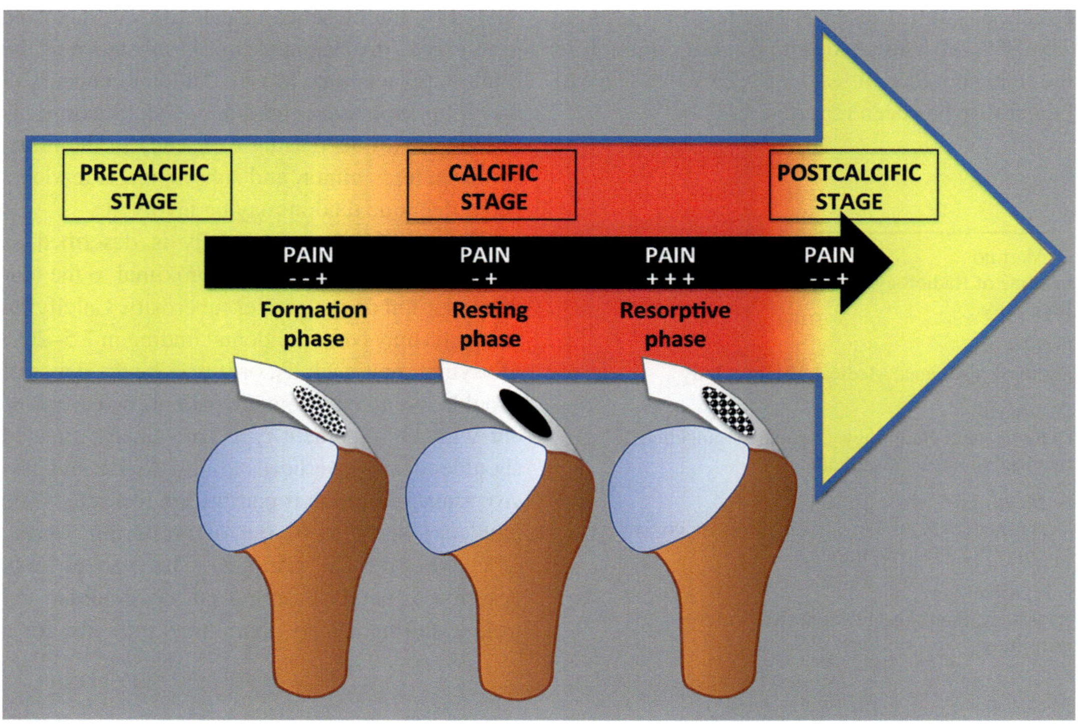

Fig. 15.1 Clinic and pathologic evolution scheme of calcific shoulder tendinitis, in accord with Uhthoff stages

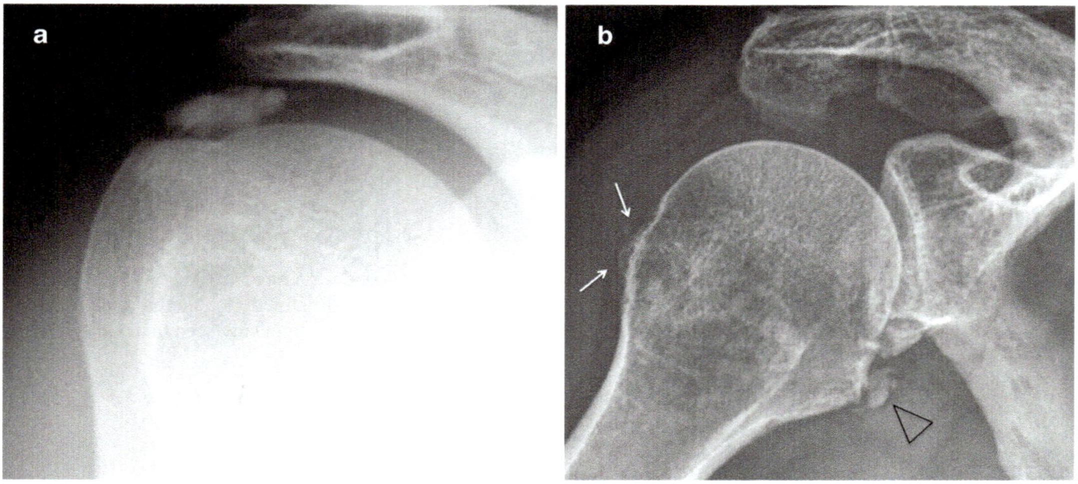

Fig. 15.2 Shoulder calcific tendinitis radiograph. (**a**) Shoulder externally rotated X-ray showing supraspinatus calcific tendinitis; (**b**) subscapularis calcific tendinitis (arrowhead), with the shoulder internally rotated; also evident are subtle enthesophytic spurs of infraspinatus tendon (arrows)

landmarks on the humeral head. External rotation consent to visualize the calcific tendinitis in the supraspinatus tendon profiles the greater tuberosity (Fig. 15.2a). Internal rotation of the humerus profiles the posterior aspect of the head on the lateral aspect of the radiograph and the anterior head medially. Calcification in the infraspinatus tendon profiles posteriorly on internal rotation (Fig. 15.2b). Calcification in the subscapularis profiles anteriorly on internal rotation (Fig. 15.2b). The regions most affected by calcific tendinitis are the critical zone of the supraspinatus tendon (80%), the lower side of the infraspinatus tendon (15%), and the pre-insertional part of the subscapularis tendon (5%).

The radiographic appearance of calcific tendinitis is as homogeneous, amorphous densities without trabeculation, which allows for differentiation from enthesopathic spurs or accessory ossicles. Most calcifications are ovoid, and margins may be smooth or ill-defined. Characterizing the shape and contour of the calcific deposit is important to classify the pathology, in order to determine the best possible treatment for the patient. It is important to be able to reliably predict the consistency of the deposit and hereby the stage of the disease by characterizing the radiological image in one of the classification systems in clinical use at present. Several radiological classifications have been proposed, based on the size or morphology, although none of them guarantee sufficient reliability and reproducibility, or reliable correlation with the radiologic picture and clinical symptoms. Gärtner and Heyer proposed a radiographic classification based on the morphological appearance of the calcification, identifying three types (Fig. 15.3a–c): (I) sharply defined and dense, (II) ill-defined/dense or sharply defined/inhomogeneous-less radiodense, and (III) translucent and cloudy appearance with vague border.

Calcifications with a well-defined, homogeneous contour are less likely to be symptomatic and may correlate with the formative or resting phase. Deposits with fluffy, hazy, ill-defined edges are often seen in patients with acute pain and may correlate with the resorptive phase of calcific tendinitis. Ultrasound is useful in both detection of rotator cuff calcium deposits and therapeutic procedures, and is also beneficial in pre- and postoperative evaluation. Its diagnostic accuracy has been reported to be similar to that of magnetic resonance imaging. Calcific plaque morphology and increased flow on power Doppler were the most useful ultrasound findings. Ultrasonography could also detect associated conditions such as rotator cuff tears, subacromial–subdeltoid bursitis, and long head of the biceps pathology and allows us to perform a dynamic evaluation to assess the subacromial

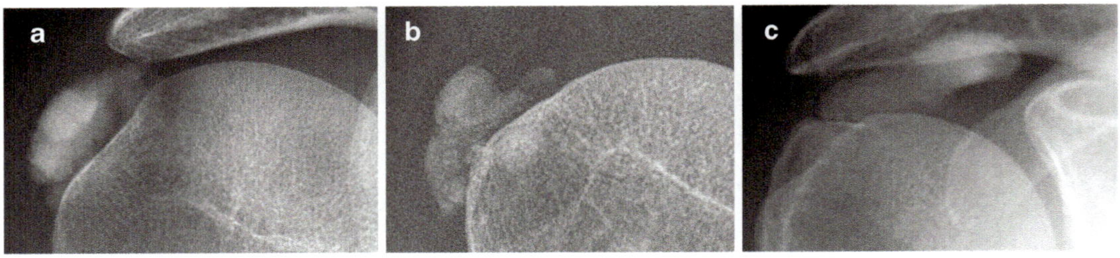

Fig. 15.3 Shoulder calcific tendinitis radiograph. (**a**) Type I calcification is well defined, with dense and homogeneous structure; (**b**) type II calcifications are depicted from less radiodense calcific deposits, with either sharp or poorly defined border (as in this case), and homogeneous or inhomogeneous structure; (**c**) type III calcification appearing as hazy, ill-defined globular area, more or less transparent in structure, typically seen in acute symptomatic patients

impingement. All three of the main rotator cuff tendons may be involved although the supraspinatus is the most common site of calcific deposits. Tendon calcifications are visible as echogenic foci usually accompanied by acoustic shadowing. With soft deposits the echogenicity may be more subtle and acoustic shadowing more variable.

Various classifications were proposed for the calcific plaques based on their location and appearance on ultrasound. Chiou et al. proposed a classification of calcific deposits into four shapes (Fig. 15.4a–d): (1) an arc shape (echogenic arc with clear shadowing); (2) a fragmented or punctate shape (two or more echogenic plaques), with or without shadowing; (3) a nodular shape (cloudy echogenic nodule without shadowing); and (4) a cystic shape (a bold echogenic wall with an anechoic area, weak internal echoes, or layering content).

There is a correlation between the ultrasound appearance of the calcified deposit, the clinical symptoms, and the three phases of histopathological findings of Uhthoff. Besides, there is an association with color Doppler ultrasonography of the rotator cuff and the calcific stage/clinical symptoms. In fact, during the resorptive phase, the deposits are surrounded by phagocytes and there was concomitant neoangiogenesis around the calcification. The combination of ultrasound and color Doppler appearance predicts more accurately formative or resorptive stage.

Severe symptoms are associated with non-arc-shape calcifications, hypervascularity, and widening of subacromial–subdeltoid bursa, suggesting resting or resorptive stage (Fig. 15.5). Identifying the resorptive phase is important for management as these deposits are nearly liquid and can be successfully aspirated. MRI is now not recommended as a first-line imaging modality, because deposits appear hypointense in all sequences, and can be missed, even though the development of new MR sequence such as susceptibility-weighted imaging (SWI) seemed to overcome this problem.

15.3 Complications: Subacromial Bursitis—Bone Involvement

A rare painful complication of calcifying tendinitis is the migration of calcium deposits from tendons, usually the supraspinatus, into the subacromial–subdeltoid bursa or into the underlying bone at the tendon attachment site (Fig. 15.6). The pathomechanism is still unknown, but seems to occur in the resorptive phase of the disease and seems to be mediated by aggressive inflammatory reaction and hyperemia at the tendon insertion and by rise of the intratendinous pressure. This can lead to secondary impingement resulting from the increased tendon size, and to rupture of the deposits into the subacromial space or into the bursa. Rarely, calcific tendinopathy eventually causes focal resorption of adjacent cortical bone, and intraosseous migration of calcic material might occur. These complications lead to severe shoulder pain and functional disability.

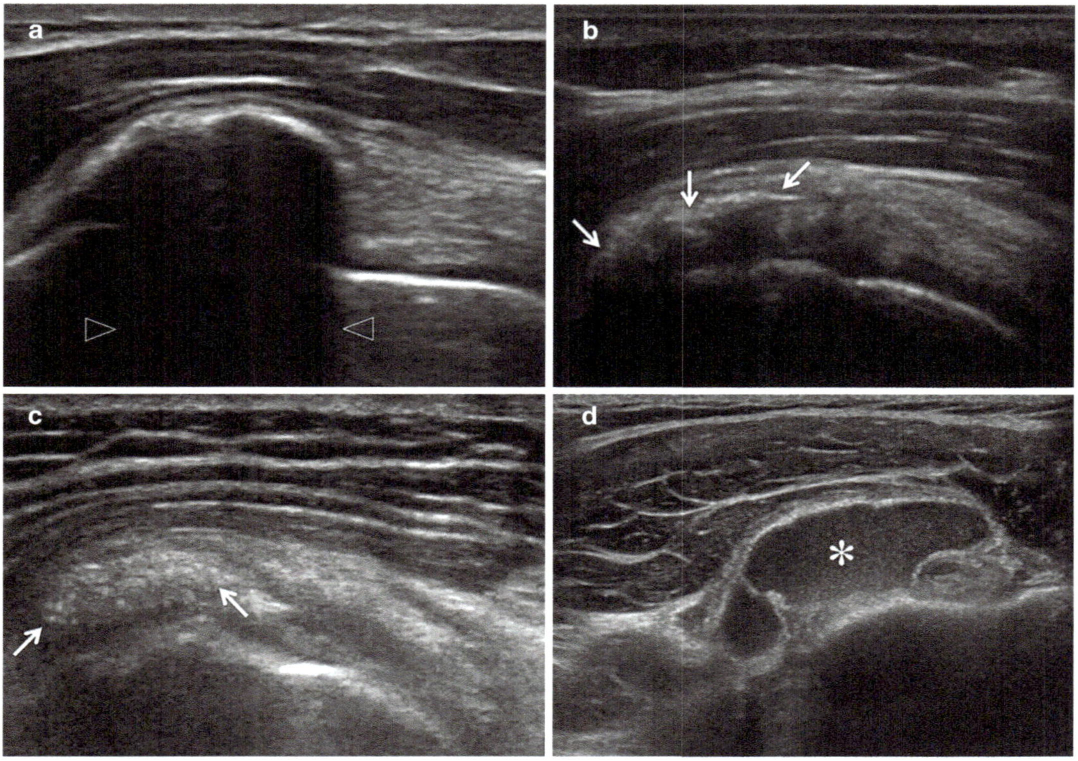

Fig. 15.4 Shoulder calcific tendinitis ultrasound. (**a**) **Arc-shaped calcification** seen as well-defined echogenic arc with deep acoustic shadowing (arrowheads) ("hard" calcification within the supraspinatus); (**b**) **fragmented shape calcification** has the appearance of fragmented and punctate echogenic profile (arrows) with or without (as in this case) acoustic shadowing; (**c**) **nodular shape calcification** that appears as ill-defined cloud-like echogenic nodule (arrows) without shadowing ("soft" calcification within the supraspinatus); (**d**) **cystic shape calcification** (white asterisk) appearing as echogenic wall with weak internal echoes

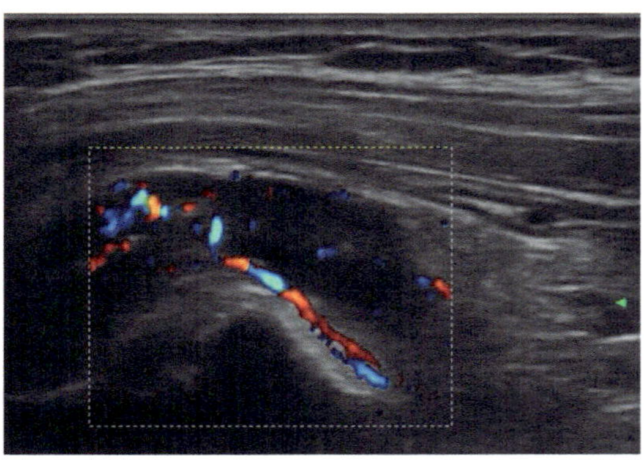

Fig. 15.5 Supraspinatus tendon calcifying tendinitis in acute resorptive phase. The color Doppler ultrasound shows hypervascularity in the subdeltoid bursa, distended by fluid

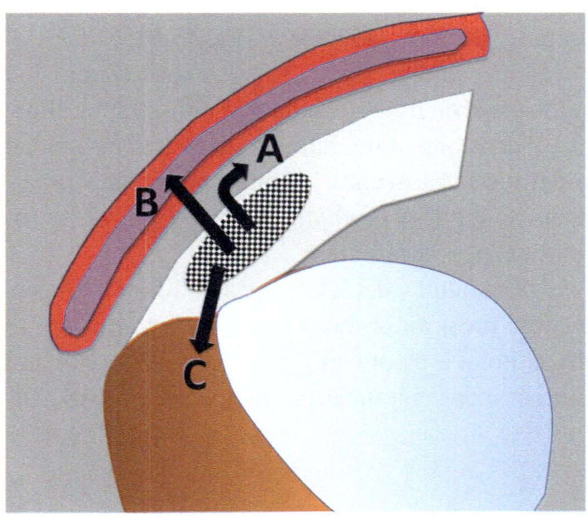

Fig. 15.6 Extratendinous calcification migration scheme: (**a**) into the sub-bursal space; (**b**) into the subacromial–subdeltoid bursa; (**c**) into the sub-insertional bone

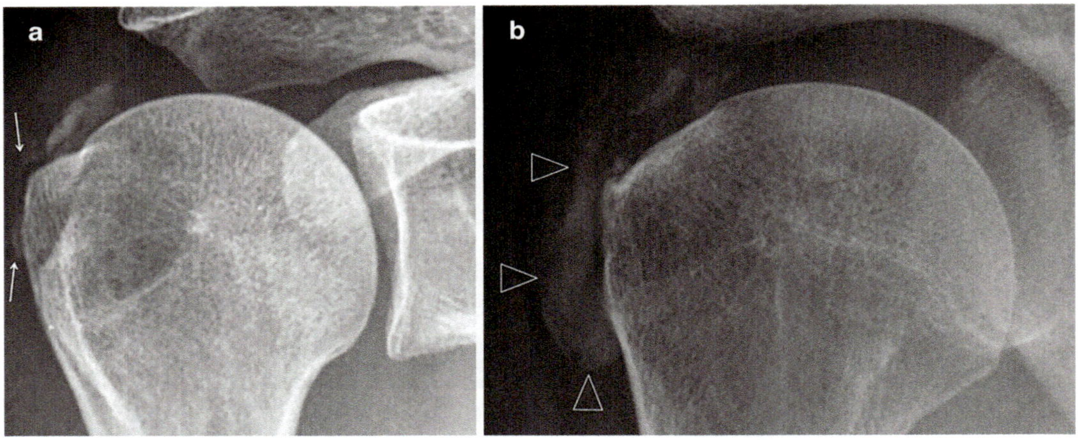

Fig. 15.7 Shoulder extratendinous calcification migration. (**a**) Shoulder X-ray showing linear calcified deposit (arrows), which surrounds the profile of the humeral trochlea, indicating the location between the tendon and the bursa; (**b**) shoulder externally rotated X-ray clearly showing supraspinatus calcific tendinitis, and migration of calcific deposits into the subacromial–subdeltoid bursa (arrowheads)

Calcium deposit migration into the sub-bursal space or into the subacromial–subdeltoid bursa appears on radiograph as ill-defined calcifications in the subacromial space (Fig. 15.7a and b). Often it is not possible to assess their exact location, whether intratendinous, sub-bursal, or intrabursal.

Ultrasound examination can visualize their exact location. Della Valle reported that in cases of intrabursal penetration of the calcification, at sonography and MRI examinations, the subacromial–subdeltoid bursa presents thickened walls and appears filled with inhomogeneous fluid containing calcium and debris (Fig. 15.8).

If the calcific deposit has migrated into the sub-insertional bone, standard radiographs show focal erosions of the humeral head and a rounded sclerotic intraosseous lesion in the greater tuberosity (Fig. 15.9), which could be mistaken for malignancy or infection.

Ultrasound depicts intratendinous hyperechoic focal amorphous calcification adjacent to focal bone erosions of the greater tuberosity and intraosseous calcification migration (Fig. 15.10).

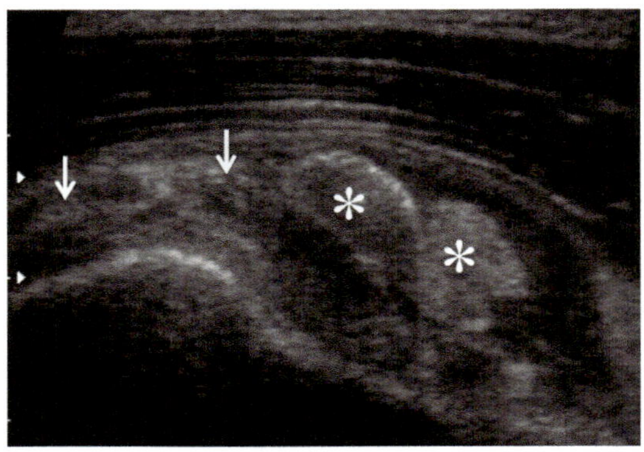

Fig. 15.8 Shoulder extratendinous calcification migration. Bursal extrusion, showing complex fluid with calcification inside the bursa, which presents thick walls. Calcifications appear as cloud-like echogenic nodules (asterisk) or minute scattered fragments (arrows)

MRI and CT are considered the best methods to demonstrate the involvement of bone marrow in calcific tendinopathy. CT is the gold standard imaging modality to depict cortical erosion of the humeral head and a rounded well-defined lytic

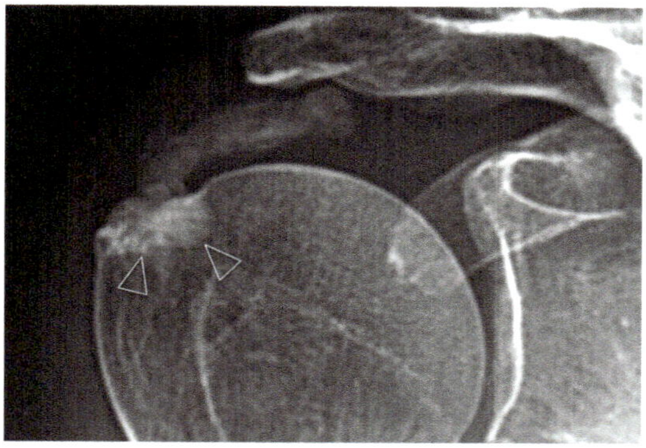

Fig. 15.9 Shoulder extratendinous calcification migration. Radiograph shows amorphous calcifications in the subacromial space and cortical erosion, with an underlying ovoid sclerotic lesion in the greater tuberosity (arrowheads)

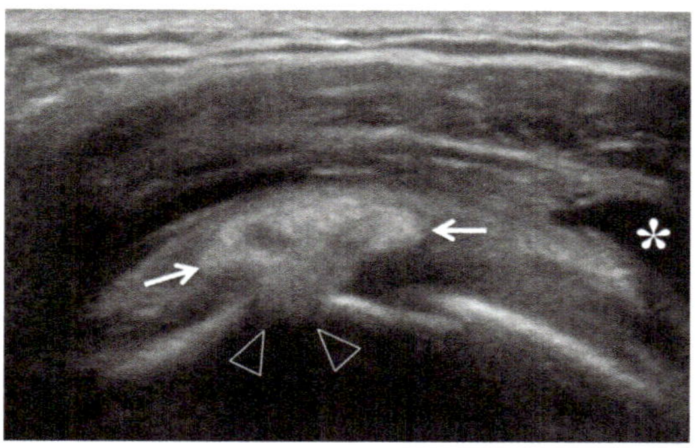

Fig. 15.10 Shoulder extratendinous calcification migration. Ultrasonography in the long axis of the supraspinatus tendon showing intratendinous calcification (arrows) associated with focal bone erosion and intraosseous calcification migration (arrowheads). Sonogram shows anechoic fluid within enlarged subacromial–subdeltoid bursa (white asterisk)

area located in the greater tuberosity (Fig. 15.11); it can also detect calcium deposit in its intraosseous location. MRI shows a cystic lesion in the greater tuberosity and humeral osteitis related to typical reactive bone marrow edema surrounding the lytic lesion (Fig. 15.12).

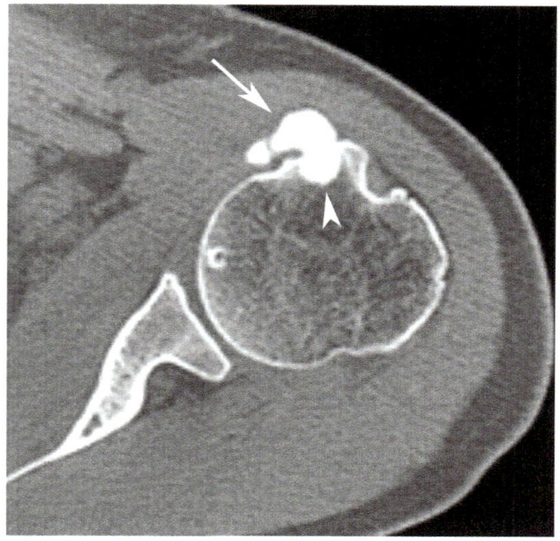

Fig. 15.11 Shoulder extratendinous calcification migration. Axial CT shows the subscapularis calcium deposit migration into the sub-insertional bone. The arrow indicates calcification, and the arrowhead indicates the subcortical bone migration in the lesser tuberosity. *Courtesy of Prof. L.M. Sconfienza*

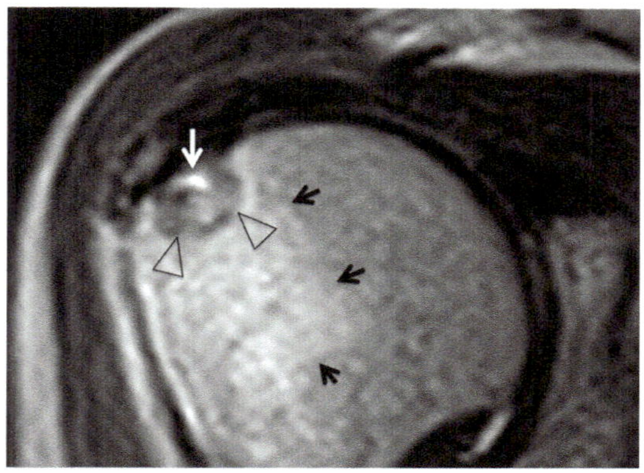

Fig. 15.12 Shoulder extratendinous calcification migration. Coronal T2-weighted sequence shows low signal intensity of the ovoid lesion in the greater tuberosity in keeping with sclerosis (arrowheads). There is a superficial focus of fluid signal (white arrow) traversing the region of cortical erosion. Ill-defined hyperintensity consistent with marrow edema (black arrows) surrounds the lesion

Further Readings

Bosworth BM. Calcium deposits in shoulder and subacromial bursitis: survey of 12,122 shoulders. JAMA. 1941;116:2477–82.

Chianca V, Albano D, Messina C, Midiri F, Mauri G, Aliprandi A, et al. Rotator cuff calcific tendinopathy: from diagnosis to treatment. Acta Biomed. 2018;89(1-S):186–96.

Chiou HJ, Chou YH, Wu JJ, Hsu CC, Huang DY, Chang CY. Evaluation of calcific tendonitis of the rotator cuff: role of color Doppler ultrasonography. J Ultrasound Med. 2002;21(3):289–95.

Codman EA. The Shoulder. 3rd ed. Boston: Thomas Todd; 1934.

Della Valle V, Bassi EM, Calliada F. Migration of calcium deposits into subacromial–subdeltoid bursa and into humeral head as a rare complication of calcifying tendinitis: sonography and imaging. J Ultrasound. 2015;18:259–63.

De Palma AF, Kruper JS. Long-term study of shoulder joints afflicted with and treated for calcific tendinitis. Clin Orthop. 1961;20:61–72.

Flemming DJ, Murphey MD, Shekitka KM, et al. Osseous involvement in calcific tendinitis: a retrospective review of 50 cases. AJR Am J Roentgenol. 2003;181:965–72.

Gärtner J, Heyer A. Calcific tendinitis of the shoulder [in German]. Orthopade. 1995;24(3):284–302.

Hamada J, Ono W, Tamai K, Saotome K, Hoshino T. Analysis of calcium deposits in calcific periarthritis. J Rheumatol. 2001;28:809–13.

Le Goff B, Berthelot JM, Guillot P, Glèmarec J, Maugars Y. Assessment of calcific tendonitis of rotator cuff by ultrasonography: comparison between symptomatic and asymptomatic shoulders. Joint Bone Spine. 2010;77(3):258–63.

Molè D, Kempf JF, Gleyze P, et al. Results of endoscopic treatment of non-broken tendinopathies of the rotator cuff. Calcifications of the rotator cuff. Rev Chir Orthop. 1993;79:532–41.

Moseley HF, Goldie I. The arterial pattern of the rotator cuff of the shoulder. J Bone Joint Surg Br. 1963;45(4):780–9.

Nogueira-Barbosa MH, Gregio-Junior E, Lorenzato MM. Retrospective study of sonographic findings in bone involvement associated with rotator cuff calcific tendinopathy: preliminary results of a case series. Radiol Bras. 2015;48(6):353–7.

Nörenberg D, Ebersberger HU, Walter T, Ockert B, Knobloch G, Diederichs G, Hamm B, Makowski MR. Calcific tendonitis of the rotator cuff: susceptibility-weighted MR imaging. Radiology. 2016;278(2):475–84.

Patte D, Goutallier D. Periarthritis of the shoulder. Calcifications. Rev Chir Orthop. 1988;74:277–8.

Porcellini G, Paladini P, Campi F, Paganelli M. Arthroscopic treatment of calcifying tendonitis of the shoulder: clinical and ultrasonographic findings at two to five years. J Shoulder Elb Surg. 2004;13:503–8.

Speed CA, Hazelman BL. Calcific tendinitis of the shoulder. N Engl J Med. 1999;340:1582–4.

Uhthoff HK, Sarkar K, Maynard JA. Calcifying tendinitis: a new concept of its pathogenesis. Clin Orthop Relat Res. 1976;118:164–8.

Uhthoff HK, Loehr JW. Calcific tendinopathy of the rotator cuff: pathogenesis, diagnosis, and management. J Am Acad Orthop Surg. 1997;5(4):183–91.

Frozen Shoulder

16

Enzo Silvestri, Davide Orlandi, Alessandro Muda, and Fabio Martino

Contents

16.1 Introduction

Frozen shoulder (FS), also known as adhesive capsulitis, is a debilitating clinical syndrome characterized by insidious onset of shoulder pain, and gradual restriction of both active and passive motion of the glenohumeral joint, without documented causes. It is a common inflammatory disorder of the shoulder, mostly affecting females in 40–70 years' group, with an incidence ranging from 2% to 5%. More frequently the disease is unilateral and the patients usually present with painful difficulty in overhead movements, getting dressed, and moving the arm behind the back. Active and passive range of motion is painful and restricted. At patient inspection, a tendency towards a winged scapula can be seen. During resisted muscle tests, reduction of movements in external rotation, internal rotation, and abduction is appreciated; another test evaluates the impossibility of abducting the humerus without lifting the shoulder when it exceeds 90° abduction. A differential diagnosis must be made with osteoarthritis, subdeltoid bursitis, Parsonage-Turner syndrome, and rotator cuff tendons pathologies.

Adhesive capsulitis is classified into two categories based on the absence or presence of concomitant shoulder disease: (1) primary, or idiopathic, refers to the disease process occurring without an identifiable cause and (2) secondary, which is clinically indistinguishable from idiopathic form, is associated with, or subsequent to, other shoulder pathologic states (trauma and immobilization, calcific tendinitis with severe subdeltoid bursitis, diabetes mellitus, hemiplegia, cervical arthritis, hyperthyroidism, Dupuytren disease). The etiology of adhesive capsulitis is not fully understood, but it is acclaimed as a cytokine-mediated inflammatory and fibrotizing problem. It is characterized by the presence of thickening and stiffness

E. Silvestri
Radiology, Alliance Medical, Genova, Italy

D. Orlandi (✉)
Department of Radiology, Ospedale Evangelico Internazionale, Genova, Italy

A. Muda
Department of Radiology, IRCCS Policlinico San Martino-IST, Genova, Italy

F. Martino
Radiology, Sant'Agata Diagnostic Center, Bari, Italy

F. Martino et al. (eds.), *Musculoskeletal Ultrasound in Orthopedic and Rheumatic disease in Adults*, https://doi.org/10.1007/978-3-030-91202-4_16

of joint capsule, associated with synovitis that often affects also the tendon sheath of the long head of the biceps brachii; the subdeltoid bursa and the rotator cuff tendons may also be involved. FS is a self-limited process in which the disease tends to resolve after a period (12–18 months) of worsening and intense pain, but recovery is generally not complete. Thus, it is a dynamic process that evolves through three distinct stages that can overlap: the **acute stage (freezing or painful stage)**, with pain at rest that increases at the extremes of movements and interruption of night sleep (3–9 months); the **adhesive stage (frozen or transitional stage)** with progressive reduction of ROMs (up to 12 months); and the **stage of resolution (thawing stage)**, with progressive pain relief and return to normal or close to normal range of movements (1–3.5 years). Management of capsulitis tends to be conservative, as most cases resolve spontaneously, although a subset of patients progress to permanent disability. Therefore, early and accurate diagnosis is crucial as adhesive capsulitis diagnosed in the later stages is more difficult to manage.

16.2 Diagnostic Imaging

Diagnosis is mainly based on clinical findings. Imaging is not imperative to diagnose frozen shoulder. However, it may help confirm the correct diagnosis even excluding other problems in painful shoulder, such as a torn rotator cuff. MRI can provide reliable imaging indicators of FS (Fig. 16.1a, b), which include joint capsule and coracohumeral ligament (CHL) thickening, presence of inflammatory tissue at the rotator interval that enhances after intravenous gadolinium injection, and obliteration of the fat triangle due to edema surrounding the CHL at the level of the subcoracoid space.

However, X-ray and ultrasound are currently considered the first-line imaging modalities. Radiography will often appear normal. The role of ultrasound is still debated; however the studies carried out indicate how there are structures involved in this disease that can be excellently evaluated with sonography. Commonly referred ultrasound findings in adhesive capsulitis are coracohumeral ligament (CHL) and joint capsule thickening. The ultrasound examination is performed on patient's shoulder placed in external rotation and in 90° abducted position, with forearm 90° flexed (Fig. 16.2a, b). In this position both CHL and joint capsule become stretched allowing the best thickness measurement. The CHL can be shown by scanning on an oblique transverse plane using the coracoid as landmark; the ligament originates from the coracoid and ends on the rotator interval (Fig. 16.3a–c). The average thickness of the CHL was significantly greater in adhesive capsulitis (3 mm) than in the asymptomatic shoulders (1.34 mm).

Placing probe in axillary cavity allows us to evaluate the joint capsule on longitudinal (when possible; if the axillary pouch stiffness consent to be stretched and the shoulder to be

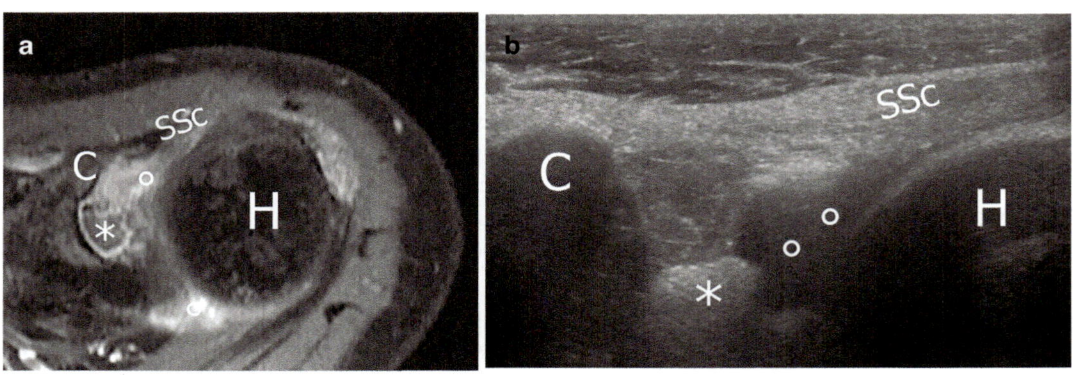

Fig. 16.1 Left frozen shoulder in acute stage. Axial T2 fat-sat magnetic resonance (MRI) scan (**a**) and corresponding ultrasound (US) scan (**b**) of shoulder adhesive capsulitis. *H* humerus, *C* coracoid, *SSc* subscapularis tendon, *asterisk* extended anterior recess edema, *circles* joint effusion

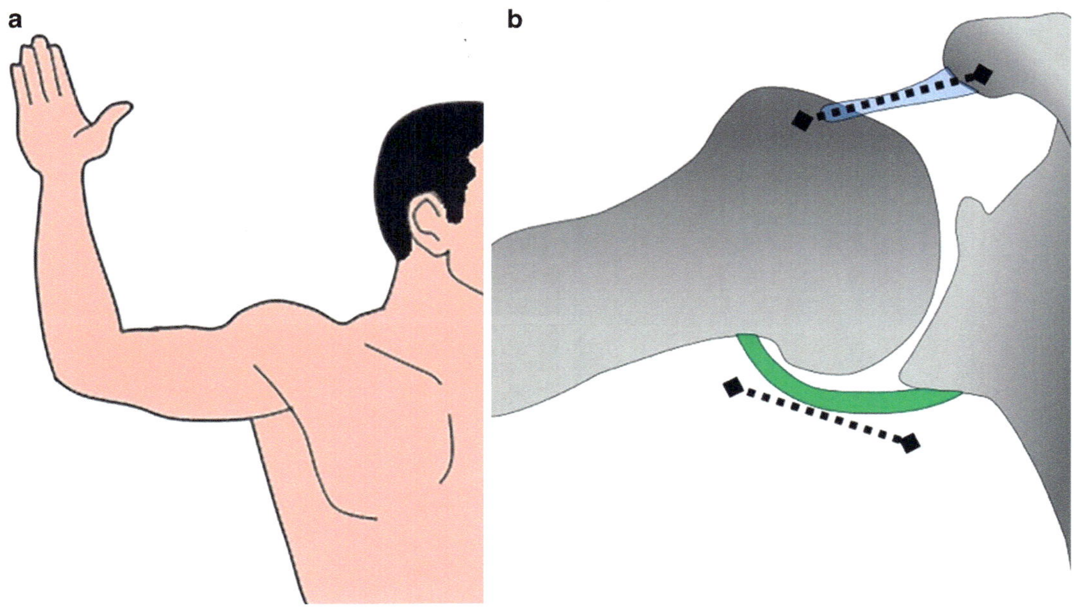

Fig. 16.2 (**a**) Patient position, with 90° abducted arm and flexed forearm. (**b**) Probe position along the coracohumeral ligament and under the capsule axillary pouch. Probe (*dotted line*); coracohumeral ligament (*blue*); capsule profile (*green*)

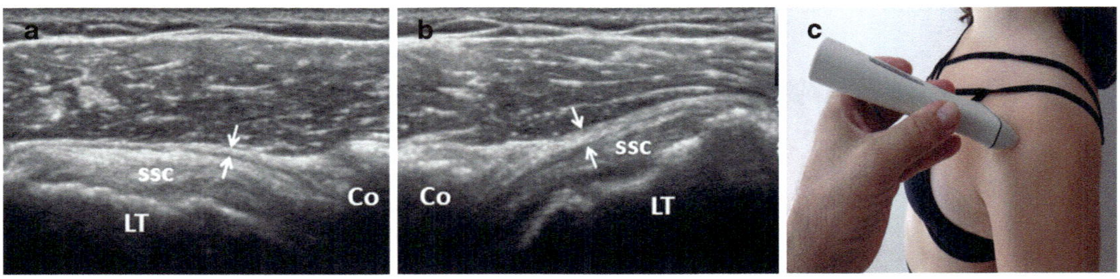

Fig. 16.3 Left frozen shoulder in adhesive stage (**b**) with respect to the normal contralateral side (**a**). The ultrasound evaluation shows the blurred thickening of the coracohumeral ligament, in a patient with painful abduction and very limited external rotation of the affected shoulder. Part label (**c**) shows correct probe position. *LT* Lesser tuberosity, *SSC* subscapularis tendon, *Co* coracohumeral ligament

abducted) (Fig. 16.4a–c) and transverse scans (more simple to place the probe) (Fig. 16.5a–c). The joint capsule thickness value is considered a combination of capsular and synovial thickness of the axillary pouch. It appears as a thin hyperechoic band which surrounds humeral neck, and is represented with linear or curved profile in longitudinal and axial views, respectively.

In symptomatic patients the joint capsule thickness greater than 2 mm measured by ultrasound can be considered indicative of frozen shoulder and correlates to MRI signs of adhesive capsulitis with high sensitivity and specificity.

The main US Doppler sign of capsulitis is the presence of hypoechoic and hyperemic synovial thickening around the biceps long head at rotator cuff interval level (Fig. 16.6). A correct conduct of the examination requires to set the system with PRF <1 KHz and low wall filter to detect small vessel flow signals, whose characteristics resemble background noise. However, diagnostic validity of this finding remains controversial due to the poor specificity.

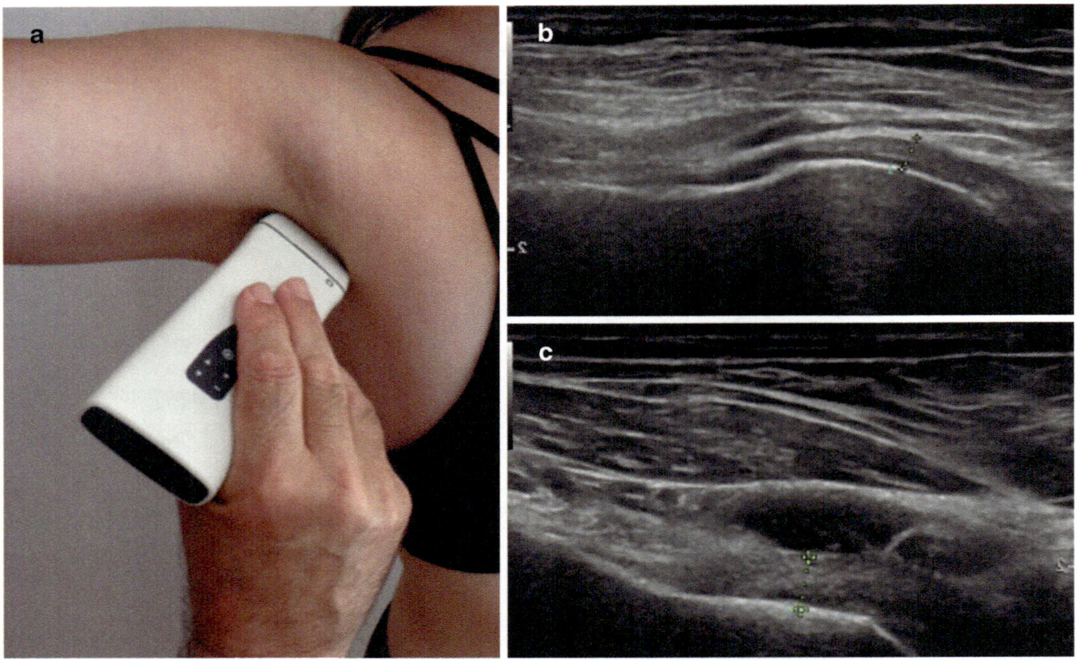

Fig. 16.4 The sonographic evaluation of axillary pouch is conducted with longitudinal scan, as shown in the model (**a**). The affected shoulder (**c**) appears thickened than normal right shoulder (**b**). The capsule thickness is delimited by calipers (courtesy of M. Zappia M.D.)

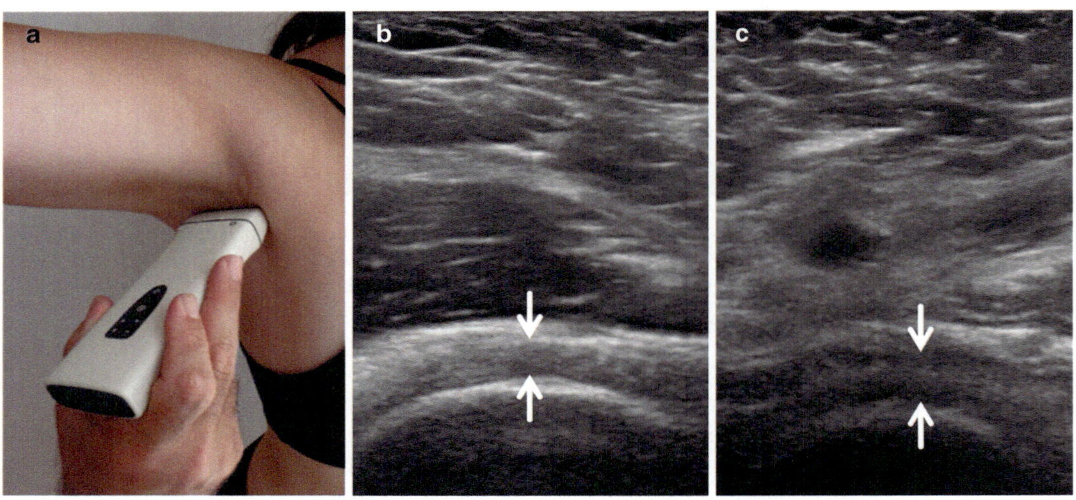

Fig. 16.5 Same patient as in Fig. 16.2. The sonographic evaluation of axillary pouch is conducted with axial scan, as shown in the model (**a**). The affected shoulder (**c**) appears thickened and more hypoechoic than normal right shoulder (**b**). The capsule thickness is delimited by *arrows*

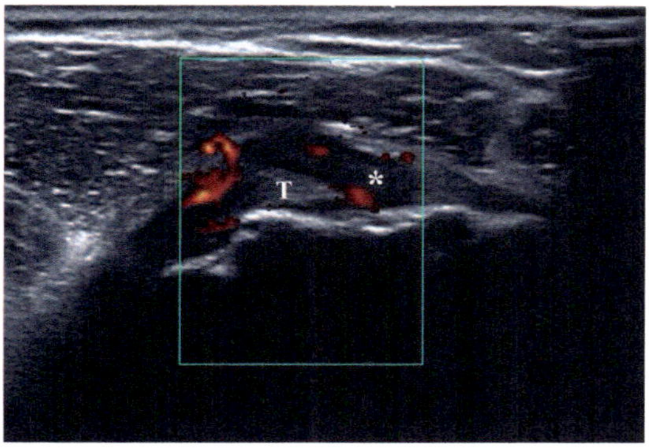

Fig. 16.6 Synovial thickening and hyperemia around the biceps long head, US transverse scan; *T* tendon, synovial effusion (*asterisk*); courtesy of E. LaPaglia M.D.

However, the diagnosis of adhesive capsulitis still substantially relies on the radiologist's observation of limited abduction or external rotation during dynamic shoulder ultrasound. The dynamic test is indicative of capsulitis if, positioning the probe on an oblique coronal plane, using the margin of the acromion as the medial reference, there is a difficulty in sliding the supraspinatus tendon and the overlying tissue plane above the bone plane during abduction. A similar test can be performed during external rotation movements by evaluating on a transverse plane the sliding of the subscapularis tendon; a decrease in the range of movement in symptomatic patients is indicative of capsulitis.

A recent study proposed the role of strain and shear-wave elastosonography of the supraspinatus and infraspinatus tendons as an aid in the diagnosis of adhesive capsulitis. The authors verified that a greater rigidity of tendon structures is possible in idiopathic adhesive capsulitis; most of the pathologies of rotator cuff tendons, such as tendinopathies, ruptures, and impingement syndromes, lead to a loss of rigidity of the tissue, while in idiopathic adhesive capsulitis a greater rigidity is observed, probably due to post-inflammatory fibrosis and response to immobilization and adaptation to muscle tension.

Currently, in symptomatic patients, sonography is recommended as the preferred first-line imaging modality due to its diagnostic accuracy, noninvasiveness, and capability to provide a dynamic comparison between the affected and unaffected sides.

Further Readings

Bunker TD. Frozen shoulder: unravelling the enigma. Ann R Coll Surg Engl. 1997;79:210–3.

Carrillon Y, Noel E, Fantino O, Perrin-Fayolle O, Tran-Minh VA. Magnetic resonance imaging findings in idiopathic adhesive capsulitis of the shoulder. Rev Rhum Engl Ed. 1999;66:201–6.

Cheng X, Zhang Z, Xuanyan G, Li T, Li J, Yin L, Lu M. Adhesive capsulitis of the shoulder: evaluation with US-arthrography using a sonographic contrast agent. Sci Rep. 2017;7:5551.

Cleland J, Durall CJ. Physical therapy for adhesive capsulitis: systematic review. Physiotherapy. 2002;88: 450–7.

Codman EA. Tendinitis of the short rotators. In: Codman EA, editor. Ruptures of the supraspinatus tendon and other lesions on or about the subacromial bursa. Thomas Todd: Boston, Mass; 1934.

Dias R, Cutts S, Massoud S. Frozen shoulder. BMJ. 2005;331:1453–6.

Emig E, Schweitzer M, Karasick D, Lubowitz J. Adhesive capsulitis of the shoulder: MR diagnosis. AJR. 1995;164:1457–9.

Homsi C, Bordalo-Rodrigues M, da Silva JJ, Stump XMGRG. Ultrasound in adhesive capsulitis of the shoulder: is assessment of the coracohumeral ligament a valuable diagnostic tool? Skeletal Radiol. 2006;35:673–8.

Jewell DV, Riddle DL, Thacker LR. Interventions associated with an increased or decreased likelihood of pain reduction and improved function in patients with adhesive capsulitis: a retrospective cohort study. Phys Ther. 2009;89:419–29.

Kline CM. Adhesive capsulitis: clues and complexities. JAMA Online. 2007:2–9.

Lee G, Briggs L, Murrell G. Ultrasound measurement of shoulder capsule thickness for diagnosing frozen shoulder. J Sci Med Sport. 2010;13(suppl 1):e75.

Lee JC, Sykes C, Saifuddin A, Connell D. Adhesive capsulitis: sonographic changes in the rotator cuff interval with arthroscopic correlation. Skeletal Radiol. 2005;34(9):522–7.

Martino F, Silvestri E, Grassi W, Garlaschi G. Musculoskeletal sonography. Milan, Berlin, Heidelberg, New York: Springer; 2006.

Park GY, Park JH, Kwon DR, Kwon DG, Park J. Do the findings of magnetic resonance imaging, arthrography, and ultrasonography reflect clinical impairment in patients with idiopathic adhesive capsulitis of the shoulder? Arch Phys Med Rehabil. 2017;98: 1995–2001.

Park J, Chai JW, Kim DH, Cha SW. Dynamic ultrasonography of the shoulder. Ultrasonography. 2018;37(3):190–9.

Ryu KN, Lee SW, Rhee YG, Lim JH. Adhesive capsulitis of the shoulder joint: usefulness of dynamic sonography. J Ultrasound Med. 1993;12(8):445–9.

Sernik RA, Vidal Leão R, Bizetto EL, Sanford Damasceno R, Horvat N, Cerri GG. Ultrasound. 2019;27(3):183–90.

Tandon A, Dewan S, Bhatt S, Jain AK, Kumari R. Sonography in diagnosis of adhesive capsulitis of the shoulder: a case–control study. J Ultrasound. 2017;20:227–36.

Van Holsbeeck M, Vanderschueren J, Shoulder WJ. Sonography in adhesive capsulitis. Chicago, USA: 83rd Annual Meeting of the Radiological Society of North America; 1997.

Walmsley S, Rivett DA, Osmotherly PG. Adhesive capsulitis: Establishing consensus on clinical identifiers for stage 1 using the Delphi technique. Phys Ther. 2009;89:906–17.

Yun SJ, Jin W, Cho NS, Ryu KN, Yoon YC, Cha JG, Park JS, Park SY, Choi NY. Shear-wave and strain ultrasound elastography of the supraspinatus and infraspinatus tendons in patients with idiopathic adhesive capsulitis of the shoulder: a prospective case-control study. Korean J Radiol. 2019;20(7):1176–85.

Zuckerman JD, Cuomo F. Frozen shoulder. In: Matsen FA, Fu FH, Hawkins RJ, editors. The shoulder: a balance of mobility and stability. Rosemont, IL: American Academy of Orthopaedic Surgeons; 1993. p. 253–67.

Septic Arthritis

17

Alessandro Muda and Fabio Martino

Contents

17.1 Introduction

In general, infectious arthritis is classified as pyogenic (septic) or nonpyogenic. Septic arthritis is a serious type of joint infection and may represent a direct invasion of joint space by various microorganisms, most commonly caused by bacteria. Nonpyogenic infective arthritis tends to be less aggressive and has a more chronic course, with causative organisms including *Mycobacterium tuberculosis,* fungi, viruses, and spirochetes.

Arthritis can develop indirectly as a result of hematogenous seeding or extension from a contiguous focus of infection. Bacterial arthritis can also arise following direct introduction, can be accidental from penetrating trauma (also from human or animal bite or from a fingernail wound), or can be iatrogenic by intra-articular injection. Joint surgery has increasingly been a source of bacterial arthritis, particularly following knee and hip arthroplasty.

A. Muda
Department of Radiology, IRCCS Policlinico San Martino-IST, Genova, Italy

F. Martino (✉)
Radiology, Sant'Agata Diagnostic Center, Bari, Italy

Septic arthritis can be theoretically caused by any bacterium; however the most common etiological agent of all septic arthritis cases is *Staphylococcus aureus*, which causes a destructive form of acute arthritis, representing a real medical emergency. Patients with a history of intravenous drug abuse, elderly, or immunocompromised people display a higher prevalence of infection by gram-negative organisms. The most common gram-negative organisms are *Pseudomonas aeruginosa* and *Escherichia coli.*

Infants and older adults are more likely to develop septic arthritis. The knees are most commonly affected, but septic arthritis can also affect the hips, shoulders, and other joints. Typically, septic arthritis affects one large joint, such as the knee or hip, and only one. Less frequently, septic arthritis can affect multiple joints simultaneously.

The infection can quickly and severely injure the cartilage and bone within the joint, so prompt diagnosis and antibiotic treatment are crucial, also to prevent permanent damage to the joint. An acute onset of monoarticular joint pain, joint

F. Martino et al. (eds.), *Musculoskeletal Ultrasound in Orthopedic and Rheumatic disease in Adults*,
https://doi.org/10.1007/978-3-030-91202-4_17

swelling by effusion, erythema, heat, and impaired range of movement, with fever and chills, should raise suspicion of sepsis. Clinical evaluation, laboratory workup, and joint fluid aspiration are the primary means of diagnosing septic arthritis. The role of imaging is to confirm the diagnosis and establish the presence and severity of joint damage.

17.2 Diagnostic Imaging

Conventional radiograph still remains as the initial imaging approach, but it has low sensitivity and specificity for acute infection. In early stages the simple radiograph can be normal and this does not rule out infection. With further development of the conditions, the typical radiological picture shows severe osteoporosis, destruction of joint cartilages with joint space narrowing, and serious damage to bones. Therefore, X-ray allows to identify late stages of the disease, when bone tissue is already damaged, and it is no more useful for therapeutic decision-making. Early recognition of the presence of intra-articular effusion in affected joint is the primary objective of diagnostic imaging, because the absence of a joint effusion essentially excludes septic arthritis. Both ultrasound and MRI can detect a joint effusion; however ultrasound is preferred for its accessibility and patient acceptance. However MRI and bone scintigraphy may be warranted to rule out adjacent osteomyelitis. Therefore, when the diagnosis of septic arthritis is presumed, ultrasonography may be mostly beneficial not only for a diagnostic confirmation, but also for simultaneous, ultrasound-guided arthrocentesis with aspiration of the purulent effusion. Ultrasonography is more sensitive for detecting effusions, particularly in challenging joints, such as the hip. This ability is especially useful in the early diagnosis of newborn septic arthritis, because of the frequent paucity of clinical signs and symptoms in these patients. Usually, when a joint effusion is found, sonography alone cannot distinguish with certainty between septic arthritis and other types of synovitis. In fact, septic arthritis demonstrates great variability in ultrasound presentation, depending on the patient age, etiological agent, evolutionary stage, and affected joint. The ultrasound appearance can range from mild echogenic articular effusion to joint destruction (Figs. 17.1 and 17.2a–e).

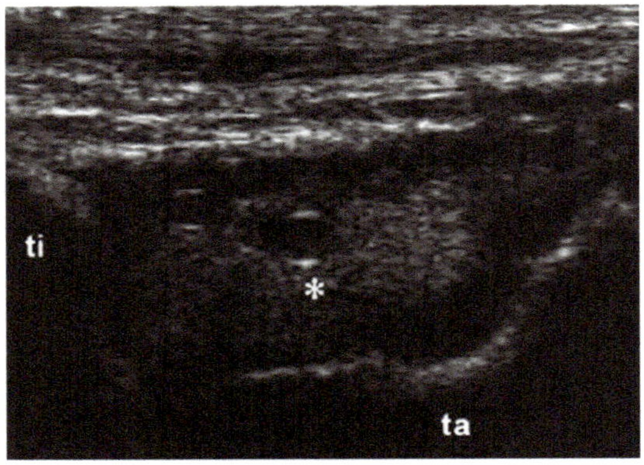

Fig. 17.1 Tibiotalar septic arthritis. Joint effusion appears inhomogeneously echogenic with turbid and sand-like appearance (*) suggestive of septic fluid collection. *ti* tibia, *ta* talus

In pediatric age, septic arthritis is relatively frequent, most commonly involving the hip joint, and can have potentially serious consequences, being considered a medical emergency. Prompt diagnosis is of paramount importance to avoid a disastrous outcome, which can lead to joint destruction when the therapy is delayed or inadequate. A classic clinical presentation of septic arthritis is a sudden onset of the pain and joint discomfort (frequently at hip), and the presence of Kocher criteria (non-weight-bearing status on the affected side; fever >38.5°; erythrocyte sedimentation rate (ESR) >40 mm/h; increase in serum white blood cell (WBC) count >12,000/mm^3). But sometimes distinguishing septic arthritis from transient synovitis or other types of arthritis of the hip in a limping child could be challenging. In fact, in the early stage of disease

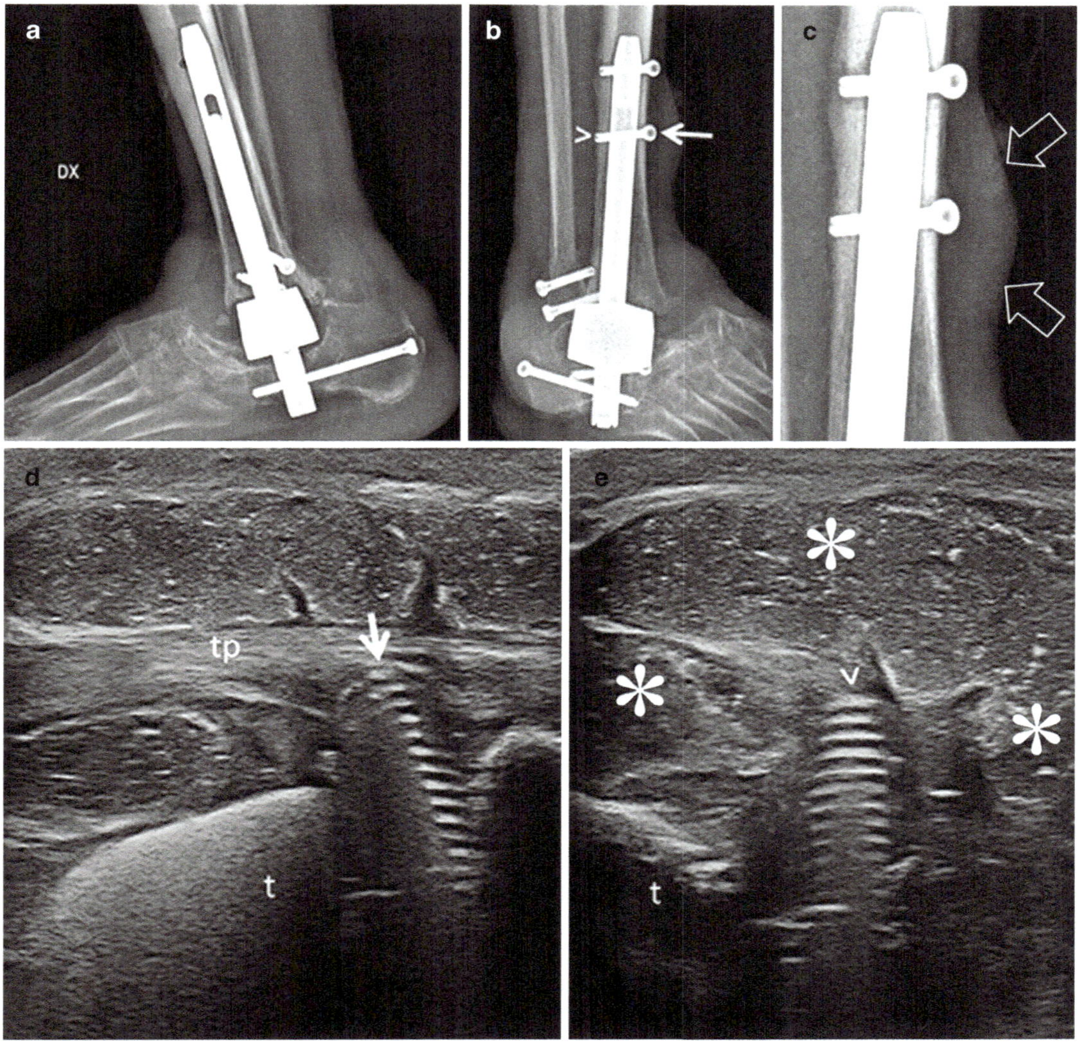

Fig. 17.2 Long-standing rheumatoid arthritis and osteomyelitis. Hot and swollen ankle for 4 weeks in a 68-year-old male, who underwent ankle arthrodesis 5 years before. Conventional radiography (**a**, **b**). Images acquired using different projections. The arrows and the arrowheads indicate the parts of the screw displayed in the ultrasound images. Radiographic detail (**c**): note soft-tissue swelling around the tibia (empty arrows), related to septic infiltrate. Ultrasound (**d**, **e**). Note the septic fluid collection (*) surrounding both screw extremities [i.e., the head (*arrow*) and the tip (*arrowhead*)] and appearing as an inhomogeneous area characterized by hyperechoic spots of different size and shape distributed in a less echogenic fluid material. *t* tibia, *tp* tibialis posterior tendon (Images courtesy of MD Cipolletta E, Ancona)

their clinical presentation could be similar but treatment and prognosis are very different. In these cases, although they are unable to provide diagnostic certainty, some echographic features may help to distinguish septic arthritis from other different types. For example, the echogenicity of exudate is usually anechoic and homogeneous in transient arthritis while in septic arthritis it often

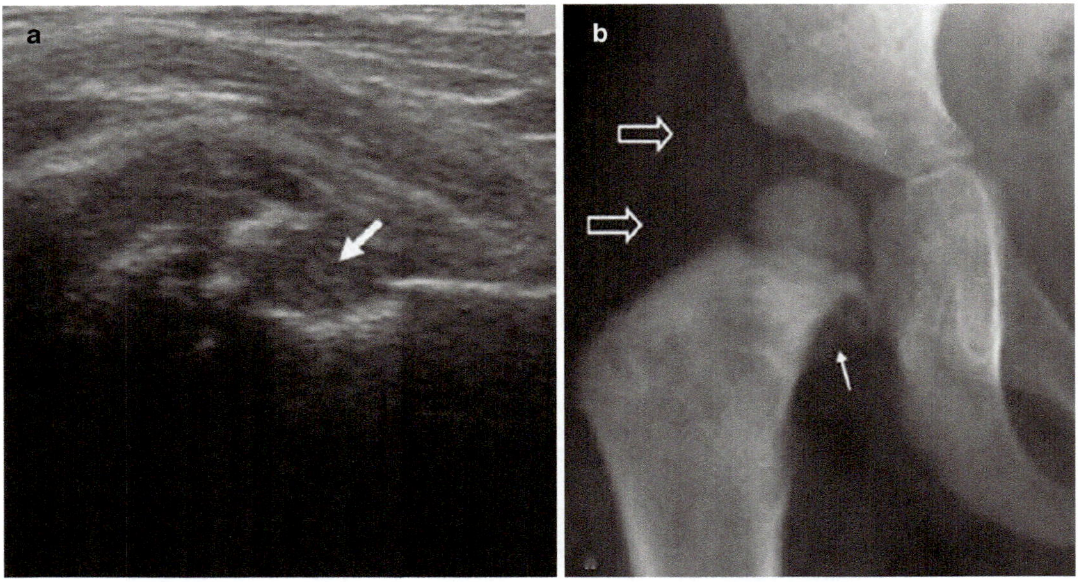

Fig. 17.3 (**a**, **b**) Septic arthritis of the hip in a limping 3-year-old child with mild hip pain. (**a**) Longitudinal US scan reveals a small effusion with inhomogeneous echogenicity and synovial thickening. Metaphyseal bone erosion is present (*large white arrow*). (**b**) X-ray in the same patient confirms the soft-tissue swelling around the involved joint, suggestive of effusion (*empty white arrows*) and bone erosion (*small white arrow*)

shows a cloudy and inhomogeneous aspect (Figs. 17.3a, b, and 17.4a–c). Synovium thickening is generally present in juvenile idiopathic arthritis (for hypertrophy), moderate in septic arthritis (for edema), and minimally evident or absent in transient arthritis. As a rule, synovial hyperemia is present at power Doppler evaluation in septic arthritis and juvenile idiopathic arthritis, while it is generally least or absent in transient arthritis.

However, we must remember that septic arthritis is a great mimic. Therefore, even if the echographic evaluation reveals a monoarticular and homogeneously anechoic effusion, and a minimal synovial thickening without hypervascularity, arthrocentesis is still mandatory if the clinical and laboratory results evoke septic involvement. Conversely, septic arthritis must always be excluded even in situations where the clinical presentation is atypical. In this way, sonography can play a useful role in differential diagnosis. In doubt, a precise and unmistakable diagnosis is only possible through arthrocentesis and isolation of the bacterium.

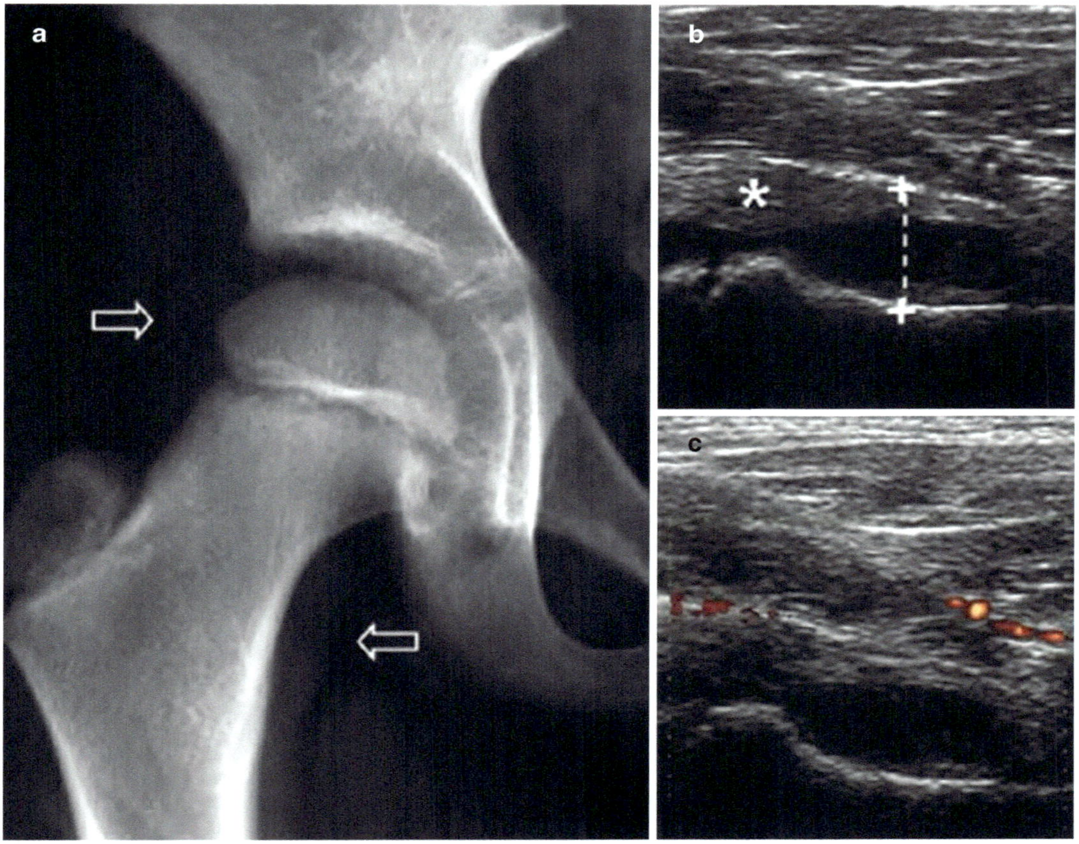

Fig. 17.4 (**a–c**) Transient synovitis in a 5-year-old child with similar clinical presentation to that of the patient in Fig. 17.2. (**a**) Frontal radiograph shows capsular swelling (*empty white arrows*). (**b**) US detects increased capsule-to-bone distance (calipers) related to joint effusion and to synovial thickening (*). (**c**) Power Doppler US demonstrates absence of intrasynovial increased flow

Further Readings

Chin TWY, Tse KS. Clinical and radiological differentiation of septic arthritis and transient synovitis of the hip. Hong Kong J Radiol. 2017;20:41–6.

Goldenberg DL. Septic arthritis. Lancet. 1998;351:197–202.

Gordon JE, Huang M, Dobbs M, et al. Causes of false-negative ultrasound scans in the diagnosis of septic arthritis of the hip in children. J Pediatr Orthop. 2002;22:312–6.

Marchal GJ, Van Holsbeeck MT, Raes M, et al. Transient synovitis of the hip in children: role of US. Radiology. 1987;162:825–8.

Martino F, Silvestri E, Grassi W, Garlaschi G. Musculoskeletal sonography. Springer: Milan, Berlin, Heidelberg, New York; 2006.

Merino R, de Inocencio J, Garcia-Consuegra J. Differentiation between transient synovitis of the hip with clinical and ultrasound criteria. An Pediatr (Barc). 2010;73(4):189–93.

Nguyen A, Kan JH, Bisset G, Rosenfeld S. Kocher criteria revisited in the era of MRI: how often does the Kocher criteria identify underlying osteomyelitis? J Pediatr Orthop. 2017;37(2):e114–9.

Ryan MJ, Kavanagh R, Wall PG, Hazleman BL. Bacterial joint infections in England and Wales: analysis of bacterial isolates over a four year period. Br J Rheumatol. 1997;36:370–3.

Shirtliff ME, Mader JT. Acute septic arthritis. Clin Microbiol Rev. 2002;15(4):527–44.

Strouse PJ, DiPietro MA, Adler RS. Pediatric hip effusions: evaluation with power Doppler sonography. Radiology. 1998;206:731–5.

Taylor-Robinson D, Keat A. Septic and aseptic arthritis: a continuum? Baillieres Best Pract Res Clin Rheumatol. 1999;13:179–92.

Zamzam MM. The role of ultrasound in differentiating septic arthritis from transient synovitis of the hip in children. J Pediatr Orthop. 2006;15:418–22.

Zieger MM, Dörr U, Schulz RD. Ultrasonography of hip joint effusions. Skelet Radiol. 1987;16:607–11.

Hemophiliac Arthropathy

18

Alessandro Muda and Fabio Martino

Contents

18.1 Introduction

Hemophilia is an X-linked recessive bleeding disorder, caused by the deficiency or absence of blood-clotting factor VIII in hemophilia A or factor IX in hemophilia B. It is a disease that affects almost exclusively males. Based on the residual coagulation factor activity level, the disease is classified as severe (<1%), moderate (1–5%), or mild (5–40%).

The most common presentation is an increased bleeding tendency; recurrent hemarthrosis is the distinctive sign of severe hemophilia and may lead to hemophilic arthropathy, a disease causing pain and affecting the patients' quality of life. Women are asymptomatic carriers and may rarely have acquired hemophilia (immunological origin).

A. Muda
Department of Radiology, IRCCS Policlinico San Martino-IST, Genova, Italy

F. Martino (✉)
Radiology, Sant'Agata Diagnostic Center, Bari, Italy

Hemorrhagic events may occur starting from the first years of life, particularly when children start to walk (this demonstrates the importance of mechanical forces in triggering the bleed).

In patients affected by hemophilia, bleeding may be spontaneous or may follow a trauma. The most common type of hemorrhage is the intra-articular one, which can take place anywhere, but the most affected areas are the large synovial joints of the knees, elbows, and ankles. The predilection for these sites is probably related to the abundant vascularization of synovial tissue and to the combination between deficiency of clotting factors and intensive mechanical forces.

After a single bleed, alterations seem to be transient, except for vascular changes that are probably irreversible and increase the risk of recurrent bleeding. Therefore, in case of repeated bleedings, the synovial cleaning capacity might be damaged, resulting in iron accumulation with deposits of hemosiderin. This event generates hemoglobin-mediated inflammation, neo-angiogenesis, synovial hyperplasia, and bone degeneration. The latter alterations are related to degenerative arthropathy and are characterized

F. Martino et al. (eds.), *Musculoskeletal Ultrasound in Orthopedic and Rheumatic disease in Adults*,
https://doi.org/10.1007/978-3-030-91202-4_18

by the development of cysts, osteophytes, subchondral sclerosis, epiphyseal enlargement, and osteoporosis.

Conservative treatment and orthopedic approach are the only therapeutic options for hemophilic arthropathy. For this reason, with the purpose of recognizing early changes in joints and preventing the progression of this disease-related arthropathy, periodic US monitoring of the joint has been recommended.

18.2 Diagnostic Imaging

Clinical confirmation of hemarthrosis and changes in synovial and osteochondral structures is essential for the selection process among the options available for the treatment of patients with hemophilia. Even when the presence of a muscle hematoma is suspected, it is essential to demonstrate its presence, undertake the most appropriate therapy, and avoid complications. Given the absence of biomarkers or other laboratory results that could help diagnose musculoskeletal abnormalities in hemophilic patients, imaging techniques are used to provide objective information on joint status and improve the efficacy and timeliness of treatment.

X-rays are widely available and may capture advanced joint changes but are insensitive to early change and unreliable for cartilage and soft-tissue evaluation. X-ray grading systems/scores include the Arnold–Hilgartner score (progressive, soft-tissue assessment included) and widely used Pettersson score (additive, soft tissue excluded). Instead, MRI and ultrasound have been shown to be particularly effective in detecting early changes in soft and osteochondral tissue in patients with hemophilia, before such changes become evident on physical examination or simple radiographs. However, MRI is not easily accessible and may require sedation in young children. The pathological conditions that can be demonstrated with sonography are synovial hyperplasia, hemarthrosis, bursal bleeding (Fig. 18.1), joint effusion, erosions of the articular cartilage (where visible), changes in the bone surface, muscle hematoma, and pseudotumor.

Spontaneous bleeding into the muscle occurs between 10% and 23% of hemorrhagic episodes in the musculoskeletal system, and may involve any muscle, even in the absence of trauma. The forearm, quadriceps, calf, and iliopsoas are most often involved, the latter having particularly severe clinical presentation (Fig. 18.2a–c).

When muscle hemorrhage is suspected, confirmation should be obtained by imaging. Hence, immediate enhanced on-demand hematological treatment must be started until the complete disappearance of the hematoma. If untreated, muscle bleeding can cause complications such as nerve injury, compartment syndrome, myositis ossificans, pseudotumor, and even infection.

Recurrent hemarthrosis can induce early villous hyperplasia of the synovium and, subsequently, a characteristic hemophilic arthropathy. Ultrasound is useful to detect early stages of hemophilic arthropathy, as opposed to conventional radiology that is not able to show synovial proliferation and initial cartilaginous damage. Ultrasound is also crucial to monitor the hem-

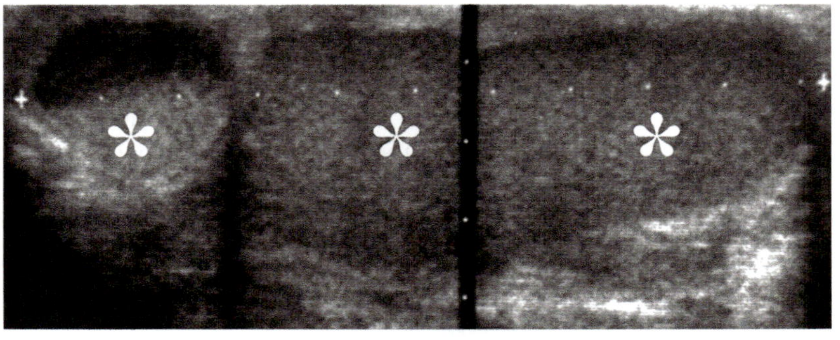

Fig. 18.1 Young male with severe hemophilia. Longitudinal US scan of the anterior aspect of the hip demonstrating enormous distention of the iliopectineal bursa (calipers) by echogenic effusion (asterisks) due to recent intra-bursal bleeding

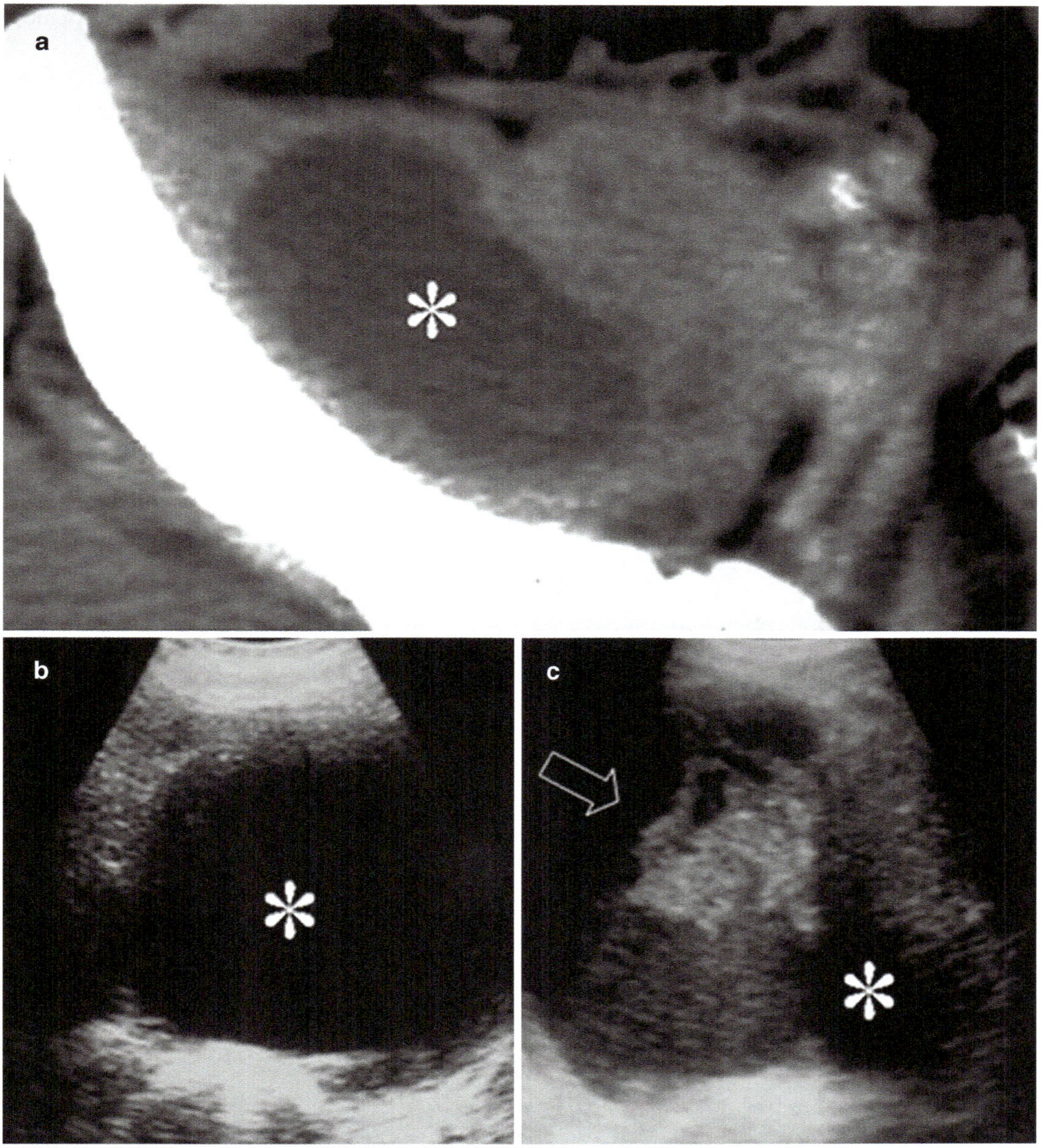

Fig. 18.2 (**a**–**c**) Patient with severe hemophilia. (**a**) Transverse non-contrast computed tomography (CT) scan detected an old iliopsoas hemorrhage, evident as an intramuscular area of hypodensity (*). (**b**) Transverse sonogram in the same patient depicts the echo-free appearance of the muscle hemorrhage (*). (**c**) Echographic control just after sudden recurrence of pain shows the presence of recent rebleeding (*empty white arrow*), which appears echogenic and easy to discriminate from the mostly reabsorbed previous hemorrhage (*)

orrhage and to investigate the response to treatment. An acute bleeding appears echogenic on sonography, because of the high reflectivity of fresh blood; another sign of acute bleeding is capsular distension (Fig. 18.3a, b).

Synovial hyperplasia can be observed as the presence of solid formations bulging in the synovial cavities (Fig. 18.4a, b). Ultrasound may also detect hemosiderin deposits that can be seen as hypoechoic areas in the context of the hypertrophied synovium, but when deposition of hemosiderin is bland it is difficult to distinguish it from the synovium.

Color and power Doppler ultrasound is used in some chronic inflammatory arthropathies to estimate disease activity by demonstrating hypervascular patterns. However, in hemophilic patients it is uncommon to observe Doppler positivity, with sporadic hypervascular "spots" indicating a moderate vascularization of this condition.

Given these considerations, the Doppler technique has low sensitivity in evaluating the vascular asset in this disease; this determines a marginal role of this technique in predicting recurrent bleeding, in orienting therapeutic choices, and in patient management in general.

Hemarthrosis can lead to excessive distension of the joint capsule, exerting compression against adjacent tissues; at elbow it may result in cubital tunnel syndrome by compression of the ulnar nerve (Fig. 18.5).

In the knee, hemarthrosis leads to joint capsule distension, mainly of the suprapatellar recess.

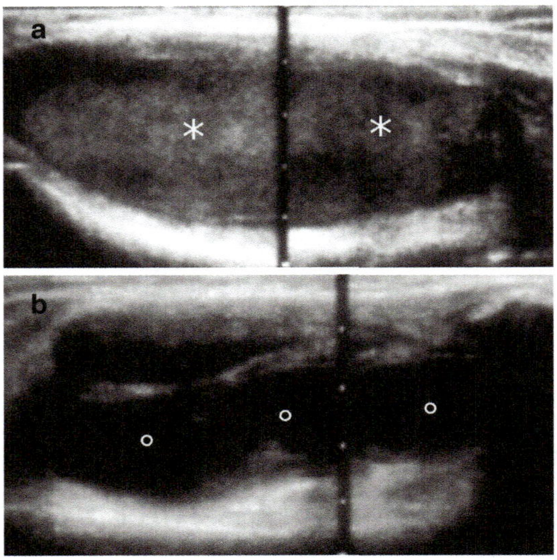

Fig. 18.3 Ultrasound view of the knee joint of 15-year-old patient with severe hemophilia. Note the acute hemarthrosis (**a**) characterized by the hyperechoic effusion (*asterisks*). A check performed after 7 days (**b**) shows the anechoic aspect of joint bleeding (*circles*)

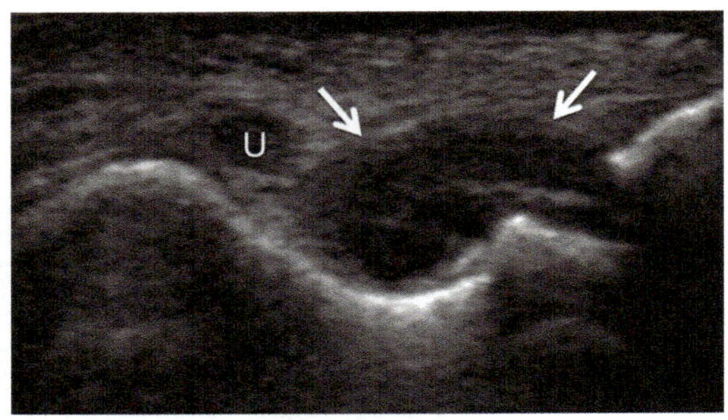

Fig. 18.5 Ultrasound of the elbow cubital tunnel showing capsular swelling (*arrows*) by chronic hemarthrosis and consequent compression and dislocation of the ulnar nerve (U)

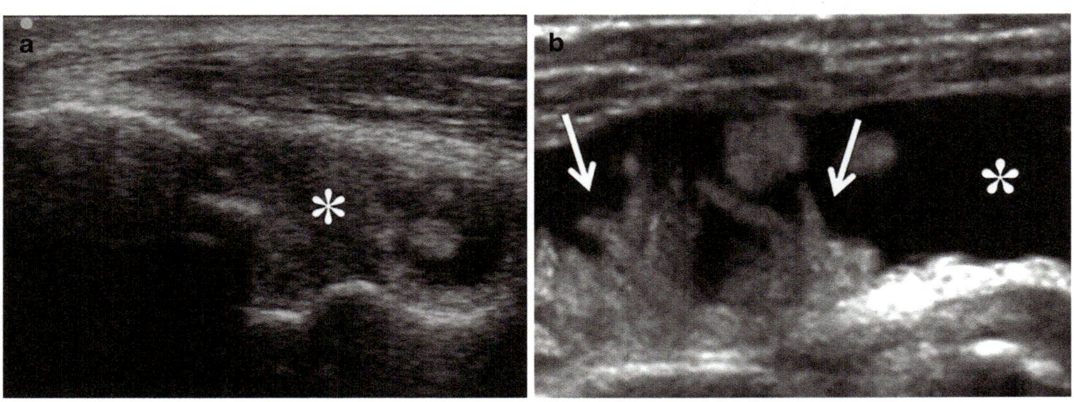

Fig. 18.4 Recurrent hemarthrosis in hemophilic patients. (**a**) Sagittal posterior scan of the elbow shows capsular swelling, filled by synovial polypoid tissue (*asterisk*). (**b**) Transverse US scan of the knee depicts the suprapatellar synovial recess which appears distended from abundant anechoic effusion (*asterisk*), related to previous hemarthrosis. Synovial villous thickening is also depicted (*arrows*) (Image courtesy of MD Martella L, Lecce)

At the beginning, the articular cartilage changes are characterized only by a decrease in its natural echogenicity, and then the persistence of the damaging insult results in loss of thickness. When the cartilage is almost completely reabsorbed, initial subchondral bone alterations might become evident. Ultrasound can detect superficial alterations in subchondral bone, such as osteophytes, surface irregularities, and cysts. Bone erosions and cysts are different; the former are in continuity with the bone surface, and the latter instead have no contact with it and can be peripheral or central. Ultrasound emerges as the most efficient tool for the early detection of arthropathy, and the HEAD-US score (scoring method for Haemophilia Early Arthropathy Detection with Ultrasound) can be used for the consistent assessment of hemophilic joints optimizing the management of destructive changes. A simplified scanning and scoring method of this procedure was proposed by Martinoli (2013). Sonography has technical limitations in detecting most of the central subchondral cysts, and in investigating the medullary bone and the surfaces deep in the joint cavity.

These weaknesses make ultrasound less comprehensive than MR imaging; nevertheless, echography has several advantages: it is faster and less expensive, it can evaluate multiple joints in the same session thanks to its quickness, it avoids ferromagnetic interactions and claustrophobia problems, it can be adapted to patients with movement limitations, and it allows dynamic study.

Further Readings

Debkowska MP, Cotterell IH, Riley AJ. Case report: acute cubital tunnel syndrome in a hemophiliac patient. SAGE Open Med Case Rep. 2019;7:1–3.

Di Minno MND, Pasta G, Airaldi S, Zaottini F, Storino A, Cimino E, Martinoli C. Ultrasound for early detection of joint disease in patients with hemophilic arthropathy. J Clin Med. 2017;6(8):77.

Doria AS, Keshava SN, Mohanta A, Jarrin J, Blanchette V, Srivastava A, et al. Diagnostic accuracy of ultrasound for assessment of hemophilic Arthropathy: MRI correlation. AJR. 2015;204(3):W336–47.

Klukowska A, Czyrny Z, Laguna P, Brzewski M, Serafin-Krol MA, Rokicka-Milewska R. Correlation between clinical, radiological and ultrasonographical image of knee joints in children with haemophilia. Haemophilia. 2001;7:286–92.

Martino F, Silvestri E, Grassi W, Garlaschi G. Musculoskeletal sonography. Milan, Berlin, Heidelberg, New York: Springer; 2006.

Martinoli C, Della Casa Alberighi O, Di Minno G, et al. Development and definition of a simplified scanning procedure and scoring method for Haemophilia early Arthropathy detection with ultrasound (HEAD-US). Thromb Haemost. 2013;109:1170–9.

Soliman M, Daruge P, Dertkigil SSJ, De Avila FE, Negrao JR, de Aguiar Vilela MS, et al. Imaging of haemophilic arthropathy in growing joints: pitfalls in ultrasound and MRI. Haemophilia. 2017;23(5):660–72.

Van Vulpen LFD, Holstein K, Martinoli C. Joint disease in haemophilia: pathophysiology, pain and imaging. Haemophilia. 2018;24(Suppl. 6):44–9.

Zhang CM, Zhang JF, Xu J, Guo YL, Wang G, Yang LH. Musculoskeletal ultrasonography for arthropathy assessment in patients with hemophilia: a single-center cross-sectional study from Shanxi Province. China Medicine (Baltimore). 2018;97(46):e13230.

Part III

Ultrasound Pathologic Findings in Orthopedic Diseases

Bone Trauma

19

Luca Cavagnaro, Davide Orlandi, Enzo Silvestri, Armanda De Marchi, and Elena Massone

Contents

19.1 Introduction

The use of ultrasound (US) in musculoskeletal medicine has evolved rapidly over the last two decades. This is due to the advantage of having introduced high-resolution linear broadband multifrequency probe and the clinical collaboration which allows an accurate management of the traumatic patient. However, despite this, US is not routinely used for fracture detection.

The normal bone appears like a hyperechoic line with posterior acoustic shadow due to the complete reflection of the US waves. This straight regular interface separates the bone from the soft tissues allowing a clear distinction between the two structures. A fracture is visualized as a break of the echogenic surface of the bony cortex. The modifications of peripheral soft tissue depend on the time when the fracture occurred (Fig. 19.1).

One cadaver study showed that US can be used to accurately detect cortical disruption as small as 1 mm. US is noninvasive; it can provide both real-time and dynamic multiple plane

L. Cavagnaro
Ortopedia e Traumatologia 2- Joint Replacement, Unit/Bone Infection Unit, Ospedale Santa Corona, Pietra Ligure, Italy

D. Orlandi (✉)
Department of Radiology, Ospedale Evangelico Internazionale, Genova, Italy

E. Silvestri
Radiology, Alliance Medical, Genova, Italy

A. De Marchi
Radiologia CIDIMU: Centro Italiano di Diagnostica Medica Ultrasonica, Torino, Italy

E. Massone
Department of Radiology, Ospedale Santa Corona, Pietra Ligure (SV), Italy

F. Martino et al. (eds.), *Musculoskeletal Ultrasound in Orthopedic and Rheumatic disease in Adults*,
https://doi.org/10.1007/978-3-030-91202-4_19

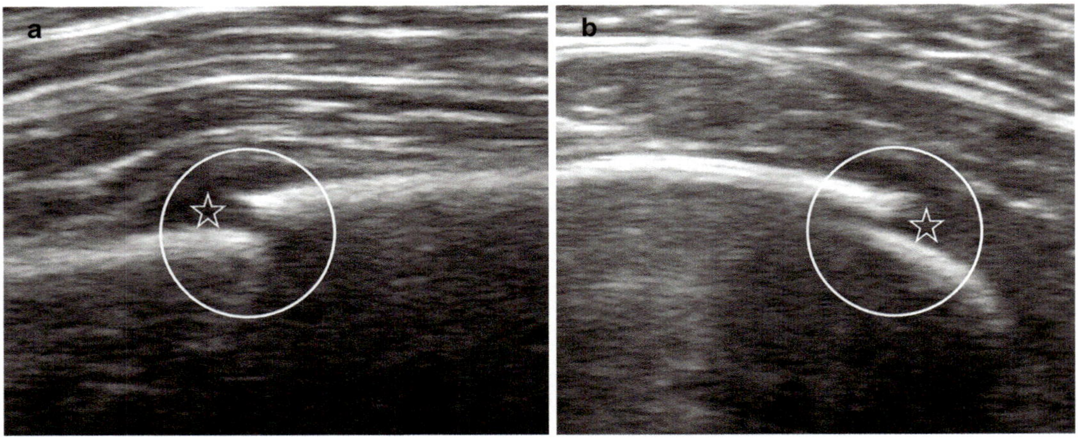

Fig. 19.1 Longitudinal (**a**) and transverse (**b**) scan of a rib. A focal disruption in the cortex line is evident (*circles*) with a small amount of hematoma in the soft tissue (*stars*)

images and does not emit ionizing radiation. The ultrasonography is performed with a high-frequency transducer 10–18 MHz for the superficial bone (e.g., metatarsal shaft) and with a lower frequency transducer (5–10 MHz) for bones with deeper localization (e.g., femur), in two-dimensional mode. This modality is particularly useful in vulnerable population such as children and pregnant women who are particularly sensible to such radiation. The clinical data like pain, swelling, ecchymosis, and/or deformity represent the important starting point in ultrasonographic examination. The probe is placed perpendicular to the region and studies each bone in longitudinal and axial planes. Some authors noted that the evaluation method involving more planes allows a circumferential view of each bone, reducing the risk of not detecting the fractures.

In some difficult anatomical regions it is useful to perform a comparative image to use as a reference. In fact in some traumatic cases, it is hard to differentiate nonpathological marginal irregularities, osteophytes, or vascular channels from fractures.

19.2 Fractures

In acute trauma, ultrasonography does not represent the first imaging modality for diagnosing bone fractures. Standard radiographs can diagnose the majority of fractures and assess the dislocation of bony ends. In particular, in complex anatomical areas diagnosis and fracture extension determination can be performed with CT. US may be useful for patients with persistent localized pain, 2–3 weeks after trauma, with negative initial radiographic examination.

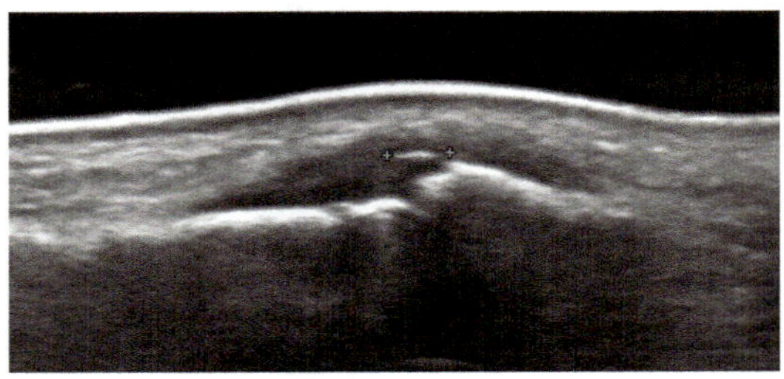

Fig. 19.2 Longitudinal US scan of the extensor region of the third finger of the hand shows a small avulsed bony fragment (*calipers*)

Ultrasonography is able to visualize irregularity, defect, and discontinuity in the cortical margin as well as small bone fragment avulsion (Fig. 19.2).

One of the most common bone defects is the Hill-Sachs lesion, an irregular depression in the posterolateral aspect of the humeral head due to anterior shoulder dislocation. US is also an efficient modality to assess the bone size and depth in a Hill-Sachs lesion (Fig. 19.3).

Compared to surgery, US has 96% sensitivity, 100% specificity, and 97% accuracy in the diagnosis. Several reports have described the usefulness of US in diagnosing nondisplaced fractures that are difficult to see on standard radiographs such as ribs, scaphoid, metatarsus, clavicle, orbit, femur, and humerus. In the chest, US can also help to differentiate rib fractures from metastases. Several articles have pointed out the utility of US for detecting fractures in pediatric population in particular in bone diagnosis of long bone fractures in children, those of the distal forearm, with good sensitivity and specificity in comparison with radiographs. In a previous study of 26

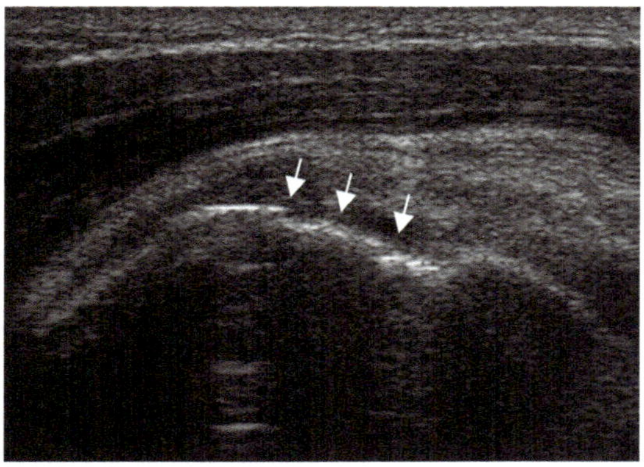

Fig. 19.3 Longitudinal scan of the humerus head: Hill-Sachs fracture shows a cortical depression in the posterior-superior portion of the humeral head (*white arrows*)

uncomplicated torus and greenstick pediatric forearms, investigators achieved 100% sensitivity and specificity in the identification of these fractures. In recent literature, in emergency department the sensitivity and specificity of distal forearm bone fractures compared with radiography were 94.4% and 96.8%, respectively.

As known in literature and as proved in another study conducted in the same emergency condition US is extremely efficient also in other anatomical sites in detecting the long bone fractures, with 100% sensitivity in humerus and femoral mid-shaft fractures. This can confirm what some authors have already suggested in previous studies that bedside US is highly specific in the detection of bone fractures. US is particularly useful for detecting fractures in the immature skeleton of children. In young sportsmen an avulsion fracture is frequently recognized when the growth plate of an apophysis is injured due to a sudden and forceful contraction of the attaching musculotendinous unit (Fig. 19.4).

Adolescents are those who usually sustain these injuries, and there is a significant male preponderance. However, in many of these studies, US was more effective in detecting fractures of large bones. In addition US was less reliable for compound injuries and fractures adjacent to joint,

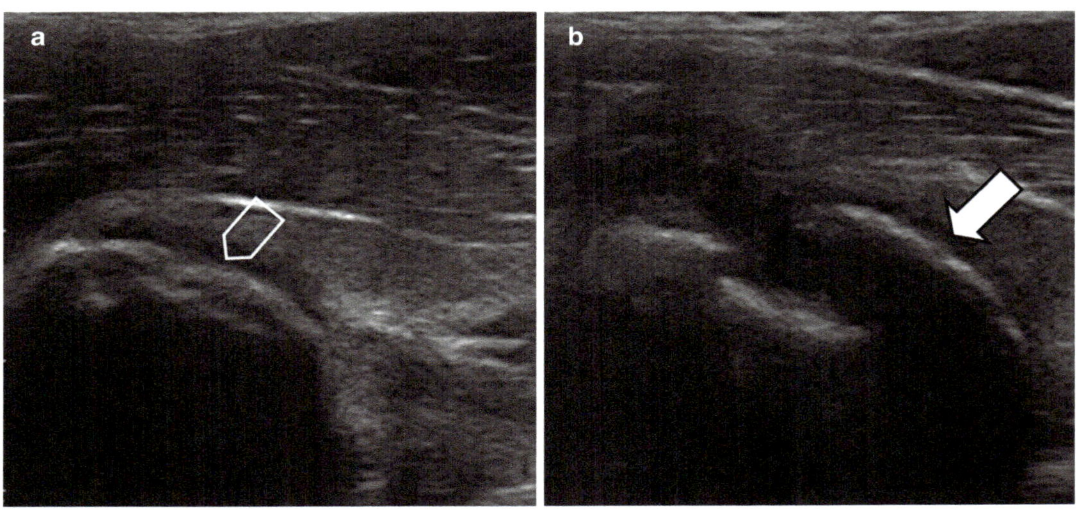

Fig. 19.4 Longitudinal scan of the anterior inferior iliac spine. (**a**) Normal US aspect (*open arrow*) and (**b**) avulsion (*white arrow*) of the anterior inferior iliac spine

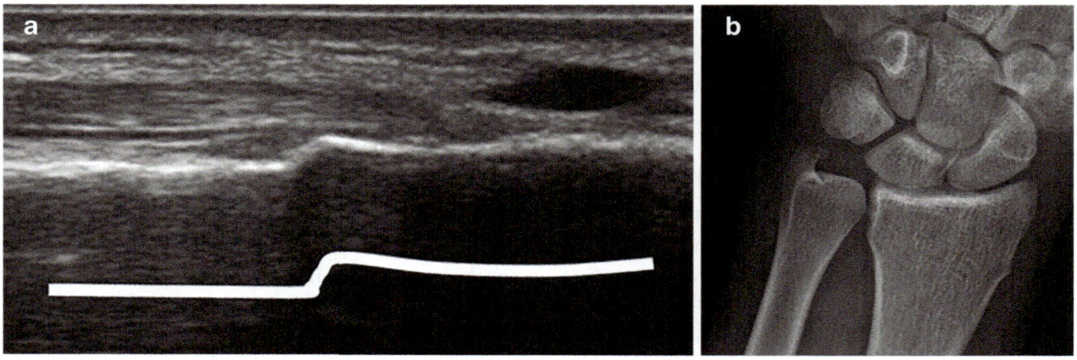

Fig. 19.5 (**a**) Longitudinal scan of the distal radius evidences a bulging of the cortex in "torus fracture" involving the distal radial metaphysis (*white line*). (**b**) Corresponding X-ray confirming the "torus fracture"

lesions of the small bone of the hand and foot, and undisplaced epiphyseal fractures. A cortical discontinuity after a direct or indirect trauma has an important diagnostic value in the management of pediatric and adult patients. The sonography can illustrate bone alignment, which is crucial also during treatment avoiding multiple attempts with conventional radiographic techniques. The sonographic monitoring can provide real-time observation that can guide and confirm the closed reduction of extra-articular distal radial fractures (Fig. 19.5a, b).

19.3 Stress Fractures

Stress fractures are caused by repetitive force, often from overuse in sportsmen: fatigue fractures. These can also develop from the normal use of a bone that is weakened by a condition such as osteoporosis: insufficiency fractures.

In stress fractures the standard radiography is negative and the fracture can only be seen once the reparative calcified callus is formed. A clinical history focused on the length, time, and mechanism of injury must be stressed. The possibility to localize and limit the examination to the site of injury represents the advantage of the US over CT and MRI.

With the development of high-resolution probes US is providing an excellent method for detecting occult fracture. Patients in whom a fracture is not suspected because no history of injury is recalled may complain pain in a swollen area. In these cases the sonographic evaluation targeted to the tender area can show a soft-tissue thickening, a focal periosteal reaction, or a cortical discontinuity and local hematoma. Also cortical irregularities and hypertrophic changes may be visualized before they are seen on plain radiographs or MRI.

The lower limbs, in particular foot and ankle, are body areas that are most commonly exposed to trauma. US can be helpful in assessing early metatarsal stress fractures. In addition according to the results of a recent paper US has high sensitivity, high specificity, negative predictive value of about 100%, and favorable likelihood ratios in the diagnosis of metatarsal fractures. However, the tibia is the most commonly implicated in runners besides metatarsal bone. In this setting, the US diagnosis of tibia stress fractures has only been reported in a few cases.

In the upper limbs, literature shows that in about 20–25% of patients with a scaphoid fracture initial radiographs are negative leading to a delayed diagnosis. The diagnostic accuracy when performing US examination always depends on a good knowledge of the normal US anatomy. In fact, concerning the scaphoid trauma, a focal US irregularity of the cortex can show the normal aspect of tuberosity.

The ultrasound may help in the diagnosis showing indirect signs of traumatic lesions like

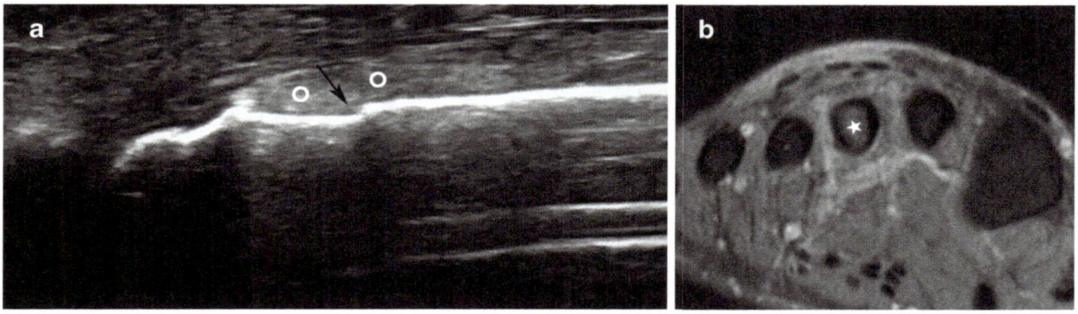

Fig. 19.6 (**a**) US longitudinal image obtained over the diaphysis of the metatarsal shows a non-displaced fracture (*black arrow*) and hyperechogenicity of the surrounding soft tissue with periosteal thickening (*white circles*). (**b**) MRI T2 axial image shows bone marrow edema (*white star*) of the third metatarsal bone with surrounding periosteal and soft-tissue reaction

an articular fluid effusion. A particular site frequently negative on radiographs is the sternal region where fractures are visible in 8–10% of patients with blunt trauma in the chest. The diagnosis of sternal radiography is often delayed. Sonography is easy to perform on a patient who is lying down. Even if several reports have described the usefulness of US in diagnosing sternal fractures some authors think that computed tomography represents the best imaging modality and is superior to sonography in sternal evaluation. In this setting, the differences in the US imaging aspect of bone injuries could be due to the different qualities of US devices used.

In more recent literature the bone stress lesion has showed different US aspects depending on the age, gender, history of repetitive sport activity, and anatomical region involved. In the site of pain the hyperechogenicity of the surrounding soft tissue indicates edema and inflammatory reaction without cortical alteration. The thickening of the periosteum, the cortical disruption, and an increased periosteal color Doppler flow in the bone lesion sites are evident signs of bone injury (Fig. 19.6).

Stress fractures are especially prominent in individuals who suddenly increase physical activity. It is important to diagnose stress fractures early to prevent bone remodeling, nonunion injuries, and loss of function. It is well known that radiographs have oftentimes yielded negative results until one callus is formed, for several reasons: the small size of the fracture, the limited movement of the patient due to pain, and the absence of significant displacement. Early diagnosis in this case depends on MRI or on bone scan scintigraphy, which is considered to be the "gold standard." The high cost of these imaging modalities, the poor accessibility of MRI, and the exposure to ionizing radiation of the scintigraphy make US the chosen imaging modality. The sonographic findings correlated well with MRI. In stress fractures, US offers dynamic images in a noninvasive, fast, and inexpensive manner. With high-quality equipment, experience, and academic ability of ultrasound operators, US can become an important and useful advantageous tool in the evaluation of fractures and occult injuries.

Further Readings

Arni D, et al. Insufficiency fracture of the calcaneum: sonographic findings. J Clin Ultrasound. 2009;37:424–7.

Backhaus M, et al. Guidelines for musculoskeletal ultrasound in rheumatology. Ann Rheum Dis. 2011;60:641–9.

Banal F, et al. Sensitivity and specificity of ultrasonography in early diagnosis of metatarsal bone stress fractures: a pilot study of 37 patients. J Rheumatol. 2009;36:1715–9.

Banal F, et al. Ultrasound ability in early diagnosis of stress fracture of metatarsal bone. Ann Rheum Dis. 2006;65(7):977–8.

Betrame V, et al. Sonographic evaluation of bone fractures: a reliable alternative in clinical practice? Clin Imaging. 2012;36:303–8.

Bodner G, et al. Sonographic findings in stress fractures of the lower limb: preliminary findings. Eur Radiol. 2005;15:356–9.

Canagasabey MD, et al. The sonographic Ottawa Foot and Ankle Rules study (the SOFAR study). Emerg Med J EMJ. 2011;28(10):838–40.

Cho KH, et al. Sonography of bone and bone-related diseases of the extremities. J Clin Ultrasound. 2004;32:511–21.

Cicak N, et al. Hill-Sachs lesion in recurrent shoulder dislocation: sonographic detection. J Ultrasound Med. 1998;17:557–60.

Engin G, et al. US versus conventional radiography in the diagnosis of sternal fractures. Acta Radiol. 2000;41:296–9.

Environmental Protection Agency. Radiation protection. 2013. http://www.cdc.gov/rpdweboo/health_effects.html. Accessed 1 Feb 2013.

Galletebeitia Laka I, et al. The utility of clinical ultrasonography in identifying distal forearm fractures in the pediatric emergency department. Eur J Emerg Med. 2019;26(2):118–22.

Graif M, et al. Sonographic detection of occult bone fracture. Pediatr Radiol. 1988;18:383–5.

Greaney RB, et al. Distribution and natural history of stress fractures in U.S. Marine recruits. Radiology. 1983;146(2):339–46.

Grechenig W, et al. Scope and limitation of ultrasonography in the documentation of fractures-an experimental study. Arch Ortop Trauma Surg. 1998;117:368–71.

Griffith JF, et al. Sonography compared with radiography in revealing acute rib fracture. AJR Am J Roentgenol. 1999;173:1603–9.

Hamer D-d, et al. Ultrasound for distal forearm fractures: a systematic review and diagnostic meta-analysis. PLoS One. 2016;11:e0155659.

Hills MW, et al. Sternal fracture: associated injuries and management. J Trauma. 1993;35:55–60.

Hodgkinson DW, et al. Scaphoid fracture: a new method of assessment. Clin Radiol. 1993;48:398.

Hubner U, et al. Ultrasound in the diagnosis of fractures in children. J Bone Joint Surg Br. 2000;82:1170–3.

Hurley ME, et al. Is ultrasound really helpful in the detection of rib fractures? Injury. 2004;35:562–6.

Jones SL, Phillips M. Early identification of foot and lower limb stress fractures using diagnostic ultrasonography: a review of three cases. Foot Ankle Online J. 2010;3:3.

Khy V, et al. Bilateral stress fracture of the tibia diagnosed by ultrasound: a case report. J Ultrasound. 2012;15:130–4.

Krestan C, Hojreh A. Imaging of insufficiency fractures. Eur J Radiol. 2009;71(3):398–405.

Lazovic D, et al. Ultrasound of diagnosis of apophyseal injuries. Knee Surg Sport Traumatol Rtrosc. 1996;3:234–7.

Marshburn TH, et al. Goal-directed ultrasound in the detection of long-bone fractures. J Trauma. 2004;57:329–32.

McNeil CR, et al. The accuracy of portable ultrasonography to diagnose fractures in an austere environment. Prehosp Emerg Care. 2009;13:50–2.

Mohsen E, et al. Diagnostic accuracy of ultrasonography in diagnosis of metatarsal bone fracture: a cross-sectional study. Arch Acad Emerg Med. 2019;7(1):e49.

Nicholson JA, et al. What is the role of ultrasound in fracture management? Diagnosis and therapeutic potential for fractures, delayed unions, and fracture-related infection. Bone J Res. 2019;8(7):304–12.

Pancione L. Diagnosis of Hill-Sachs lesion of the shoulder. Comparison between ultrasonography and arthro-CT. Acta Radiol. 1997;38:523–6.

Papalada A, et al. Ultrasound as a primary evaluation tool of bone stress injuries in elite track and field athletes. Am J Sports Med. 2012;40:915–9.

Patel DS, et al. Stress fracture: diagnosis, treatment, and prevention. Am Fam Physician. 2011;83:39–46.

Patten RM, et al. Nondisplaced fractures of the greater tuberosity of the humerus: sonographic detection. Radiology. 1992;182:201–4.

Pohl M, et al. Biomechanical predictors of retrospective tibial stress fractures in runners. J Biomech. 2008;41:1160–5.

Romani WA, et al. Identification of tibial stress fractures using therapeutic continuous ultrasound. J Orthop Sports Phys Ther. 2000;30:442–52.

Sayed A, et al. Ultrasonography of occult fractures: a pictorial essay. Can Assoc Radiol J. 2001;52(5):312–21.

Sofka CM. Imaging of stress fractures. Clin Sport Med. 2006;25:53–62.

Tai-Chang C, et al. Sonography of monitoring closed reduction of displaced extra-articular distal radial fractures. J Bone Joint Surg Am. 2002;84(2):194–203.

Warden S, et al. Stress fractures: pathophysiology, epidemiology, and risk factors. Curr Osteoporos Rep. 2006;4:103–9.

Weinberg ER, et al. Accuracy of the clinician performed point of care ultrasound for the diagnosis of fractures in children and young adults. Injury. 2010;41:862–8.

Williamson D, et al. Ultrasound imaging of forearm fractures in children: a viable alternative? J Accid Emerg Med. 2000;17:22–4.

Wook Jin MD, et al. Diagnostic value of sonography for assessment of sterna fractures compared with conventional radiography and bone scan. J Ultrasound Med. 2006;25:1263–8.

Muscle Injury

20

Giulio Pasta, Davide Orlandi, Enzo Silvestri, Biagio Moretti, Lorenzo Moretti, Davide Bizzoca, Piero Volpi, and Gian Nicola Bisciotti

Contents

G. Pasta
Specialista in Radiologia e Diagnostica per Immagini, Studio Associato di Radiologia Dr. Pasta, Emilia-Romagna, Italy

D. Orlandi (✉)
Department of Radiology, Ospedale Evangelico Internazionale, Genova, Italy

E. Silvestri
Radiology, Alliance Medical, Genova, Italy

B. Moretti · L. Moretti · D. Bizzoca
Orthopedic & Trauma Unit, Department of Basic Medical Sciences, Neuroscience and Sense Organs, University of Bari "Aldo Moro", AOU Consorziale "Policlinico", Bari, Italy

P. Volpi
IRCCS Humanitas Research Hospital, Milano, Italy

G. N. Bisciotti
Kinemove Rehabilitation Centers, Pontremoli (SP), Italy

20.1 Introduction

Muscle injuries are frequently related to sport activities but also to daily and working life. Muscle injuries represent the most common traumatic event in the field of sports medicine, which account for up to 30% of all sports-related pathology. For example, considering professional football players, the most frequently affected anatomical area by "time-loss injuries" (e.g., all those accidents that force the athlete to stop practicing the sport, causing a significant impact on the team) is the thigh (with hamstrings being the most commonly involved muscle group), followed by the knee, ankle, and groin.

When facing a muscle injury, a diagnostic hypothesis could be formulated looking at the clinical data (patient history and physical examination). Then, a complete patient history collec-

F. Martino et al. (eds.), *Musculoskeletal Ultrasound in Orthopedic and Rheumatic disease in Adults*,
https://doi.org/10.1007/978-3-030-91202-4_20

tion (symptoms, mechanism of trauma, previous accidents) and a thorough physical examination (ecchymosis and swelling, muscle palpation, and positivity to clinical tests), together with proper diagnostic imaging, allow to reach a precise diagnosis.

Considering the high incidence of muscle injuries in sports, efforts have been made in order to reduce the number of these accidents. The first step in this direction has been the attempt to establish an unequivocal, universally recognized classification of muscle injuries.

In the last century, several classifications were proposed:

- O'Donoghue, 1962.
- Ryan, 1969.
- American College of Sports Medicine,1980.
- Takebayashi, 1995.
- Stoller, 2007.

Nowadays, especially in Italy, the most commonly used classification is the one proposed in 2000 by the **Isokinetic** group of Dr. Nanni, which is very practical, functional, and schematic, based on the pathogenesis, clinics, and imaging.

However, by the end of 2012 some new classifications emerged that revolutionized the field of muscular injury classifications.

The first classification, proposed by **Maffulli-Chan**, is more anatomy-oriented and based on echo-MR imaging, allows to accurately define the anatomical site of the injury, and therefore is more precise in terms of prognosis and healing times, which is extremely important for professional sports teams (although it is advisable to integrate imaging with clinical data). The authors believe that imaging is important not only to understand which athletes can be submitted to surgical intervention in case of high-grade musculotendinous lesions, but also to anticipate when the athlete will be able to return to the field.

Later in 2012, the so-called **Munich consensus classification** was proposed, similarly based on echo-MRI. This classification, more clinically oriented than the previous one, divides muscle lesions into various subgroups based on clinical and imaging features. The relevance of this classification lies in the fact that the previous classifications lacked subgroups and therefore muscle lesions with different etiology, clinics, treatment, and prognosis were classified into the same group.

If on the one hand the Maffulli-Chan classification was important because of its anatomical accuracy (that allows to discriminate between the different locations of lesions and therefore understand that, for example, a lesion in the proximal third of the hamstrings is more severe than a lesion in the distal third and requires a longer recovery time), on the other hand it could have the limitation of not being very clinical, while the Munich classification is very precise in clinical, but not anatomical, terms.

Hence, the I.S.Mu.L.T. decided to integrate these two classifications to produce a classification that in the near future could be universally recognized as an aid to the diagnostic and therapeutic process and:

- Allows a faster return to activity.
- Reduces complications.
- Minimizes relapses.

If we look at this new I.S.Mu.L.T. classification from an ultrasound imaging point of view, muscular lesions are divided into two broad categories depending on the mechanism of injury (Table 20.1):

- From direct trauma.
- From indirect trauma.

20.2 Imaging of Muscle Injuries

The two main techniques used for studying muscular lesions are ultrasound (US) and magnetic resonance imaging (MRI). These two techniques should be considered complementary and not mutually exclusive; however, it is clear that being able to always perform both is utopic, especially in the world of nonprofessional sports. Therefore, the best way forward is to use ultrasound as the first-level examination, considering MRI when US is inconclusive, when there is a mismatch between clinical examination and US, and for the assessment of severe injuries with tendon involvement.

Table 20.1 Classification of muscle injuries according to the I.S.Mu.L.T guidelines

Injury	Division	Type	Classification	Definition	US/MRI
Indirect	Nonstructural injury	I: Muscle disorder related to overexertion	1A: Fatigue induced 1B: DOMS (delayed-onset muscle soreness)	Sore, circumscribed increase of tone within a muscle. 1B: Widespread increase in muscle tone and pain that appears a few hours after physical activity	Ultrasound negative or with hypo/hyperechogenic zone that disappears after 3–5 days and negative power Doppler. MRI negative or with limited edema
		II: Neuromuscular disorder	2A: Neuromuscular related to vertebral column disorders and/or pelvis 2B: Neuromuscular related to muscle		
	Structural injury	III: Partial muscle injury	3A: Minor partial injury	Injury of one or more primary bundles within a secondary bundle	Positive for fiber ruptures. Intramuscular hematoma
			3B: Moderate partial injury	Injury of at least one secondary bundle, with an area of rupture involving <50% of the muscle surface	Positive for significant fiber rupture, including probable retractions. Lesions of the fascia and intermuscular hematoma
		IV: (sub)total muscle injury	4: Subtotal or total injury or tendon avulsion	Lesion involving >50% of the muscle surface (subtotal) or involving the whole muscle (total) or the osteotendinous junction	Subtotal or total musculotendinous discontinuity. Possible retraction and wavy tendon morphology. Lesions of the fascia and intermuscular hematoma
Direct		Contusion	Mild: >1/2 ROM Moderate: <1/2 and > 1/3 ROM Severe: <1/3 ROM	Direct trauma that causes diffuse or limited hematoma and causes pain and decreased ROM	Diffuse or circumscribed hematoma of variable size
		Tear			

Ultrasound is a valid tool in the identification and staging of muscle lesions, in the assessment of their evolution, and in the detection of complications thanks to its intrinsic characteristics (cheap, quick, repeatable, best anatomical detail of superficial structures, real-time dynamic imaging, easy vascularity assessment).

However, US also suffers from some disadvantages:

- Limited view (some sites are inaccessible because they are too deep or hidden or their morphology is difficult to study).
- Early assessment of tears is limited by a significantly reduced sensibility.
- Minor lesions could be undetectable.

These problems are solved with MRI, because of its intrinsic advantages:

- Multiparametricity (there are multiple sequences and in this case sequences with a high intrinsic contrast (fluid sensitive) are of particular importance, for example STIR and T2 that allow to discriminate even minor alterations).
- Sensitivity of 92%, compared to 76% of US.
- Panoramic view, based on the possibility to have a wider view on the affected area, also allowing exploration of sites that were inaccessible with US.

Even the current literature lacks consensus on which of the two exams is the gold standard and when is the best moment to perform imaging, also considering that MRI tends to overestimate the muscle tear assessment in its early phase and moreover that it is a static exam that cannot directly assess muscle tear stability. On the contrary, US slightly underestimates muscle tear size but is able to perform a dynamic assessment of the injury by performing a direct compression on the patient skin or asking to perform an active contraction of the affected muscle. This is essential, since it allows to examine the separation and dislocation of tertiary bundles and to evaluate the true extension of the lesion (Fig. 20.1).

Generally speaking, considering that the edematous-hemorrhagic fluid collection is greatest after 24 h and starts to decrease after 48 h, the best moment to perform muscle tear imaging is thought to be between 24 and 48 h from the trauma.

Another advantage of US is the possibility to use **color** and **power Doppler**. Doppler US is a technique that allows to visualize the main blood vessels and to study their blood flow thanks to real-time association of a bidimensional US image with a pulsed Doppler signal.

Essentially, color Doppler allows us to visualize the movement of blood inside the venous and arterial vessels and estimate how much blood reaches a certain structure or organ.

Power Doppler is similar to color Doppler but it measures the energy of the frequency of the examined structures, therefore producing a more sensitive signal (Fig. 20.2).

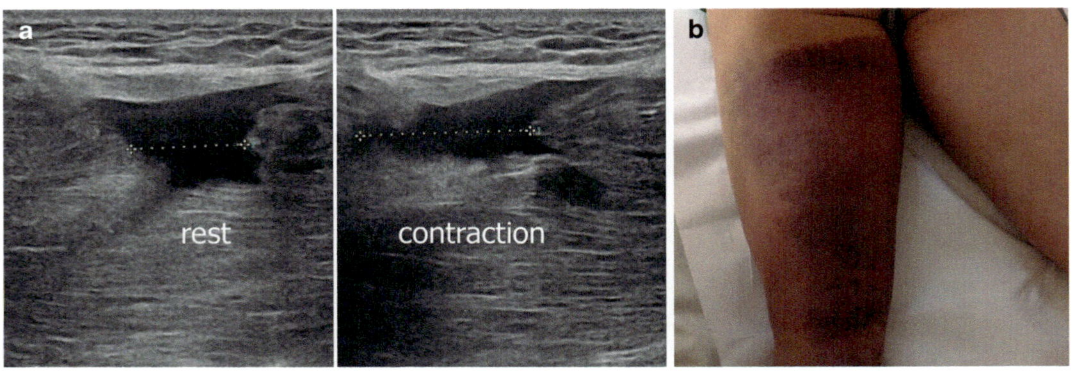

Fig. 20.1 Third-degree lesion at the proximal myotendinous junction (MTJ) of the left hamstring. (**a**) US performed during muscle relaxation and contraction, showing an increase in the gap. (**b**) Appearance of the injured thigh after a fall during an enduro race

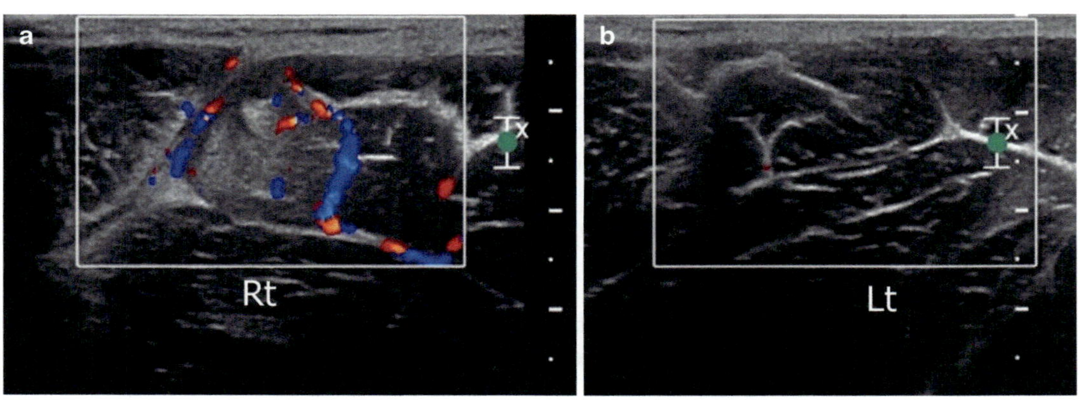

Fig. 20.2 Use of color Doppler for monitoring a second-degree lesion of the right proximal adductor longus. Notice the hypervascularization of the injured area (**a**) compared with the contralateral side (**b**)

Also sonoelastography (USE) can be useful in the follow-up of a structural lesion, even though this technique is still under development and the studies performed until now are still experimental and preliminary.

USE measures tissue distortion in response to an external force, assuming that the distortion will be less in harder tissues compared to softer tissues.

This technique is based on the comparison of ultrasound radio-frequency waves obtained before and after a slight tissue compression with a normal probe. Color pixels are assigned to the USE image based on the degree of dislocation with a range varying in a specific color which can be selected by the operator (e.g., from red (soft tissues) to blue (hard tissues)) (Fig. 20.3).

Let us see some examples of US examination in different types of muscle injuries:

- **Nonstructural injury.** US findings are negative or at most we can observe a slightly hyperechoic area due to edematous imbibition or a hypoechoic and suffused area, which disappears in 3–5 days (Fig. 20.4).

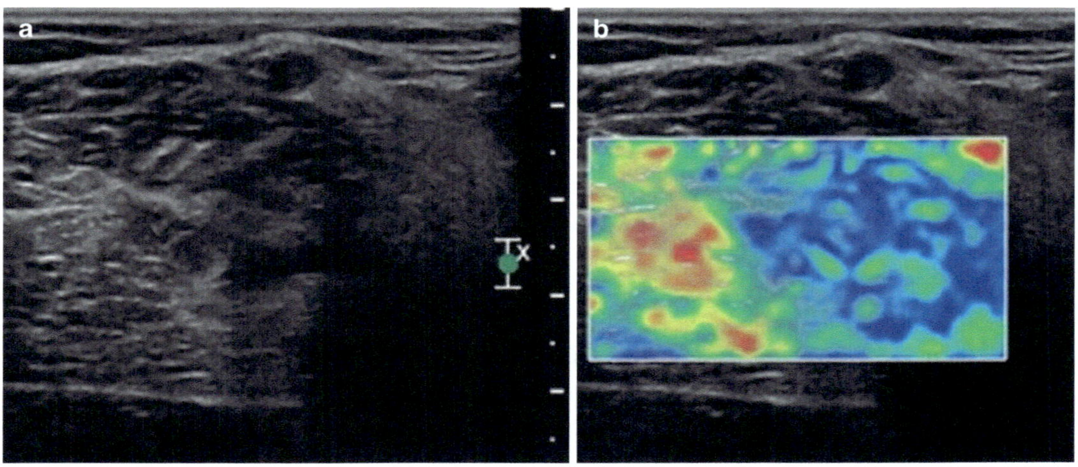

Fig. 20.3 Fibrosis of the semimembranosus. B-mode US scan (**a**) and corresponding real-time sonoelastography (**b**)

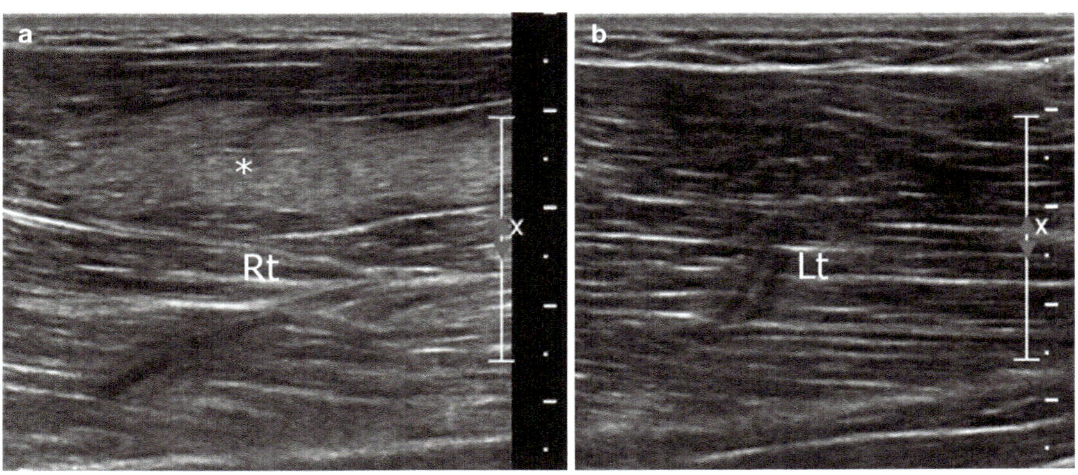

Fig. 20.4 US of a nonstructural alteration of the right semimembranosus (**a**). Note the increased echogenicity of the affected muscle fibers (*asterisk*) compared to the healthy contralateral muscle (**b**)

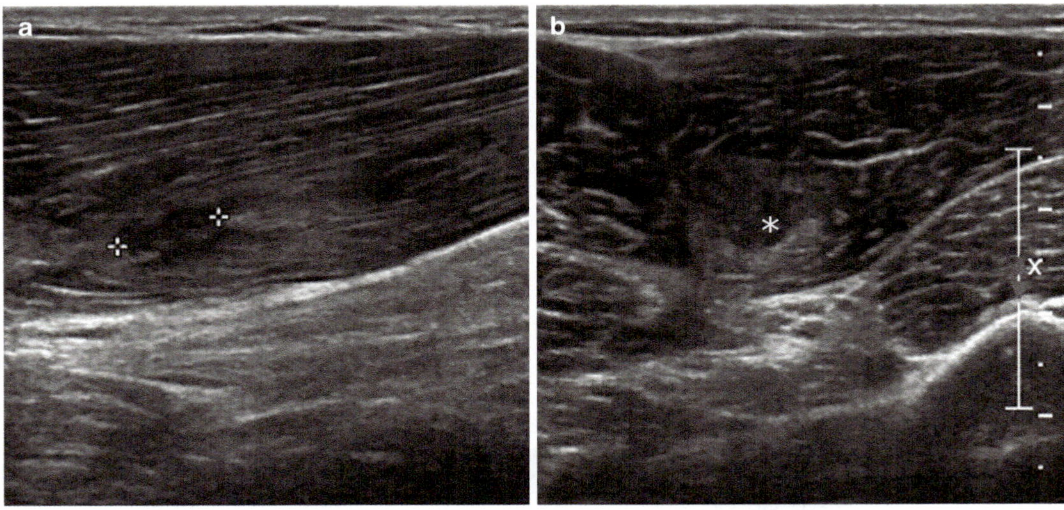

Fig. 20.5 Longitudinal (**a**) and transverse (**b**) US scan showing a small intramuscular anechoic area (asterisk) due to a minor partial lesion (3A) of the biceps femoris muscle

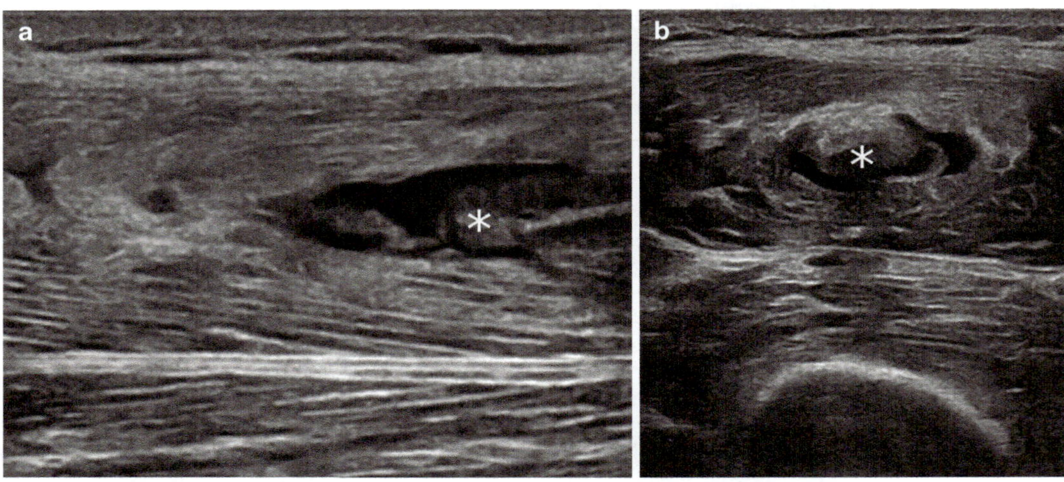

Fig. 20.6 Longitudinal (**a**) and transverse (**b**) US scan showing a moderate partial lesion (3B) of the rectus femoris muscle (*asterisk*)

- **Structural injury.** The ultrasound study shows the discontinuity of the muscle bundles, reactive edema, and hematoma. In case of complete rupture of the muscular belly, the retracted muscle bundles appear on the ultrasound with the typical bell-clapper image, surrounded by a hypoanechoic hematoma (Figs. 20.5, 20.6 and 20.7).

20.3 Classification of Muscle Injuries

As previously mentioned, it is becoming increasingly important to have a common terminology, which should be as international and as shared as possible, and should start from the classification of accidents and eventually help to establish a

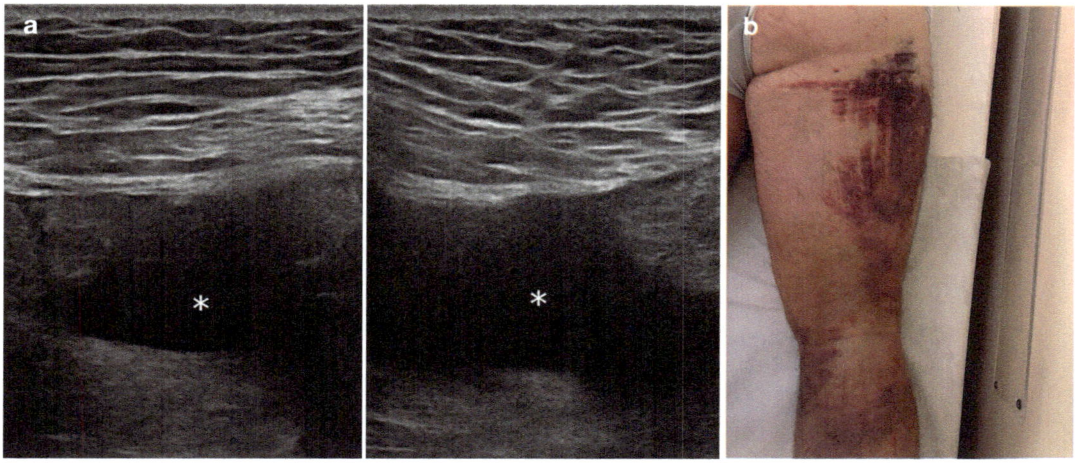

Fig. 20.7 Transverse (**a**) and longitudinal (**b**) US scan of a complete lesion (grade 4) of the proximal musculotendinous junction of the semimembranosus with a large hematoma (*asterisk*). Appearance of the injured thigh after a fall during a water-ski race

clear diagnosis, a precise prognosis, and an appropriate therapy.

The classification should therefore be precise, complete, and accessible also, and above all, by those who are not familiar with dealing with these accidents. We hereby consider the new I.S.Mu.L.T. classification for the next paragraph (Table 20.1).

20.3.1 Injuries from Direct Trauma

Injuries from direct trauma are caused by an external force acting against the muscle. The thigh muscles are most frequently affected (for example vastus intermedius muscle). They include (Table 20.2):

- Contusion, very common in athletes, caused by an external compressive force applied against the muscle (for example impact with an opponent).
- Laceration, rare in athletes, caused by a direct cut injury (impact against a structure with sharp edges, against opponent's soccer studs, etc.) involving the epimysium and the underlying muscle.

Table 20.2 Classification of muscle injuries from direct trauma (ROM: range of motion)

Contusion	**Mild:** >1/2 physiological ROM **Moderate**: <1/2 and >1/3 physiological ROM **Severe**: <1/3 physiological ROM	Direct trauma that causes diffuse or circumscribed hematoma, pain, and decreased ROM
Tear		

Lacerations are not classified into subgroups; the necessary therapy is surgical suturing and recovery times depend on the extent and depth of the lesion (Fig. 20.8).

Contusions are classified as mild, moderate, or severe (Fig. 20.9) depending on the functional impotence that derives from them, which is assessed as the ability to actively perform a movement at the level of the corresponding joint (the knee for the quadriceps, the hip for the gluteus maximus, etc.). It is worth mentioning that the athlete must be re-examined after 24 h to better evaluate the injury, because often, immediately after a contusion, the pain is so disabling that there would be the risk of classifying them all as severe contusions.

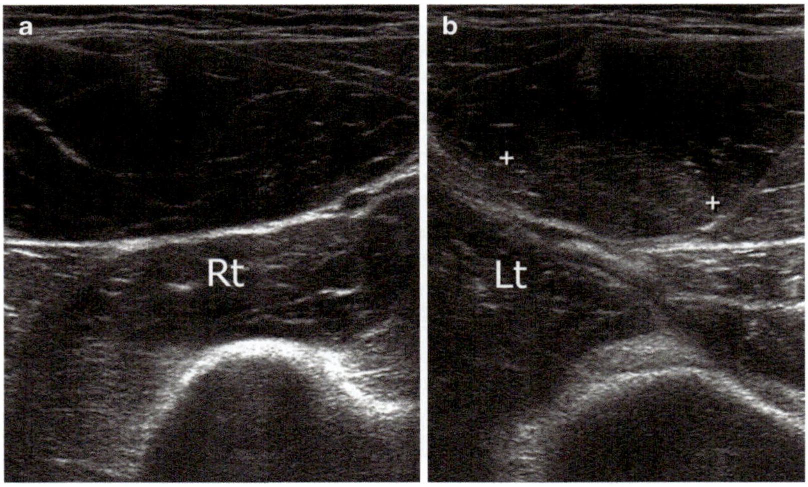

Fig. 20.8 (**b**) B-mode US scan of a submuscular and fascial skin laceration of the left rectus femoris (*asterisk*) compared with the contralateral side (**a**)

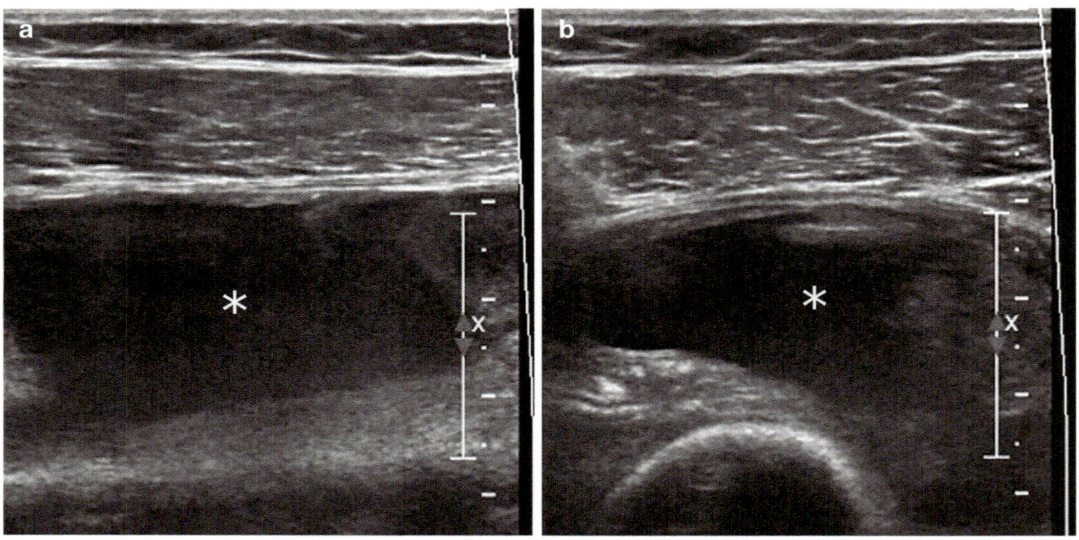

Fig. 20.9 Longitudinal (**a**) and transverse (**b**) US scan showing severe contusion of the left vastus intermedius muscle with a large hematoma (*asterisk*)

20.3.2 Injuries from Indirect Trauma

Injuries from indirect trauma derive from an intrinsic force generated by a sudden energetic muscle contraction. These accidents occur without contact with the opponent or other blunt structures or equipment: the athlete hurts himself/herself.

The most frequently affected muscles are the biarticular ones and those with a greater amount of high-speed contraction fibers (hamstrings, rectus femoris).

They are divided into two broad categories:

- Nonstructural muscle injuries.
- Structural muscle injuries.

In the former, there are no anatomical lesions of the muscle fibers, and they are divided into four subgroups. The latter are instead characterized by a true anatomical lesion of muscle fibers, even if small, and they are classified into three subgroups.

20.3.2.1 Nonstructural Muscle Injuries

In this type of injury there is no muscle fibers damage. They are the most numerous category, but also the most insidious one to diagnose and treat. In football, they make up 70% of muscle injuries and, while not presenting any muscle lesion, they are responsible for over 50% of absences from sports due to muscle injuries.

If neglected they can result in structural injuries. They are divided into four subgroups (Table 20.3):

US is often negative or, at most, shows a transient hyperechogenicity or hypoechogenicity (3–5 days). Power Doppler is negative. MRI is often negative or sometimes can demonstrate a limited edema. The gold standard examination is MRI because it often allows to detect even mild edema; this means that the sensitivity for these lesions goes from 76% of ultrasound to 92% of MRI. It is important in this sense to use the appropriate intrinsic high-contrast sequences.

Subgroup 1A is caused by fatigue and favored by continuous changes in the type of exercise or playing surfaces or by training with excessive workloads.

Subgroup 1B is caused by an excessive number of exercises and eccentric stresses (Fig. 20.10).

Subgroup 2A is caused by problems of the spine that may be difficult to diagnose, such as minor intervertebral defects (MID) that irritate the corresponding spinal nerve causing an altered control of the tone on the "target" muscle. In these cases, the resolution of the muscle lesion also depends on the treatment of the spine problem.

Table 20.3 Classification of nonstructural muscle injuries

Nonstructural injury	I: Muscle disorder related to overexertion	1A: Fatigue-induced 1B: DOMS (delayed-onset muscle soreness)	Sore, circumscribed increase of tone within a muscle. 1B: Widespread increase in muscle tone and pain that appears a few hours after physical activity
	II: Neuromuscular disorder	2A: Neuromuscular related to vertebral column and/or pelvis disorders 2B: Neuromuscular related to muscle	

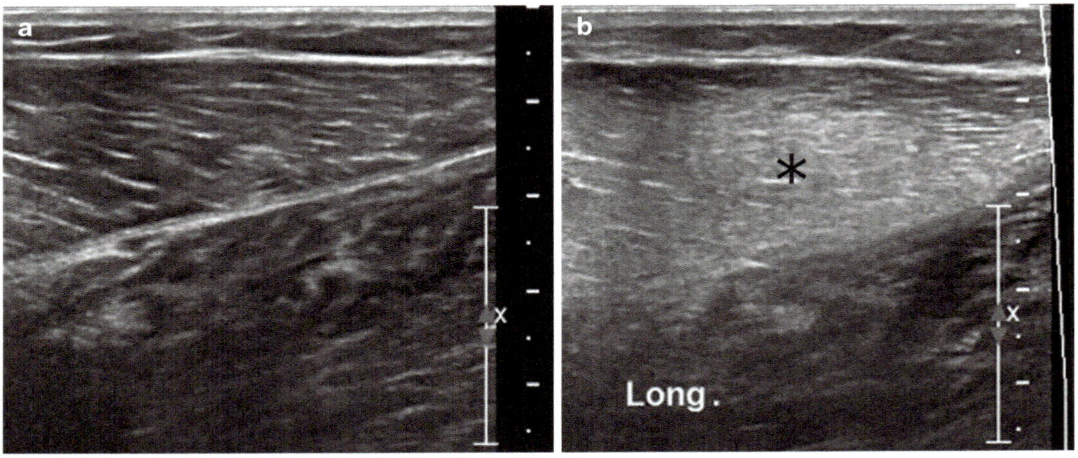

Fig. 20.10 (**b**) B-mode US scan of a type 1B nonstructural injury of the medial gastrocnemius (asterisk) compared with the contralateral side (**a**)

Subgroup 2B arises from an imbalance in neuromuscular control, especially of the mechanism of reciprocal inhibition originating from muscle spindles. Keep in mind that muscle tone is mainly under the control of the gamma circuit (stretch reflex) and the activation of alpha motor neurons is mainly under the control of the descending motor pathways. Sensory information from the muscle is carried by ascending pathways to the brain. The afferent signals enter the spinal cord through the alpha motor neurons of the associated muscle, but they also give off branches capable of stimulating interneurons in the spinal cord that inhibit the alpha motor neurons of the antagonist muscles.

A dysfunction of these neuromuscular control mechanisms can lead to significant impairment of normal muscle tone and can cause muscle disorders, especially when the inhibition of antagonist muscles is altered (e.g., decreased) and the agonist contracts excessively to compensate.

20.3.2.2 Structural Muscle Injuries

They are divided into three subgroups according to the extent of the anatomical lesion within the muscle (Table 20.4):

- 3A: Minor partial injury: injury of one or more primary fascicles within a secondary fascicle
- 3B: Moderate partial injury: injury of at least one secondary fascicle with an area of rupture less than 50% of the section surface of the muscle in that location
- 4: Subtotal injury, i.e., injury greater than 50% of the section surface of the muscle at that location, or total injury, i.e., injury with rupture of the entire muscle or bone-tendon junction.

Table 20.4 Classification of structural muscle injuries

Nonstructural injury	III: Partial muscle injury	3A: Minor partial injury	Injury of one or more primary fascicles within a secondary fascicle
		3B: Moderate partial injury	Injury of at least one secondary fascicle with an area of rupture <50% of the muscle surface in that location
	IV: (Sub) total muscle injury	4: Subtotal or total injury or tendon avulsion	Injury of >50% of the muscle surface (subtotal) or of the entire muscle (total) or of the tendon-bone junction

The classification of structural injuries also includes defining the location where the injury occurs in the muscle: proximal (P), medium (M), or distal (D). In fact, the lesions that occur at the proximal level of the hamstring and rectus femoris have a more severe prognosis than those of the same size that occur in other areas of the muscle.

As regards the triceps surae, instead, injuries that occur distally have a more severe prognosis compared to those with proximal involvement.

The classification of these structural muscle injuries is based, as we can see, on the anatomical extent of the lesion. It is not easy to distinguish a minor partial lesion from a small moderate one, and MRI can overestimate the extent of the lesion. Ultrasound and MRI are therefore still not precise enough in determining structural damage; often, for example, the liquid seen on the MRI can lead to an overestimation of the damage, so this will be one of the most important topics to continue studying in the upcoming years.

- **Partial minor injury 3A**: The ultrasound, in the acute phase, shows a slightly hyperechoic area which then turns into a nonhomogeneously hypoechoic area with initial echostructural subversion, in the context of which a small intramuscular anechoic focal area is demonstrated (Fig. 20.11).
- **Moderate partial injury 3B:** The acute-phase ultrasound shows a hyperechoic area that transforms into a very uneven area with evident structural subversion, in the context of which a large intra- and intermuscular anechoic area is demonstrated (Fig. 20.12).
- **Partial subtotal or total injury 4:** In the acute phase, ultrasound shows a highly disorganized iso-hyperechoic area, which turns into a very inhomogeneous area with evident structural alterations, bell-shaped stump

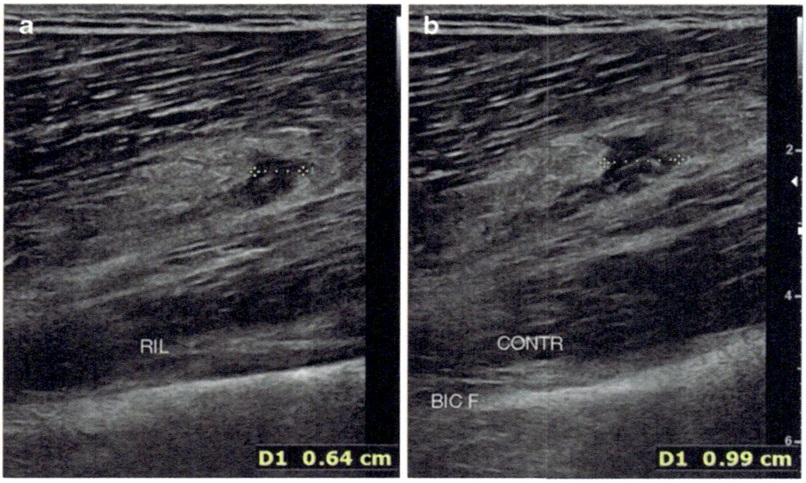

Fig. 20.11 B-mode US scan of a minor partial injury (3A) of the right femoral biceps at rest (**a**) and during contraction (**b**) showing only minor instability at the injury site (calipers)

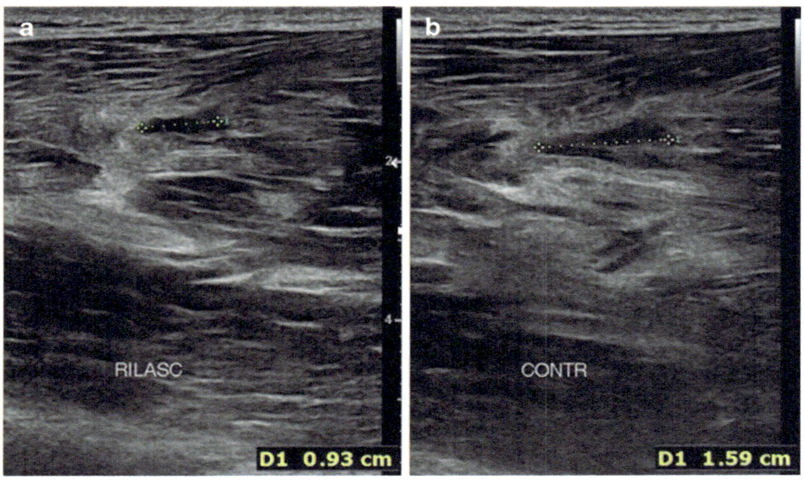

Fig. 20.12 B-mode US scan of a moderate partial injury (3B) of the hamstring at rest (**a**) and during contraction (**b**) showing clear instability at the injury site (calipers)

retraction, and a large anechogenic intra- and intermuscular area (Fig. 20.13).

20.3.3 Complications

Ultrasound is very important not only for the identification of muscle lesions and for their classification but also for monitoring them and therefore for identifying any complications. In this chapter we will only deal with the acute complications, namely intermuscular fluid collections and serum-blood cysts.

- **Intermuscular fluid collection:** a fluid collection, mostly bloody, that occurs between two muscle groups a few days after direct or indirect trauma. Most often they develop

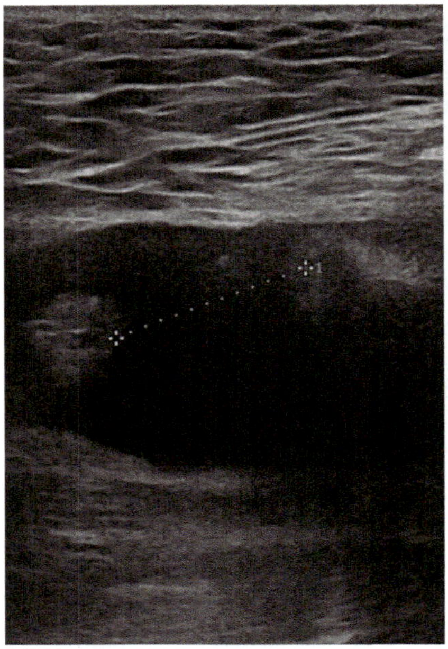

Fig. 20.13 Fourth-degree injury of the muscle-tendon junction of the semimembranosus (calipers) with a large hematoma

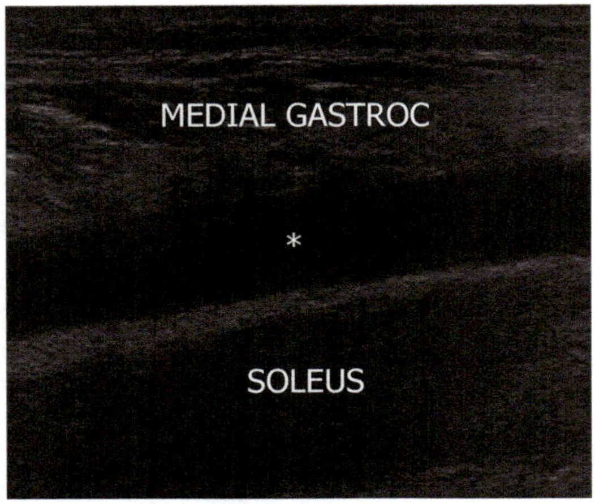

Fig. 20.14 Fluid collection (*asterisk*) between medial gastrocnemius and soleus muscles

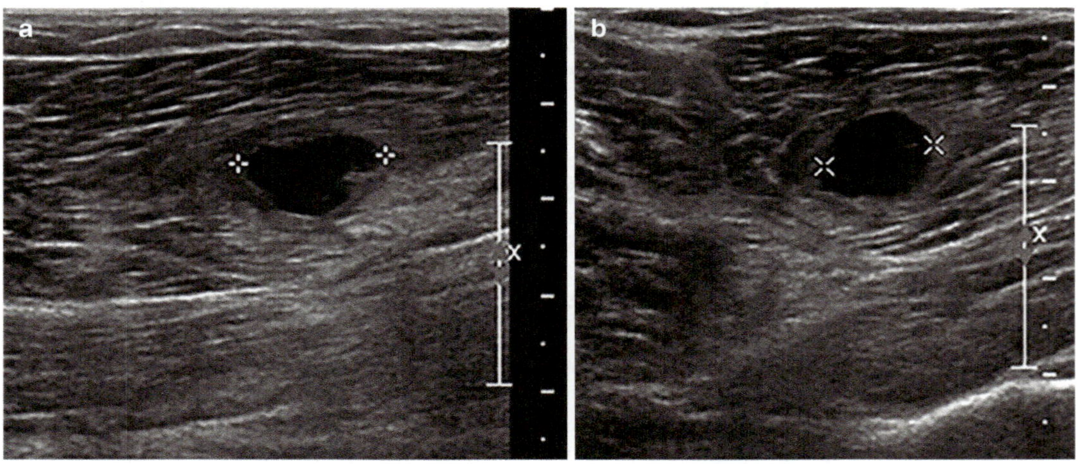

Fig. 20.15 Longitudinal (**a**) and transverse (**b**) US scan showing a serohemorrhagic cyst of the biceps femoris

between the rectus femoris and the vastus intermedius or between the medial gastrocnemius and the soleus, where the muscle fasciae are robust and not very extensible (Fig. 20.14).

- **Serohemorrhagic cyst**: complication that occurs when the hematoma, not completely reabsorbed, is encapsulated by fibrous tissue and the blood collection remains fluid.
- It is encountered most frequently in the calf muscles and it can be the consequence of blunt trauma or treatment errors in the acute phase (Fig. 20.15).

Further Readings

Askling C, Tengvar M, Saartok T, et al. Sports related hamstring strains – two cases with different etiologies and injury sites. Scand J Med Sci Sports. 2000;10(5):304–7.

Bisciotti GN, Volpi P, Alberti G. Italian Consensus Statement (2020) on return to play after lower limb muscle injury in football (soccer). BMJ Open Sport Exerc Med. 2019;5(1):e000505. https://doi.org/10.1136/bmjsem-2018-000505.

Bisciotti GN, Volpi P, Amato M, et al. Italian consensus conference on guidelines for conservative treatment on lower limb muscle injuries in athlete. BMJ Open Sport Exerc Med. 2018;4(1) https://doi.org/10.1136/bmjsem-2017-000323.

Bryan DJ. Gastrocnemius vs. soleus strain: how to differentiate and deal with calf muscle injuries. Curr Rev Musculoskelet Med. 2009;2(2):74–7.

Chan O, Del Buono A, Best TM, Maffulli N. Acute muscle strain injuries: a proposed new classification system. Knee Surg Sports Traumatol Arthrosc. 2012;20(11):2356–62.

Corazza A, Orlandi D, Baldari A, et al. Thigh muscles injuries in professional soccer players: a one year longitudinal study. Muscles Ligaments Tendons J. 2013;3(4):331–6. http://www.ncbi.nlm.nih.gov/pubmed/24596698. Accessed 19 Jan 2020

De Smet AA. Magnetic resonance findings in skeletal muscle tears. Skelet Radiol. 1933;22:479–84.

Dierking JK, Bemben MG, Bemben DA, et al. Validity of diagnostic ultrasound as a measure of delayed onset muscle soreness. J Orthop Sports Phys Ther. 2000;30:116–22.

Fornage BD. Muscular trauma. Clin Diagn Ultrasound. 1995;30:1–10.

Hashimoto BE, Kramer DJ, Wiitala L. Applications of musculoskeletal ultrasound. J Clin Ultrasound. 1999;27:293–318.

Itoh A, Ueno E, Tohno E, et al. Breast disease: clinical application of US elastography for diagnosis. Radiology. 2006;239:341–50.

Kolouris G, Connell D. Evaluation of the hamstring muscle complex following acute injury. Skelet Radiol. 2003;32:582–9.

Maffulli N, Nanni G, Pasta G, et al. I.S.Mu.L.T. Guidelines for muscle injuries. MLTJ. 2013;3(4):241–9.

Megliola A, Eutropi F, Scorzelli A, et al. Ultrasound and magnetic resonance imaging in sports-related muscle injuries. Radiol Med. 2006;111:836–45. https://doi.org/10.1007/s11547-006-0077-5.

Mueller-Wohlfahrt HW, Haensel L, Mithoefer K, et al. Terminology and classification of muscle injuries in sport: the Munich consensus statement. Br J Sports Med. 2013;47(6):342–50.

Noonan TJ, Garrett WE. Muscle strain injury: diagnosis and treatment. J Am Acad Orthop Surg. 1999;7:262–9.

Pasta G, Manara M. Diagnostic imaging in muscle injury. Muscle Injuries Sports Med J. 2013;3:97–134.

Peter B, Sydney KK. Brukner & Khan's clinical sports medicine. 2nd ed. Australia: McGraw-Hill; 2002.

Rubin SJ, Feldman F, Staron RB, et al. Magnetic resonance of muscle injury. Clin Imaging. 1995;19:263–9.

Speed C. A systematic review of shockwave therapies in soft tissue conditions: focusing on the evidence. Br J Sports Med. 2014;48(21):1538–42. https://doi.org/10.1136/bjsports-2012-091961.

Takebayashi S, Takasawa H, Banzai Y, et al. Sonographic findings in muscle strain injury: clinical and MR imaging correlation. J Ultrasound Med. 1995;14:899–905.

Volpi P. Medico del calcio: Il manuale. Edra spa, 2018.

Wohlfahrt M, Ekstrand J, Orchard J, et al. Terminology and classification of muscle injuries in sport: the Munich consensus statement. Br J Sports Med. 2012;47:342–50.

Tendon Trauma

21

Umberto Viglino, Davide Orlandi,
Alberto Aliprandi, and Elena Massone

Contents

21.1 Introduction

Tendon injuries include multiple conditions from acute rupture to chronic tendon degeneration. Inflammatory conditions usually affect the peritenon of anchoring tendons (paratenonitis), the synovial sheath of sliding tendons (tenosynovitis), or the osteotendinous junction (enthesitis). The etiological factors of these conditions could be intrinsic (sex, age, biomechanics) or extrinsic (sports or occupational functional overload, repetitive traumatism, etc.) but a combination of both is very common. Such conditions can be classified as acute (<6 weeks), subacute (6–12 weeks), and chronic (>12 weeks).

21.2 Tendinosis

Tendinosis is a degenerative condition of anchoring and sliding tendons, usually associated with mild painful symptoms.

The tendinosis process is characterized by fibroblast activation with production of high-molecular-weight collagen and proteoglycans, which can contain a lot of water with consequent diffuse edema. Necrosis and fibrinous exudation show up progressively with possible fibrocartilaginous metaplasia and precipitation of calcium deposits.

U. Viglino
Postgraduate School of Radiology, Genoa University, Genova, Italy

D. Orlandi (✉)
Department of Radiology, Ospedale Evangelico Internazionale, Genova, Italy

A. Aliprandi
Responsabile Servizio di Radiologia, Istituti Clinici Zucchi, Monza (MB), Italy

E. Massone
Department of Radiology, Ospedale Santa Corona, Pietra Ligure (SV), Italy

F. Martino et al. (eds.), *Musculoskeletal Ultrasound in Orthopedic and Rheumatic disease in Adults*,
https://doi.org/10.1007/978-3-030-91202-4_21

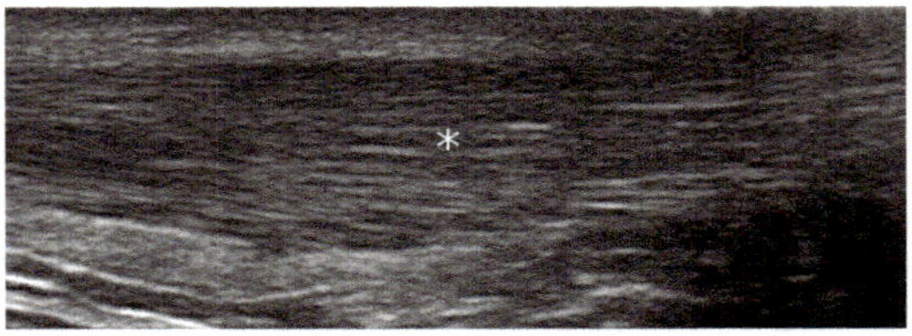

Fig. 21.1 Low-grade tendinosis. Note the typical fibrillar echogenicity fragmentation (*)

In this setting, diagnostic imaging has an essential value for diagnostic evaluation because a complete and realistic assessment of tendinous condition could not be based on anamnesis and clinic exam only. Ultrasound (US) can detect very early tendon alterations, showing mild tendon thickening and fragmentation of normal fibrillar echogenicity as first US signs of tendinosis (Fig. 21.1).

The typical early tendinosis US pattern is represented on long-axis scans by complete alteration of tendon echogenicity with fusiform tendon thickening, at which corresponds a "rounding" aspect on short-axis scans, with typical ventral concavity loss.

In severe tendinosis appear focal hypoechoic areas and expressions of mucoid degeneration (Fig. 21.2) with disorganization of collagen fibers and with micro- or macro-calcifications (hyperechoic spots). Large calcifications have posterior acoustic shadow and are expression of focal intratendinous osseous-calcific metaplasia (Fig. 21.3).

Color or power Doppler evaluation could be useful in order to highlight vascular signal spots within the degenerative site, which could be expression of angiogenetic activation, with potential restoring of the damaged area. The absence of vascular signal within these areas, on the contrary, could indicate the evolution of the degenerated area toward necrosis. However in daily clinical practice there are frequent cases of simultaneous presence of degenerative (tendinosis) and flogistic (paratenonitis) alterations, characterized by complex color and power Doppler patterns which anyway can increase the accuracy and reliability of B-mode US (Fig. 21.4a, b).

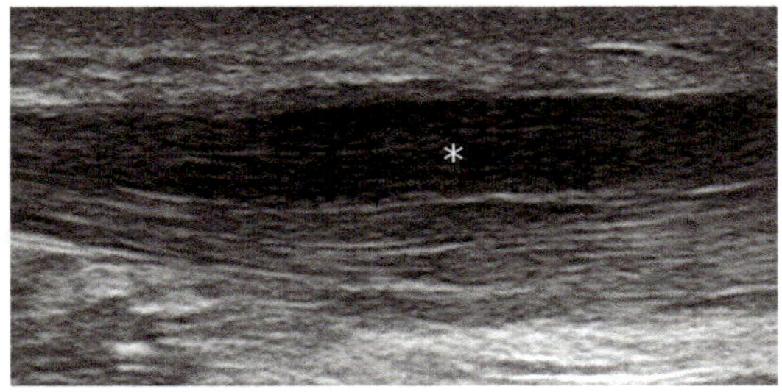

Fig. 21.2 Achilles tendinosis. The tendon appears thickened, diffusely dishomogeneous with wide focal hypoechoic area (*), expression of focal mucoid degeneration

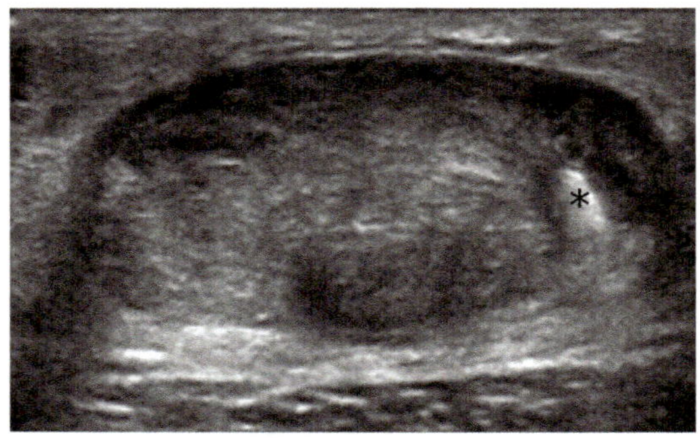

Fig. 21.3 Transverse scan of Achilles tendon. The tendon is thickened and dishomogeneous in a case of tendinosis with a small site of osseous calcification (*asterisk*)

There are some biomechanical and anatomic predisposing conditions to the developing of tendinosis. Giving an example, the presence of a megalic posterior-superior calcaneal tubercle (Haglund syndrome) can cause friction with the preinsertional aspect of the Achilles tendon causing subsequent tendinopathy. In these cases, ultrasound shows the presence of flogistic and degenerative alterations, with tendon thickening and loss of fibrillar echotexture, frequently associated with precalcaneal and retrocalcaneal bursitis (Fig. 21.5a, b).

21.3 Enthesopathy

Enthesopathy or insertional tendinopathy is a flogistic-degenerative condition affecting the osseous-tendinous junctions and is typical of anchoring tendons subjected to intense and repet-

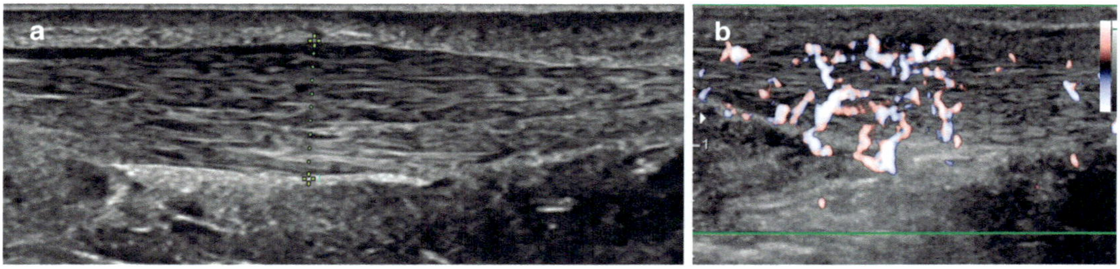

Fig. 21.4 (**a**) Longitudinal US scan of Achilles tendon. The tendon appears thickened, dishomogeneous, with fibrillar structure loss due to tendinosis; (**b**) power Doppler shows a concomitant hypervascularity caused by the hyperemic-flogistic condition

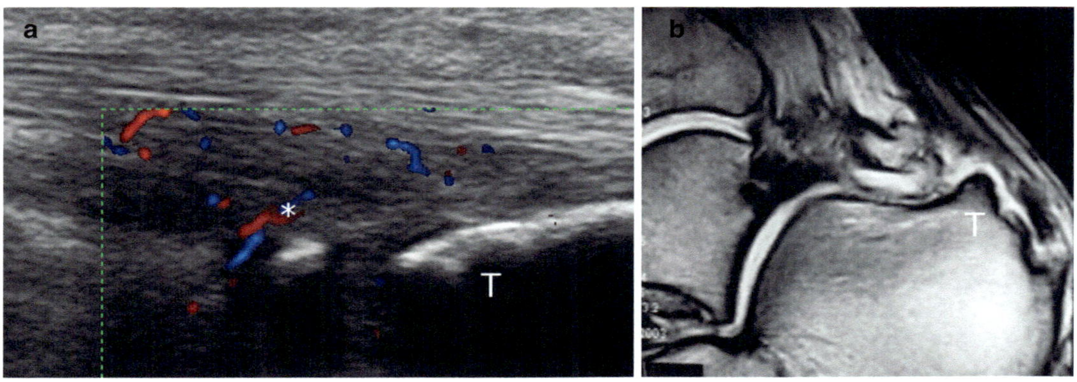

Fig. 21.5 Haglund syndrome. (**a**) The longitudinal US scan shows thickening and dishomogeneity of preinsertional tract of Achilles tendon with retrocalcaneal bursitis and concomitant hypervascularity with flogistic peri-intratendinous vascular signals at power Doppler examination (*). (**b**) MR exam (GE T2w sequence) in the same patient confirms ultrasound alterations and shows in addition the megalic posterior-superior calcaneal tubercle (T)

itive mechanical stress, being directly related with functional overload.

The most commonly affected structures are Achilles and patellar tendon (e.g., jumper's knee) and the common extensor and flexor tendons of the elbow (e.g., tennis elbow).

Normal enthesis is formed by the combination of tendon fibers and fibrocartilage. Blood vessels are present but, because of low blood speed and flow, are detectable only with the most advanced microvascular power Doppler tools.

The first detectable anatomic-pathologic alterations in enthesopathies are enthesis thickening with local hyperemia and neoangiogenesis; Doppler evaluation can show the early increment of tendon vascularity without actual altered collagen matrix.

Tendon structural dishomogeneity with focal hypoechoic areas and insertional calcification may be present, and these are expressions of intratendinous myxoid degeneration typical of severe infection (Fig. 21.6). Frequently associated are the flogistic reaction of the adjacent bursae and the presence of erosions and irregularities of the cortical surface in the insertional area.

US appearance of bone erosions is represented by discontinuity of the echogenic profile of the bony surface; however, MRI evaluation is essential for a complete evaluation of advanced cases of enthesopathy because it is the only technique that can detect the presence of bone marrow edema using high-contrast sequences (Fig. 21.7).

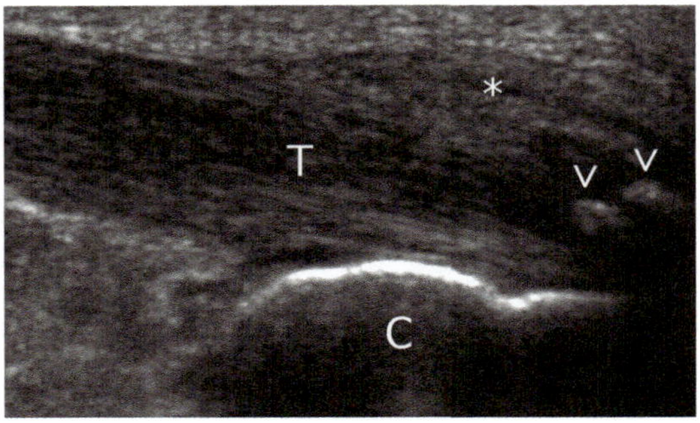

Fig. 21.6 Longitudinal scan of Achilles tendon (T) in a case of enthesopathy. Note the diffuse alteration of inner tendon echostructure with insertional calcifications (arrowheads) and thickening of precalcaneal soft tissues (*asterisk*). *C* calcaneus

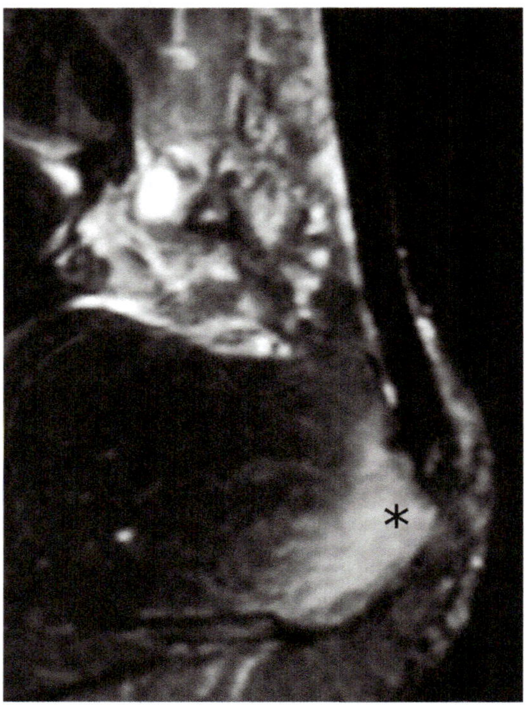

Fig. 21.7 MRI exam of the ankle, sagittal scan (fat-sat technique) shows bone marrow edema of calcaneal bone in correspondence with Achilles tendon insertion (*)

21.4 Tendon Rupture

Tendon rupture can be caused by acute trauma or can occur spontaneously as a complication of tendinosis. Mechanic overload, if excessive and persistent, can progressively induce partial or complete tears inside the degenerate tendon structure. Frequently, these ruptures are incomplete but they can alter the tendon homogeneity, continuity, and function with different degrees of severity.

At US evaluation, the rupture is represented by a hypo/anechoic gap that interrupts the fibrillar continuity of the tendon (Fig. 21.8a, b). In complete ruptures US can show the fiber discontinuity with diastasis of tendon stumps and blood effusion. In these cases, dynamic evaluation is important for a more precise description of the site and extension of rupture.

In some anatomical locations tendon rupture evaluation needs a more precise classification. This is particularly evident when evaluating rotator cuff tendons; tears can be divided, using extension and site criteria, into the following:

- *Partial tear*, which can be divided into ***bursal sided*** when the tear is limited to the tendon surface in contact with subacromial-subdeltoid bursa (Fig. 21.9); ***articular sided*** when it is limited to the tendon surface in contact with the glenohumeral articular surface; and ***intratendinous***. Intratendinous partial tear is characterized by anechoic intra-substance tendon delamination (Fig. 21.10).
- *Full-thickness tear*: when the full thickness of the tendon is involved (mild, moderate, wide) (Fig. 21.11), with possible stump diastasis, but with part of the tendon still intact.
- *Complete tear*: when the whole tendon is involved, with different grades of stump diastasis (Fig. 21.12).

In wide complete tears with tendon stump retraction there is humeral head exposure and subacromial space reduction which can progressively lead to a new pseudo-articulation between humeral head and acromion (Fig. 21.13).

Tendon rupture repair is a gradual process that needs from a few days to some months to obtain the full tendon healing and it develops through a three-step process: inflammatory phase (about a week, there is recruit of macrophages and tendon fibroblast by increased concentrations of cyto-

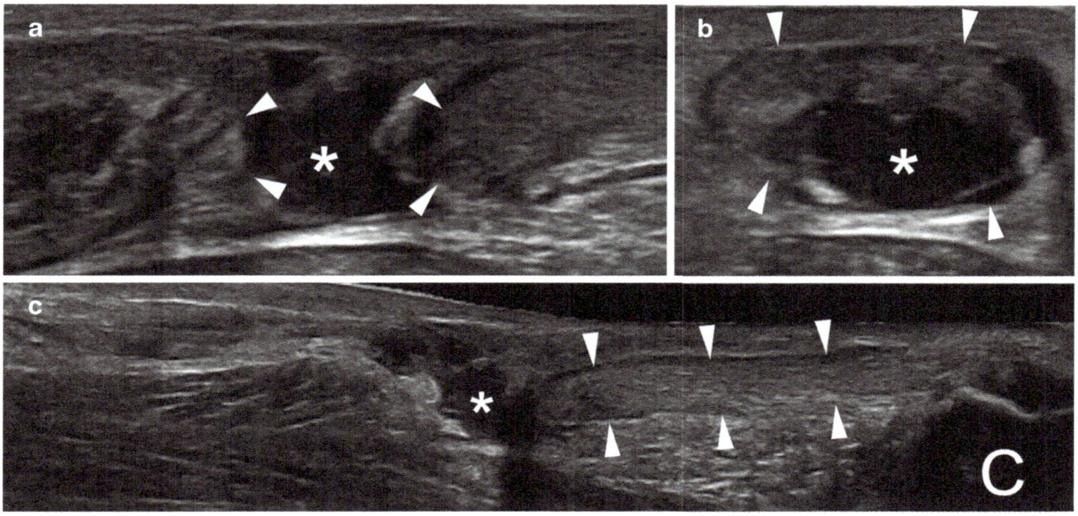

Fig. 21.8 (**a**) Longitudinal, (**b**) axial, and (**c**) extended field-of-view longitudinal US scan of a complete tear of the Achilles tendon at its middle third. Arrowheads show the tendon stumps divided by a gap (asterisk). *C* calcaneus

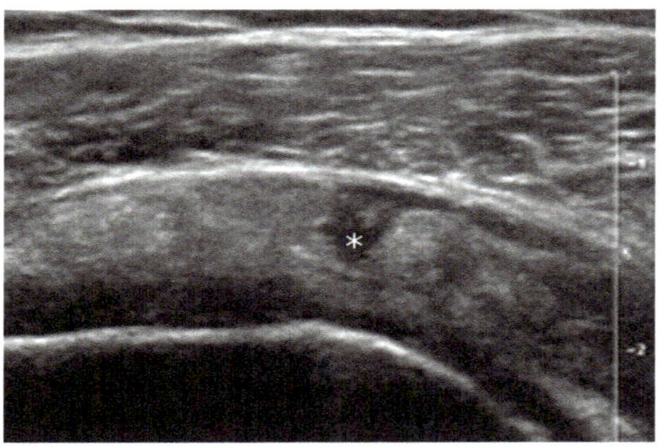

Fig. 21.9 Partial tear (*) on the bursal side of supraspinatus tendon

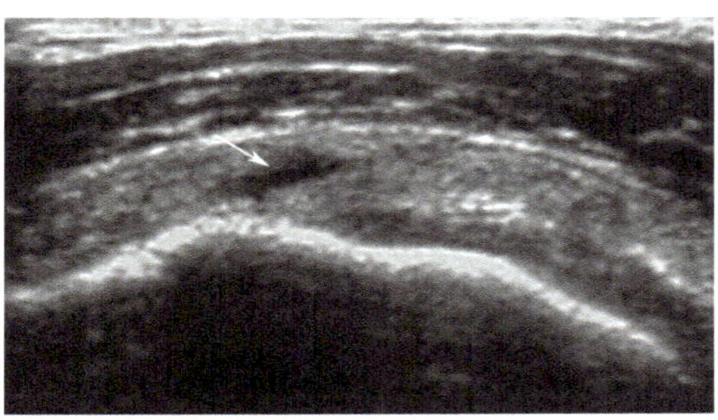

Fig. 21.10 Intratendinous partial tear (*arrow*) of supraspinatus tendon

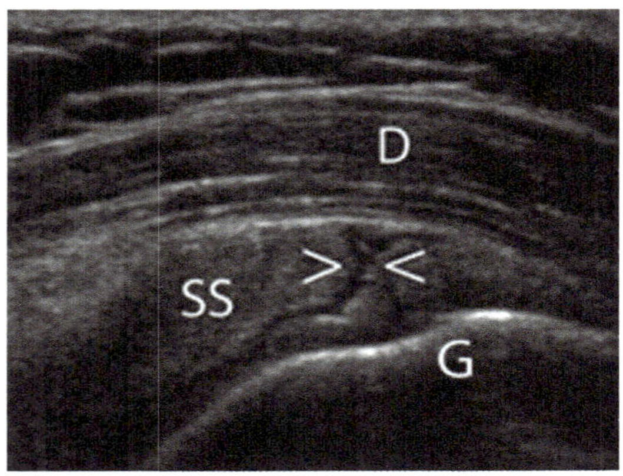

Fig. 21.11 Full-thickness tear of supraspinatus tendon (*arrowheads*) extending from the bursal to the articular side of the tendon. *SS* supraspinatus tendon, *D* deltoid muscle, *G* great tubercle of humerus

kines), proliferative phase (production of collagen), and remodeling phase (reorganization of new collagen with correct orientation and cross-linkage of collagen fibers).

In this reparative remodeling process are involved different cytotypes (including marrow-derived mesenchymal stem cells, fibroblasts, and inflammatory cells) and many growth factors like platelet-derived growth factor (PDGF-BB), trans-

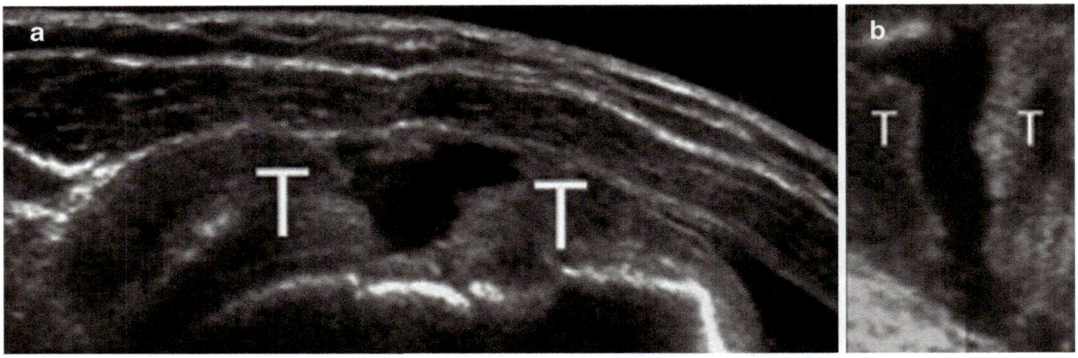

Fig. 21.12 (**a**) Complete tear of supraspinatus tendon with moderate diastasis of tendon fibers (T) on a highly degenerate matrix. (**b**) MPR reconstruction shows rupture "from above" on a coronal plane. *T* tendon stumps

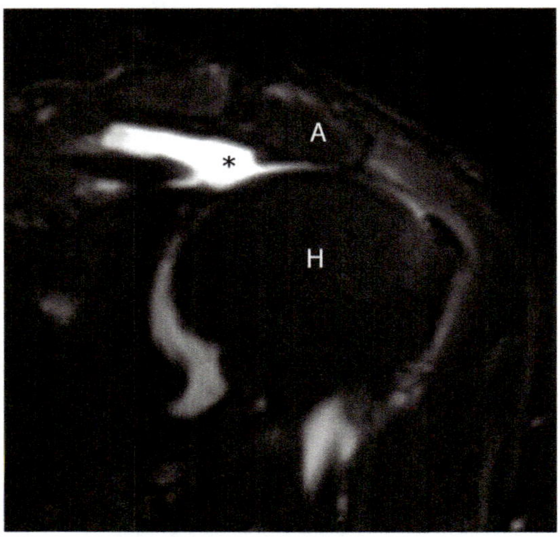

Fig. 21.13 Chronic massive tear of the rotator cuff with pseudo-articulation between humeral head (H) and acromion (A) and concomitant joint effusion (*)

forming growth factor β (TGF-β), vascular endothelial growth factor (VEGF), and basic fibroblast growth factor (bFGF).

21.5 Tendon Dislocations

Sliding tendons can have bending along their course with spatial misalignment as compared to the normal functional axis of the muscle. To assure correct articular biomechanics, the anatomical structures such as muscle belly and tendons, with their corner points and lever fulcrums, must be in the physiological position in osseous-fibrous channels. The anatomical structures designated to keep these structures in the correct position are **retinacula**, transverse thickenings localized in the deep muscular fascia and firmly fastened to bone eminences. Their integrity is crucial to allow a solid stabilization. When it is reduced, the tendon will dislocate determining an instability condition. There are different severity grades on tendon instabilities: in mild conditions tendon dislocates only following certain movements, and in more severe conditions the subluxation and dislocation are more frequent, and sometimes a fixed dislocation could be observed. Moreover, in case of congenital absence or retinacula hypoplasia, dislocation could be spontaneous. In this setting high-resolution US, performed with dedicated dynamic maneuvers, represents the "gold standard" technique for the diagnosis of tendon instability.

Even though tendon instability is not a frequent pathological condition, it could be frequently associated with ligament sprains and its presence must be considered because early diagnosis is of key importance to prevent the developing of tendinosis or tendon rupture.

The tendons more prone to develop instability are the long head of biceps brachii (LHBB) at the humerus biceps groove in the shoulder and the peroneal tendons at the peroneal groove in the ankle.

LHBB can dislocate following a rupture of transverse ligament or coracohumeral ligament and can be associated with the rupture of subscapularis tendon. In addition, there are genetically predisposing anatomical conditions such as a flat bicipital groove that could lead to spontaneous dislocation.

US shows the empty bicipital groove and the tendon dislocated medially, above or under the subscapularis tendon (Fig. 21.14). In order to demonstrate the instability, a dynamic US evaluation of the LHBB performed with arm extra-rotation by 90° with flexed elbow could be useful.

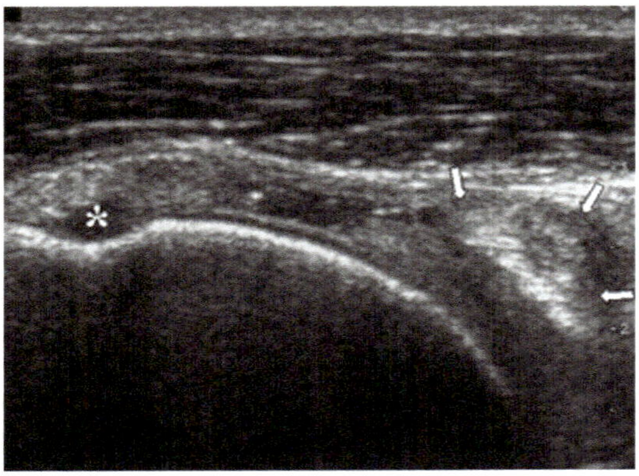

Fig. 21.14 Transverse scan of the shoulder that shows medial dislocation of long head biceps brachii tendon (*arrows*) after subscapularis tendon rupture. Note the empty bicipital groove between humeral tuberosities (*asterisk*)

In the ankle, peroneal tendons are held in physiological position by superior and inferior peroneal retinacula, located, respectively, over and under the deflexion site at the level of the peroneal groove of the lateral malleolus.

Traumatic instability is caused by the lesion of the superior retinaculum with consequent tendency to anterior dislocation of peroneal tendons over peroneal malleolus. In addition, there are genetically predisposing anatomical conditions such as a flat peroneal groove that could lead to peroneal instability.

US dynamic maneuver for peroneal instability demonstration is performed placing the transducer on tendons' short axis in correspondence of deflexion site and, during dorsiflexion of the foot, observing the tendon dislocation over lateral malleolus (Fig. 21.15).

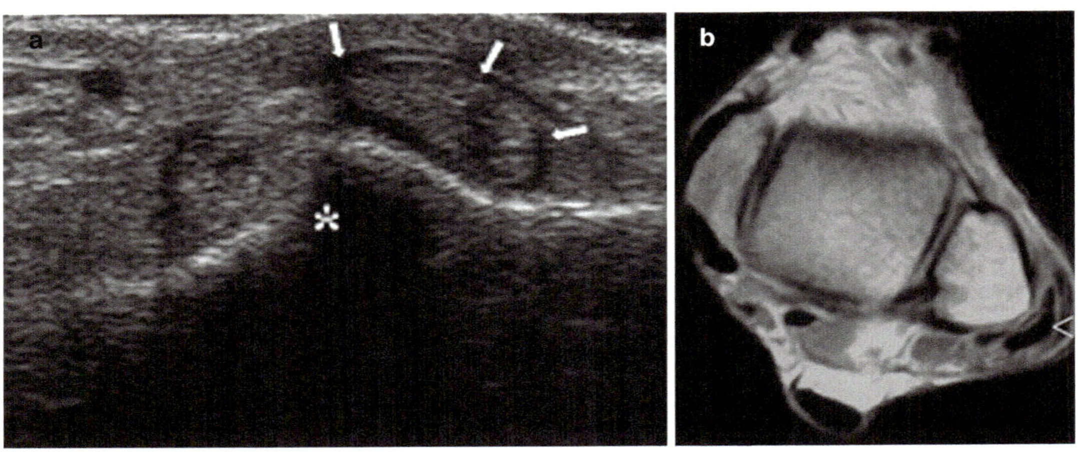

Fig. 21.15 (**a**) Transverse scan of lateral compartment of the ankle that shows peroneal tendon dislocation (*arrows*) over peroneal malleolus (*asterisk*). (**b**) Same patient, the MRI exam (axial scan, SE T1-weighted technique). Arrowhead = peroneal tendons

Further Readings

Bianchi S, Martinoli C. Ultrasound of the musculoskeletal system. Milan: Springer; 2007.

Freedman BR, Sarver JJ, Buckley MR, Voleti PB, Soslowsky LJ. Biomechanical and structural response of healing Achilles tendon to fatigue loading following acute injury. J Biomech. 2014;47(9):2028–34. https://doi.org/10.1016/j.jbiomech.2013.10.054.

Maffulli N, Wong J, Almekinders LC. Types and epidemiology of tendinopathy. Clin Sports Med. 2003;22(4):675–92.

Martino F, Silvestri E, Grassi W, Garlaschi G. Ecografia dell'apparato osteoarticolare Anatomia, semeiotica e quadri patologici. Milan: Springer; 2006.

Scott A, Backman LJ, Speed C. Tendinopathy: update on pathophysiology. J Orthop Sports Phys Ther. 2015;45(11):833–41.

Silvestri E, Muda A, Sconfienza LM. Normal ultrasound anatomy of the musculoskeletal system a practical guide. Milan: Springer; 2012.

Thomopoulos S, Parks WC, Rifkin DB, Derwin KA. Mechanisms of tendon injury and repair. J Orthop Res. 2015;33:832–9. John Wiley and Sons Inc. https://doi.org/10.1002/jor.22806.

Superficial Interosseous Ligament Injury

22

Enzo Silvestri, Davide Orlandi, Elena Massone, and Ernesto La Paglia

Contents

22.1 Introduction

Interosseous ligaments are connective and fibrous reinforcing and stabilizing structures of the joint capsule with hyperechogenic fibrillar ultrasound pattern. Since they are superficial structures their optimal evaluation is obtained with high-frequency linear probe. Depending on the biomechanics with which the trauma occurs, we may have pure ligamentous lesions or lesions with avulsions of the ligament insertion bone bract and consequent instability of the reference joint. The former result in an ultrasound picture of loss of the regular fibrillar echostructure with possible diastasis of the stumps and with various degrees of edematous hemorrhagic infarction of the peri-ligamentous soft tissues, and the others associate these findings with the presence of parcellar detachment of cortical bone tract from the cortical profile ligament insertion. Dynamic ultrasound imaging can also provide additional information about ligament dislocation and joint diastasis during stressful maneuvers. Ultrasonography also affords quick comparative imaging of the uninjured side.

E. Silvestri
Radiology, Alliance medical, Genova, Italy

D. Orlandi (✉)
Department of Radiology, Ospedale Evangelico Internazionale, Genova, Italy

E. Massone
Department of Radiology, Ospedale Santa Corona, Pietra Ligure (SV), Italy

E. La Paglia
Department of Radiology, Humanitas Cellini, Torino, Italy

F. Martino et al. (eds.), *Musculoskeletal Ultrasound in Orthopedic and Rheumatic disease in Adults*,
https://doi.org/10.1007/978-3-030-91202-4_22

22.2 Superficial Interosseous Ligament Injuries

The main upper and lower limb superficial interosseous ligament lesion sites will be examined.

22.2.1 Stener Lesion

A Stener lesion is a complete tear of the ulnar collateral ligament from the thumb proximal phalanx at the level of the metacarpophalangeal joint with its dislocation superficial to the adductor pollicis aponeurosis, leading to interposition of the aponeurosis between the UCL and the MCP joint. The distal dislocation of the UCL and its interposition beneath the adductor aponeurosis distinguish the Stener lesion from other UCL injuries and it is particularly important as it impedes healing, thereby conducting patient to surgery (Figs. 22.1 and 22.2).

Biomechanics leading to Stener injury is hyperabduction and hyperextension of the first MCP joint (typically an acute lesion occurs from a fall onto the ground with an abducted thumb with a ski pole in hand, but the same mechanism can also occur from sports such as hockey, soccer, handball, basketball, and volleyball).

In addition to being noninvasive, cost effective, and less time consuming, ultrasound has been shown to have from 83% to 100% sensitivity and specificity in discerning between non-displaced and displaced tears, showing the anatomic relationship of the UCL as it pertains to adductor aponeurosis. The appearance of a Stener lesion on ultrasound has been called the "tadpole sign" or yo-yo on a string sign. Ridley et al. note, "*The head of the tadpole is formed by the retracted proximal fragment of the UCL which displaces to be adjacent to the head of the metacarpal. The tail of the tadpole is formed by the adductor aponeurosis which is often thickened and lies deep to the retracted UCL fibers.*"

The "yo-yo on a string sign" appearance presents by the small mass displaced superficial to the adductor pollicis from the torn ligament fibers that retracted proximally (Fig. 22.3).

22.2.2 Scapholunate Ligament Disruption

The interosseous scapholunate ligament extends from the lunate to the scaphoid bones and, especially the dorsal band which is the thickest and functionally most important part, contributes to

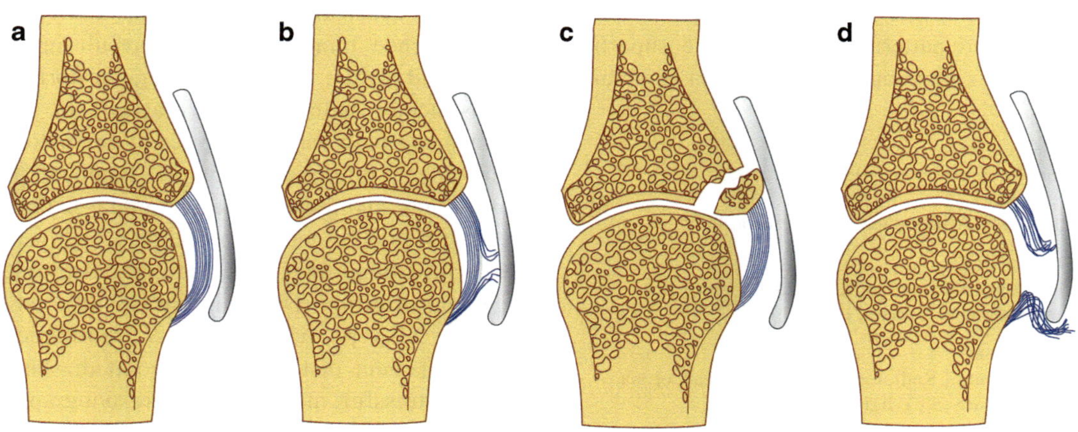

Fig. 22.1 (**a**) Normal aspect of ulnar collateral complex of the thumb; (**b**) middle third partial ulnar collateral ligament lesion without any dislocation vs. the adductor aponeurosis; (**c**) avulsion lesion of distal insertion of ulnar collateral ligament with cortical bone fragment's production; (**d**) Stener lesion as a complete tear of the ulnar collateral ligament from the thumb proximal phalanx at the level of the metacarpophalangeal joint with its dislocation superficial to the adductor pollicis aponeurosis

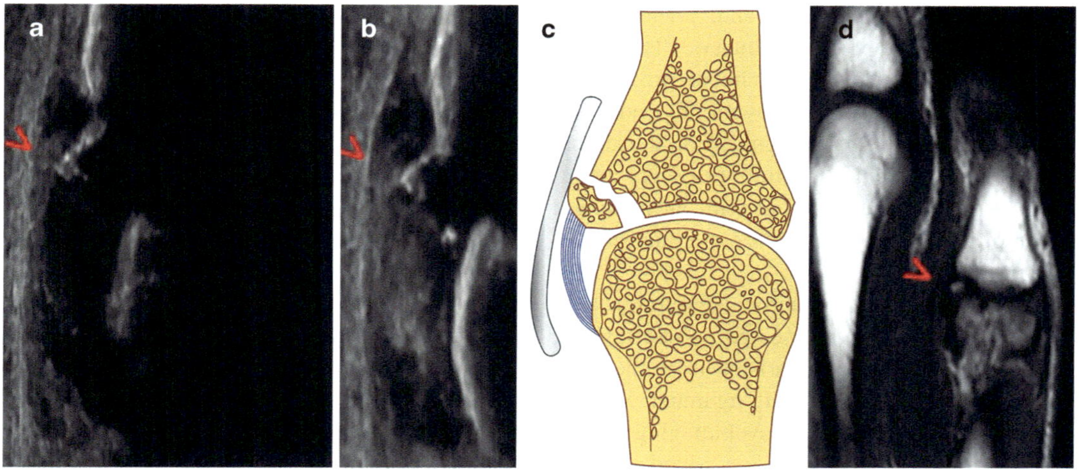

Fig. 22.2 US longitudinal view of the thumb (**a**, **b**), anatomical Scheme (**c**), and T1w coronal MRI (**d**) showing an avulsion lesion of distal insertion of ulnar collateral ligament with cortical bone fragment's production at the basis of the thumb proximal phalanx at the level of metacarpophalangeal joint (*red arrowheads*)

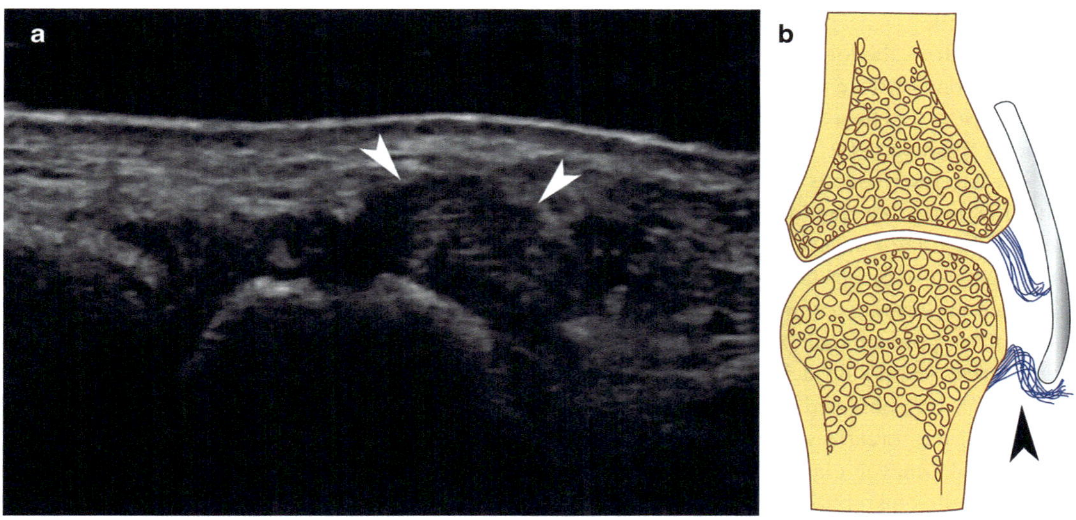

Fig. 22.3 Stener lesion appearance on ultrasound (**a**) and corresponding anatomical Scheme (**b**) showing the so-called tadpole sign. The head of the tadpole is formed by the retracted proximal fragment of the UCL (*arrowheads*) which displaces to be adjacent to the head of the metacarpal. The tail of the tadpole is formed by the adductor aponeurosis which is often thickened and lies deep to the retracted UCL fibers

the stability of the interposed segment of the carpus.

A disruption of this ligament may lead to a dorsal or volar instability of interposed segment which can be demonstrated with a complete radiological approach (standard radiographs—four views) associated with an US examination in order to get an early diagnosis and minimize the potential for inappropriate or delayed treatment.

The injury mechanism most commonly involves a combination of hyperextension and radial deviation stresses with an impact on the thenar eminence. The intact dorsal band of the SLL appears as an echogenic fibrillar structure (mean thickness 1.1 mm and mean length 4.2 mm) in the scapholunate interval. The evaluation with a high-frequency linear probe (15–18 MHz) and dynamic maneuvers can lead to the demonstration of a discontinuity of the dorsal band of the ligament in neutral position or a non-visualization of the ligament with an increased width of the scapholunate space in ulnar inclination of the wrist.

Ancillary findings are cortical disruption, subperiosteal hematoma, radiocarpal joint effusions, and carpal ganglion cysts arising from the anterior band of the scapholunate ligament. When a lesion is suspected, second-level imaging such as MRI arthrography should be performed.

22.2.3 Coracohumeral Ligament

Bicipital pulley is a capsuloligamentous complex which stabilizes the long head of bicipital tendon in the bicipital groove and the whole anatomical space is known as the rotator interval: the coracohumeral ligament—the roof of the rotator interval—is an interosseous band which, together with the superior glenohumeral ligament (the floor of the rotator interval) forms a sling around the long head of biceps tendon.

When performing a shoulder US examination a complete approach to the evaluation of the rotator interval should be achieved by the use of dynamical tests obtained while intra- and extra-rotation of the forearm while keeping the elbow flexed. Habermeyer classified various types of bicipital pulley disruption involving also the subscapularis tendon and the supraspinatus tendon. Isolated pulley injuries with the only involvement of the coracohumeral ligament (type 1 Habermeyer) lead to 7.1% of the cases.

Dynamic maneuvers performed during ultrasonography show, as an indirect sign of lesion of the SGHL and integrity of CHL, an empty bicipital groove and the long head of bicipital tendon dislocated close to the subscapularis insertion of the CHL (Fig. 22.4).

When a lesion is suspected, second-level imaging such as MRI arthrography should be performed (Fig. 22.5).

22.2.4 Coracoclavicular Ligaments

The coracoclavicular ligaments (trapezoid and conoid) are responsible for acromioclavicular joint (ACJ) stability and are known as suspensory ligament of the shoulder: the trapezoid ligament leads from the inferior aspect of the clavicular epiphysis to the superior aspect of the coracoid while the conoid ligament extends from the inferior aspect of the conoid tuberculum at the clavicular diaphysis to the basis of the coracoid.

ACJ injuries' etiology is a fall with direct impact to the shoulder, while the arm is adducted. The Rockwood classification is based on the radiographic analysis of the ACJ and leads from a normal aspect with no displacement (grade 1) to displacement of >100% of the height of the ACJ and clavicle displaced inferiorly and anteriorly with trapezius and deltoid muscles' damage (grade 6).

Ultrasound can be combined with radiography for the diagnostic workup of ACJ injuries in the acute phase. Ultrasound can be performed in the neutral position as it is better tolerated by patients.

The lesion of the ACJ can be associated with the lesion of the coracoclavicular ligaments ranging from normal coracoclavicular ligaments (grade 1) to distended coracoclavicular ligaments, enlarged and with loss of echogenic appearance on US (grade 2), to ruptured coracoclavicular ligaments and ligament stump located at bone insertion (grade 3).

22.2.5 Ankle Interosseous Ligaments

Ankle is the most commonly injured major joint in the body and ankle ligamentous sprains are extremely common in biomechanics of eversion (85%) and inversion (15%) with respective involvement of ligamentous bands of lateral complex, medial/deltoid complex, and syndesmosis.

The ankle ligaments are best evaluated with high-frequency transducers (preferably from 15 to 18 MHz) in the long axis, with short-axis imaging for problem-solving. Similar to other

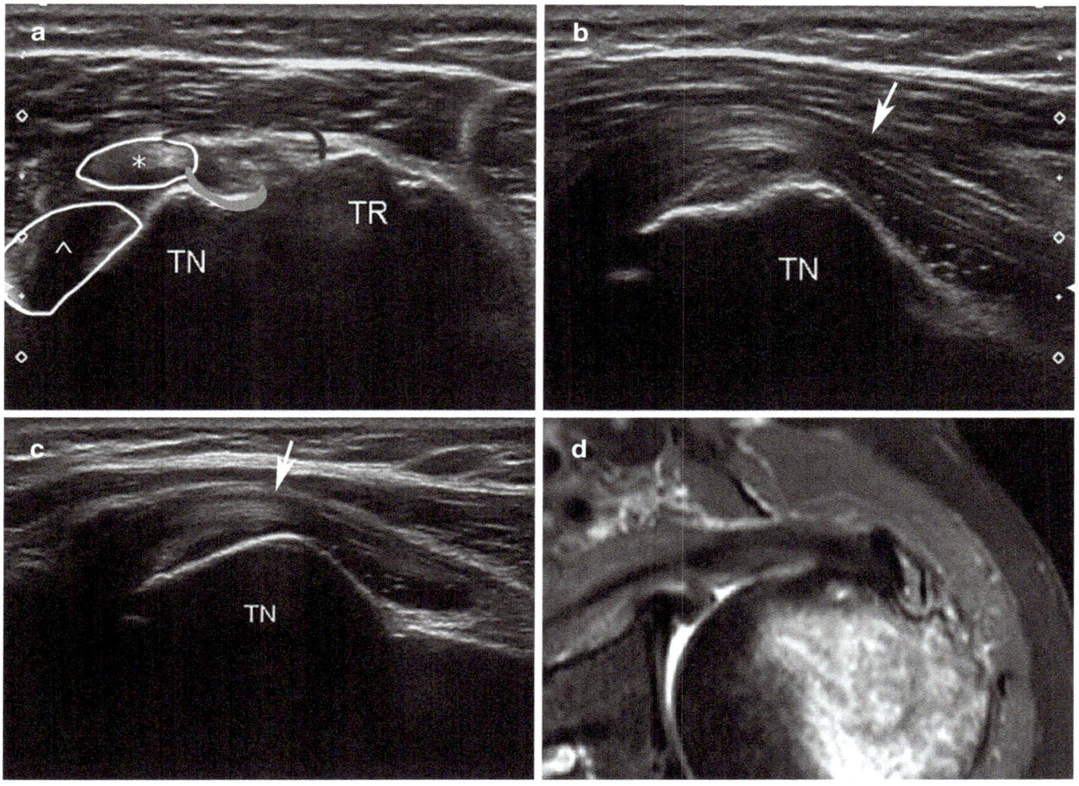

Fig. 22.4 Axial and sagittal US scan of the bicipital pulley and bicipital groove (**a–c**) and fat-sat T2w axial MRI (**d**) of the same site showing a dislocation of the bicipital tendon (*asterisk*) close to the subscapularis insertion of the CHL (*dark gray curved line*) as an indirect sign of superior glenohumeral ligament lesion. *Arrowhead:* subscapularis tendon; *bright gray curved line:* bicipital groove; *TN:* lesser tuberosity of the humerus; *TR:* greater tuberosity of the humerus; *white arrow:* vertical portion of the long head of the biceps brachii tendon (LHBBT)

ligaments, the ankle ligaments should appear as echogenic with a more compact fibrillar structure than tendons, most commonly connecting two osseous structures.

A general consideration regarding patient positioning is that the ligament should be slightly taut during evaluation to eliminate redundancy. The transducer should be angled so that the ligament fibers are perpendicular to the sound beam to eliminate anisotropy.

Normal thickness of the ankle ligaments ranges from 2 to 5 mm. Some general principles apply when it comes to the US appearance of ligament injuries. Acute partial-thickness ligament tears typically appear as hypoechoic thickening with preservation of some continuous fibers (Fig. 22.6).

Acute full-thickness ligament tears typically present as discontinuity, non-visualization of the ligament, or visualization of hypoechoic or heterogeneous material representing a torn ligament and hemorrhage (Fig. 22.7).

A chronic injury may appear as ligamentous thickening, attenuation, or non-visualization. Avulsion injuries may show tiny echogenic shadowing fragments of bone. Dynamic US may show lack of normal tendon tightening during stress maneuvers in complete tears: in the evaluation of anterior talo-fibular ligament the anterior drawer test is useful to distinguish a partial from a complete tear by placing the patient prone with the foot hanging over the edge of the examination table while pulling the forefoot anteriorly when in plantar flexion and inversion. When the

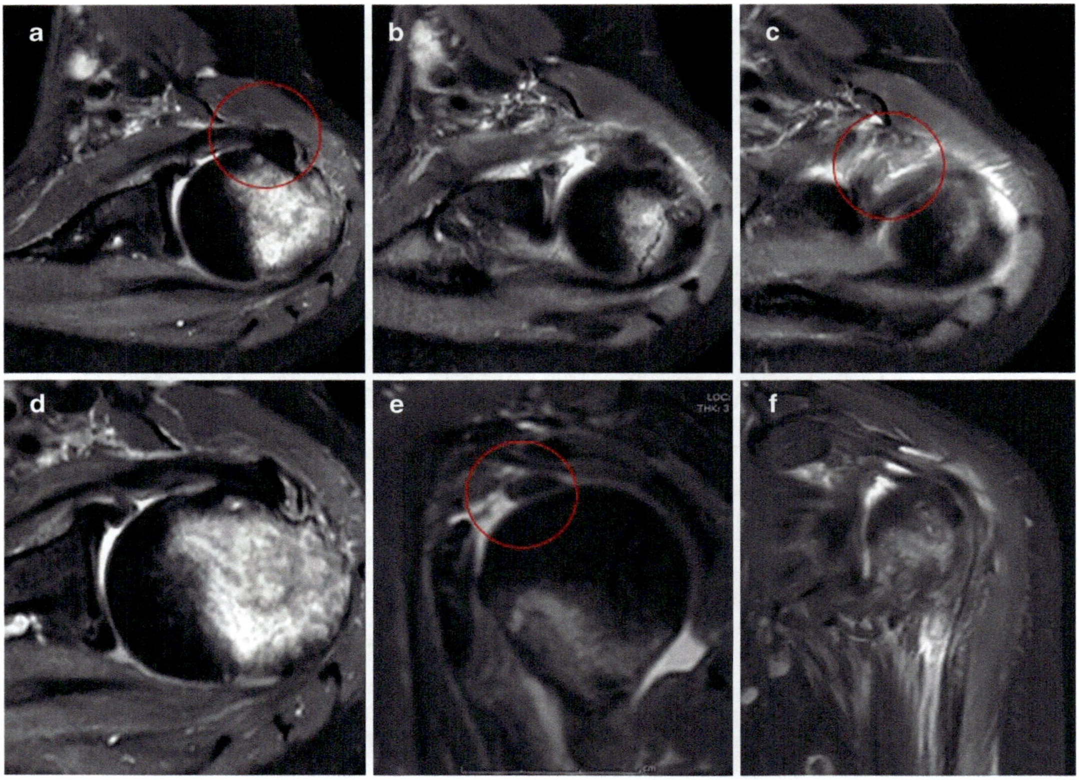

Fig. 22.5 MR arthrography of the shoulder showing (from **a** to **f**) dislocation of the bicipital tendon close to the subscapularis insertion of the CHL and disruption of superior glenohumeral ligament (*red circles*). Note the empty bicipital groove (*asterisk*) on the fourth axial image (**d**)

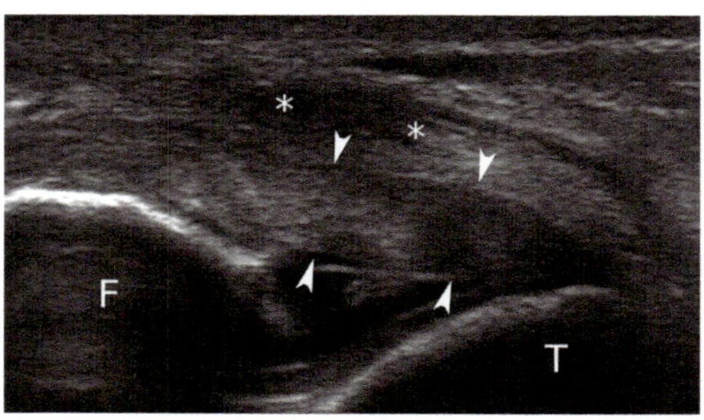

Fig. 22.6 Acute partial-thickness tear of the anterior talo-fibular ligament (ATFL) showing hypoechoic thickening of the ligament (*arrowheads*) and surrounding edema (*asterisks*). *F* fibula, *T* talus

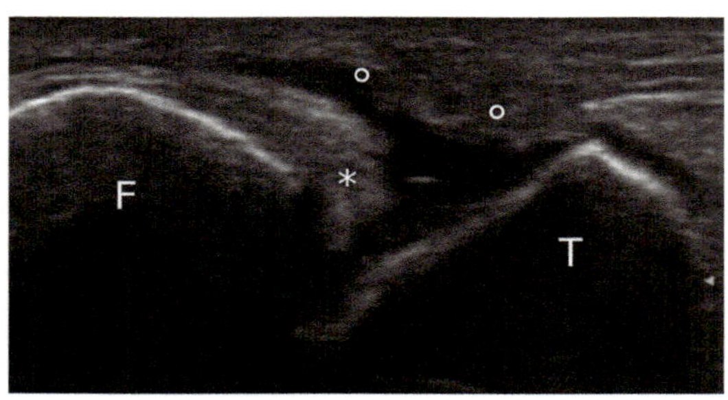

Fig. 22.7 Acute full-thickness tear of the anterior talofibular ligament (ATFL) showing ligament fibers' discontinuity (*asterisk*) with surrounding hemorrhage and edema (*circles*). *F* fibula, *T* talus

ligament is torn, the anterior shift of the talus against the fibula will open the gap in the substance of the ligament.

Dynamic US may also be useful to better evaluate the integrity of calcaneo-fibular ligament (CFL); by full dorsiflexion of the foot this ligament becomes taut and peroneal tendons are lifted up. Lack of elevation of the peroneal tendons with dorsiflexion is an indirect indicator of a CFL tear. Complete CFL tears may be accompanied by fluid in the overlying peroneal tendon sheath.

Further Readings

Alves T, et al. Normal and injured ankle ligaments on ultrasonography with magnetic resonance imaging correlation. J Ultrasound Med. 2019;38:513–28.

Baumann B, et al. Arthroscopic prevalence of pulley lesions in 1007 consecutive patients. J Shoulder Elb Surg. 2008;17(1):14–20.

Bilfeld MF, et al. US of the coracoclavicular ligaments in the acute phase of an acromioclavicular disjunction: comparison of radiographic, ultrasound and MRI findings. Eur Radiol. 2017;27:483–90.

Ebrahim FS, et al. US diagnosis of the UCL tears of the thumb and Stener lesions: technique, pattern-based approach and differential diagnosis. Radiographics. 2006;26(4):1007–20.

Hung CY, et al. Gamekeepers thumb (skiers, ulnar collateral ligament tear). Treasure Island (FL): StatPearls Publishing; 2019.

Lucerna A, Rehman UH. Stener lesion. Treasure Island (FL): StatPearls Publishing; 2019. PMID: 31082048

Martinoli C, et al. Musculoskeletal ultrasound: technical guidelines. Insights Imaging. 2010;1:99–141.

Mattox R, et al. Sonographic diagnosis of an acute Stener lesion: a case report. J Ultrasound. 2016;19(2):149–52.

Meyer P, et al. Imaging of wrist injuries: a standardized US examination in daily practice. J Belg Soc Radiol. 2018;102(1):9.

Morvan G, et al. Ultrasound of the ankle. Eur J Ultrasound. 2001;14:73–82.

Nakata W, et al. Bicipital pulley: normal anatomy and associated lesions at MR arthrography. Radiographics. 2011;31(3):791–810.

Peetrons P, et al. Sonography of ankle ligaments. J Clin Ultrasound. 2004;34:491–9.

Ridley LJ, et al. Tadpole sign: Stener lesion. J Med Imaging Radiat Oncol. 2018;62(Suppl 1):162.

Rockwood C, et al. Acromioclavicular injuries. In: Fractures in adults. Philadelphia, PA: Lippincott-Raven; 1996. p. 1341–413.

Sconfienza LM, et al. Dynamic high-resolution US of ankle and midfoot ligaments: normal anatomic structure and imaging technique. Radiographics. 2015;35:164–78.

Tauber M. Management of acute acromioclavicular joint dislocations: current concepts. Arch Orthop Trauma Surg. 2013;133(7):985–95.

Peripheral Entrapment Neuropathies

23

Salvatore Guarino, Davide Orlandi, Enzo Silvestri, and Marcello Zappia

Contents

S. Guarino
Department of Radiology, Monaldi Hospital, AORN Ospedali dei Colli, Naples, Italy

D. Orlandi (✉)
Department of Radiology, Ospedale Evangelico Internazionale, Genova, Italy

E. Silvestri
Radiology, Alliance Medical, Genova, Italy

M. Zappia
Musculoskeletal Radiology Unit, Istituto Diagnostico Varelli, Napoli, Italy

Dipartimento di Medicina e Scienze della Salute, Università degli Studi del Molise (CB), Campobasso, Italy
marcello.zappia@unimol.it

F. Martino et al. (eds.), *Musculoskeletal Ultrasound in Orthopedic and Rheumatic disease in Adults*,
https://doi.org/10.1007/978-3-030-91202-4_23

23.1 Introduction

Entrapment neuropathies are a group of mononeuropathy syndromes due to compression/impingement of a single peripheral nerve.

Regardless of the cause of compression, the nerves react to this irritative stimulus with the same characteristics and the ultrasound (US) appearance of the entrapped nerve has constant features:

- Crushing of the nerve at the compression site, associated with its focal thickening proximally to the pathological site, due to edema and vascular congestion.
- Loss of the normal "honeycomb" fascicular pattern of the nerve, which shows a homogeneously hypoechoic internal aspect.
- Swelling of the fascicles.
- Intraneural echogenic fibrotic areas in chronic entrapments.
- Hypoechoic appearance due to the edema of the epineurium with poorly defined margins of the nerve.
- Echogenic concentric or asymmetric halo, representing a thickening of the outer nerve sheath.
- Increasing vascularity, at color/power Doppler evaluation.
- Hyperechoic aspect with reduction of the mass of the innervated muscles.

23.2 Entrapment Neuropathies of Upper Limb

23.2.1 Suprascapular Nerve

The suprascapular nerve (SSN) arises from the upper trunk of the brachial plexus with contributions from the C5 and C6 nerve roots and inconstantly the C4 nerve root. The nerve runs posteriorly to the clavicle to the superior border of the scapula, where it passes into the suprascapular notch, a variable depression on the superior border of the scapula. Through this notch, the SSN traverses the upper border of the scapula under the superior transverse scapular ligament (Fig. 23.1). The nerve then runs roughly medially to the posterior glenoid rim entering in the spinoglenoid notch where it passes, with the adjacent artery, under the spinoglenoid (inferior transverse scapular) ligament (Fig. 23.2). Before entering in the spinoglenoid notch the SSN most commonly supplies two motor branches to the supraspinatus muscle and, exiting from the spinoglenoid notch, supplies two branches to the infraspinatus muscle. The SSN also supplies up to 70% of the sensation of the shoulder, with nerve branches to the glenohumeral joint, acromioclavicular joint, and coracoacromial ligament as well as to the skin.

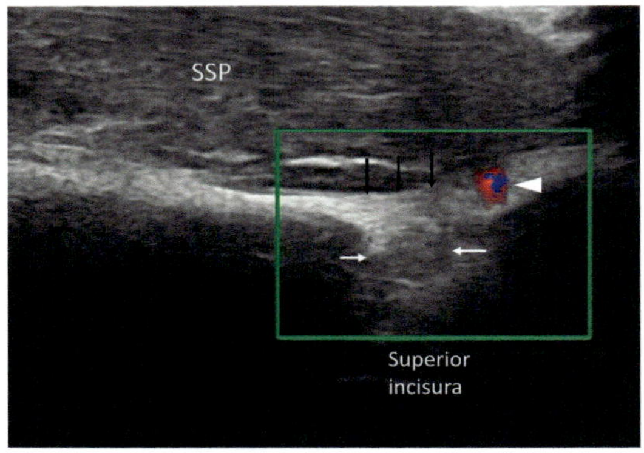

Fig. 23.1 Suprascapular notch. Transverse US image of suprascapular nerve (*white arrows*) in suprascapular notch (or superior incisura) of the scapula. The nerve passes in the suprascapular notch, beneath the superior transverse scapular ligament (*black arrows*). In the superior incisura the suprascapular artery (*arrowhead*) runs outside this tunnel. *SSP* supraspinatus muscle

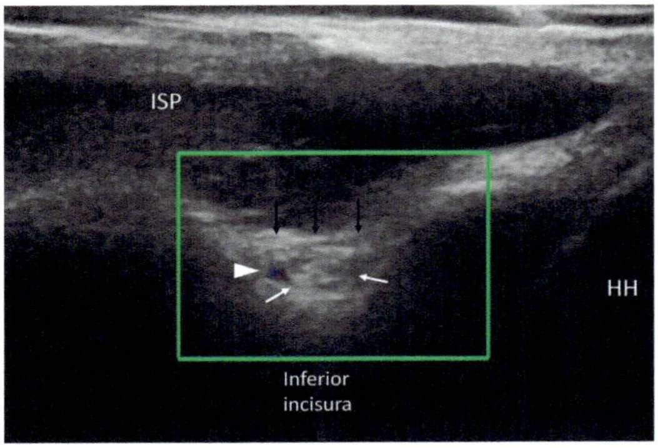

Fig. 23.2 Spinoglenoid notch. Transverse US image of suprascapular nerve (*white arrows*) in spinoglenoid notch (or inferior incisura) of the scapula. The nerve passes in the spinoglenoid notch, beneath the inferior transverse scapular ligament (*black arrows*). In the inferior incisura the suprascapular artery (*arrowhead*) runs inside this tunnel. *ISP* infraspinatus muscle *HH* humeral head

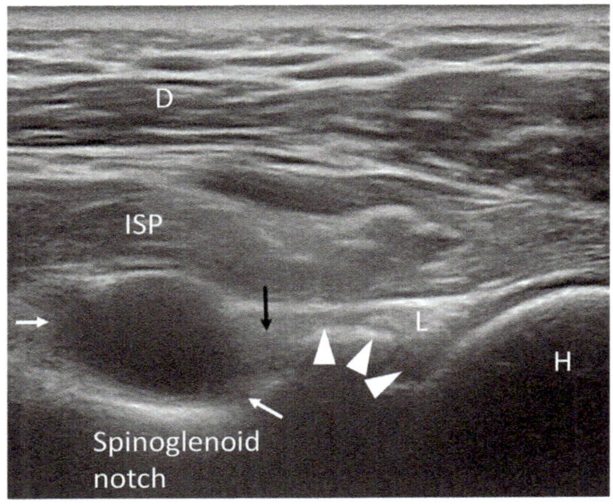

Fig. 23.3 Glenoid paralabral cyst. Transverse US image of posterior glenohumeral recess shows a large paralabral cyst (*white arrows*) occupying the spinoglenoid notch. A thin amount of fluid (*arrowheads*) shows the cyst communication with the joint cavity due to the SLAP injury. The suprascapular nerve (*black arrow*) is not well identifiable as it is compressed between the cyst and the notch floor. *ISP* infraspinatus muscle, *L* labrum, *H* humeral head, *D* deltoid muscle

The SSN entrapment may occur at three levels: the suprascapular notch (also known as scapular notch or supraspinous notch or superior incisura), the spinoglenoid notch (inferior incisura), and along its course in the osteofibrous tunnel located in subfascial position between the two incisurae.

Numerous bony morphological variants of the suprascapular (superior) notch have been described.

In the less frequent SSN entrapment in the spinoglenoid notch, potential predisposing morphological features have been evocated: V-shaped, narrow, or "deep" suprascapular notch; a band-shaped, bifurcated, or completely ossified superior transverse scapular ligament; and particular arrangements of the suprascapular nerve and vessels at the suprascapular notch. These morphologies are assessable during US examination.

The spinoglenoid (inferior) notch is the most common site of SSN entrapment. Usually the nerve is compressed from a ganglion paralabral cyst due to a SLAP lesion. US well depict the paralabral cysts as round or oval hypoechoic lesions with well-defined margins within the spinoglenoid notch. The cyst may contain hyperechoic areas due to the gas bubbles within it. The continuity of the cyst with a defect in the posterior labrum can be identified (Fig. 23.3).

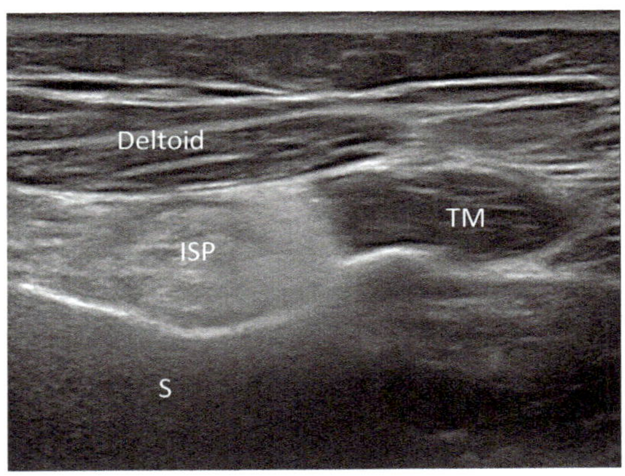

Fig. 23.4 Infraspinatus muscle atrophy. Transverse US image of posterior cuff muscles shows the atrophy of infraspinatus (ISP) due to suprascapular nerve entrapment. The infraspinatus muscle appears hyperechoic with respect to the teres minor (TM) muscle with the "black and white" effect. *D* deltoid muscle, *S* scapula

US scan of the posterior rotator cuff muscles is also helpful in identifying the compression site. Isolated atrophy of the infraspinatus muscle indicates SSN compression within or at the exit of the spinoglenoid notch (Fig. 23.4). Conversely, if both the supraspinatus and the infraspinatus muscles are involved, the compression is located proximal to the notch.

23.2.2 Musculocutaneous Nerve

The musculocutaneous nerve (MCN) is one of the main terminal branches of the brachial plexus and it supplies the muscles of the anterior compartment of the arm (the coracobrachialis, biceps brachii, and brachialis muscles) and the skin on the lateral aspect of the forearm. Typically, the MCN arises from the lateral cord of the brachial plexus; it pierces the coracobrachialis muscle and it descends distally between the biceps brachii and brachialis muscle. Just below the elbow, it pierces the deep fascia lateral to the biceps tendon.

US can identify the MCN from its origin from the lateral cord in the axilla, to the distal third of the arm. The MCN mean cross-sectional area at the level of the arm is 2.5 ± 0.4 mm^2.

Most of the mechanical MCN neuropathies are due to trauma or stretching microtraumas. Entrapment MCN neuropathies are rare. Neuropathy after excessive exercises and after long head biceps tenotomy has been described.

23.2.3 Axillary Nerve

The axillary nerve originates from the spinal cord at the C5 and C6 levels with occasional contribution from C4. It is derived from the posterior cord of the brachial plexus and travels below the coracoid process, obliquely along the anterior surface of the subscapularis, and then travels posteriorly, adjacent to the inferomedial capsule passing through the quadrilateral space. The quadrilateral space is delimited by the long head of the triceps medially, the humeral shaft laterally, the teres minor muscle superiorly, the teres major and latissimus dorsi muscles inferiorly, and the subscapularis muscle anteriorly. This is the anatomical main region of compression of the axillary nerve.

First described by Cahill and Palmer in 1983, the quadrilateral space syndrome (QSS) can lead to poorly localized shoulder pain, discrete tenderness to palpation and teres minor, and deltoid denervation. These symptoms are typically exacerbated in abduction and external rotation position.

The most common cause of compression of the axillary nerve is the presence of a fibrous band within the quadrilateral space, but paralabral cysts, bony spurs/fragments, and benign tumors have also been reported.

Although the axillary nerve can be identified, the nerve compression remains difficult to directly assess with US. Otherwise, the denervation of teres minor muscle often allows the first sign for QSS diagnosis. Atrophy of the teres minor can be easily assessed by comparing the US appearance of this muscle with that of the adjacent infraspinatus.

Dilated posterior circumflex humeral artery at the quadrilateral space can be another important sign for quadrilateral space diagnosis.

Paralabral cysts or other space-occupying lesions in quadrilateral space can be identified, too.

23.2.4 Radial Nerve

The radial nerve is the largest nerve in the upper limb. It is a branch of the brachial plexus arising from the posterior cord with fibers originating from the C5, C6, C7, C8, and T1 roots. After entering the axillary region, it runs distally, in the posterior aspect of the upper arm, passing in a spiral groove found in the posterior cortex of the humerus. Anterior to the lateral epicondyle, the radial nerve divides into superficial and deep branches.

The superficial branch is purely sensory and its entrapment syndrome at proximal wrist (called Wartenberg's syndrome) is uncommon.

The deep, purely motor, branch of the radial nerve is called posterior interosseous nerve (PIN) and it runs between the two heads of the supinator muscle, innervates it, then enters the forearm, and supplies the majority of the forearm and hand extensors. In its most proximal part the supinator muscle forms a fibrous arc called arcade of Fröhse, which is a common site of PIN compression.

23.2.4.1 Spiral Groove Syndrome

Spiral groove syndrome is often caused by a fracture of the humerus at this level. Radial palsy can be caused by (1) the injury of the nerve that passes adjacent to the cortical bone; (2) entrapment of the nerve between the skeletal segments or in the callus; (3) impingement between radial nerve and screws; and (4) entrapment of the nerve between the humerus and the surgical hardware. US is recommended in the algorithm for the management of radial nerve palsy associated with the fracture of the shaft of the humerus. In case of radial nerve palsy after a surgically treated humeral fracture, US is useful in determining the type of nerve damage. In case of injury, at US the nerve may appear thickened and hypoechoic or interrupted (Fig. 23.5). In case of fractures, the radial nerve appears displaced by the bone fragments or pinched between them. In the postoperative period, the radial nerve may be found stretched over or pinched by the orthopedic hardware used for osteosynthesis (Figs. 23.6 and 23.7).

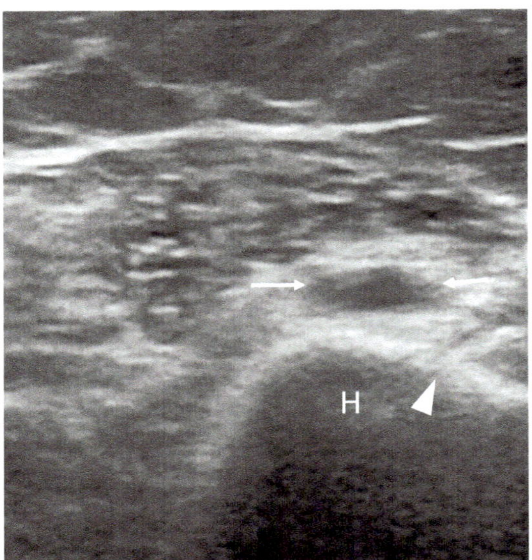

Fig. 23.5 Radial nerve injury. Transverse US image shows the radial nerve (*white arrows*) hypoechoic and swollen due to the direct trauma of the previous humeral fracture (*arrowhead*). No nerve entrapment is visible. *H* humerus

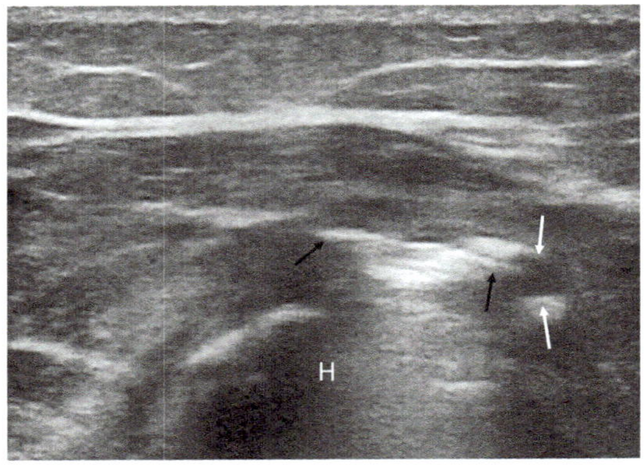

Fig. 23.6 Radial nerve entrapment in a fixation screw spiral after surgical osteosynthesis of humeral shaft fracture. Transverse US image shows the radial nerve (*white arrows*) entrapped and partially injured by the lightly extruded surgical screw (*black arrows*). *H* humerus

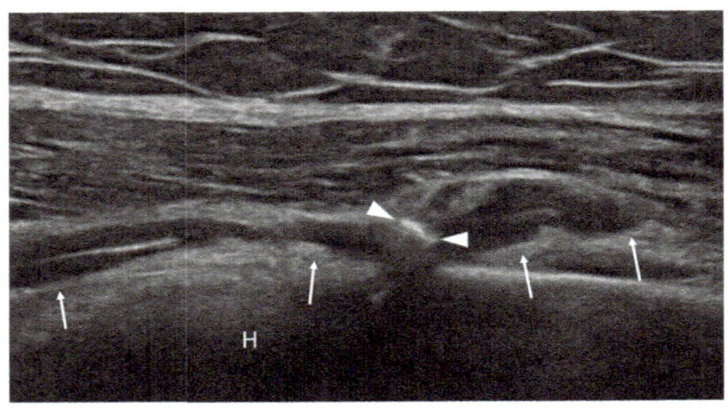

Fig. 23.7 Radial nerve entrapment under the hardware after surgical osteosynthesis of humeral shaft fracture. In the longitudinal US image the radial nerve (*arrows*) appears pinched between humeral cortex and osteosynthesis hardware (*arrowheads*) with hourglass aspect of the nerve. *H* humerus

23.2.4.2 Posterior Interosseus Syndrome

The posterior interosseus syndrome, also called supinator syndrome or radial tunnel syndrome, is a rare compression neuropathy of the upper limb affecting the deep branch of the radial nerve.

Supinator syndrome appears in two forms, a truly neurogenic, paralytic form and a painful form. The painful form is often difficult to distinguish from lateral epicondylitis.

The true neurogenic form is different from a lesion of the main trunk of the radial nerve,

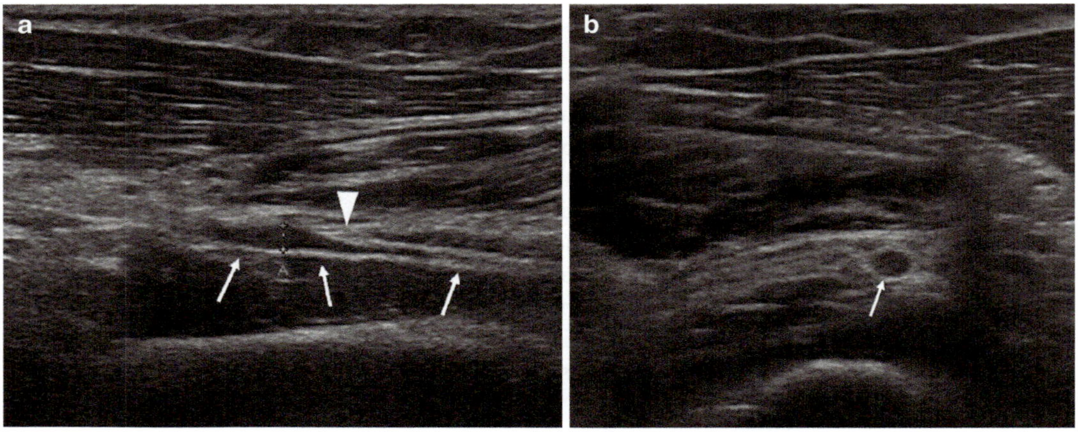

Fig. 23.8 (**a**, **b**) Posterior interosseus nerve (PIN) entrapment in the arcade of Fröhse. Longitudinal (**a**) and transverse (**b**) US images demonstrate the PIN (*arrows*) compressed by the hyperechoic and thickened Fröhse's arcade (*arrowhead*). The PIN appears hypoechoic and swelling (between calipers) just proximally to the compression site

because there are no sensory symptoms and the patient has usually a finger drop rather than the wrist drop of a radial neuropathy because the extensor carpi radialis muscle is spared, although this clinical feature is not constant.

PIN syndrome can be caused by extrinsic effects, such as compression on the PIN from adjacent structures, or by intrinsic lesions of the nerve. The arcade of Fröhse is the most common cause of extrinsic compression. The arcade of Fröhse can be classified as tendinous and membranous and the tendinous type is considered a significant risk factor for PIN syndrome. Repeated pronation and supination could be aggravated by the compression, as the nerve is "fixed" in the supinator muscle, resulting in its elongation and rotation during these movements. Compression and proximal hypoechoic swelling of the PIN at the entrance into the supinator canal are typically US appearance in Fröhse arcade compression cases (Fig. 23.8a, b).

The PIN may also be compressed by soft-tissue masses (such as lipomas, deep ganglia, and synovitis), radial head fracture, and Monteggia fracture-dislocation (Fig. 23.9). In addition, the nerve in that area is more susceptible to post-traumatic injuries and swelling of the

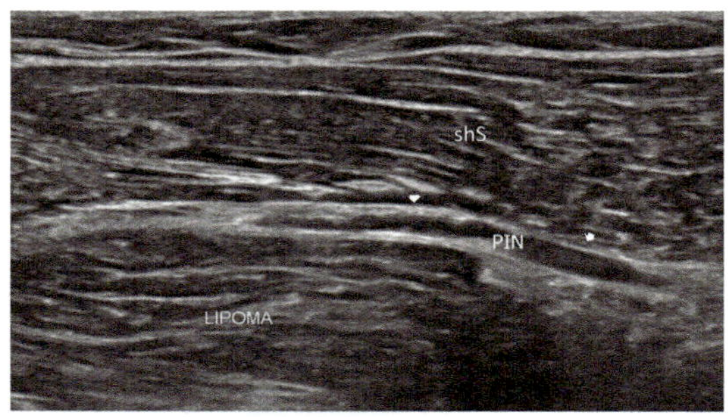

Fig. 23.9 Posterior interosseus nerve (PIN) entrapment. Longitudinal US image demonstrates the PIN compressed between a lipoma of deep head and superficial head of supinator muscle (shS). The PIN (*arrows*) shows hourglass aspect. The patient was suffering from isolated finger drop of the index

PIN is usually found distally to the Fröhse arcade (Fig. 23.10)

23.2.5 Ulnar Nerve

Potential ulnar nerve entrapment can occur at five sites around the elbow: the arcade of Struthers, the medial intermuscular septum, the medial epicondyle, the cubital tunnel, and the deep flexor pronator aponeurosis. The most common site of entrapment is the cubital tunnel.

23.2.5.1 Cubital Tunnel Syndrome

Cubital tunnel syndrome involves compression and irritation of the ulnar nerve at the elbow, where the nerve passes through the cubital tunnel under Osborne's ligament. It is considered the second most common upper extremity nerve entrapment after carpal tunnel syndrome.

Compression of the nerve at this level can be caused by numerous causes both congenital and acquired, including an anconeus-epitrochlearis muscle, bone deformities, ganglion cysts, and other space-occupying lesions.

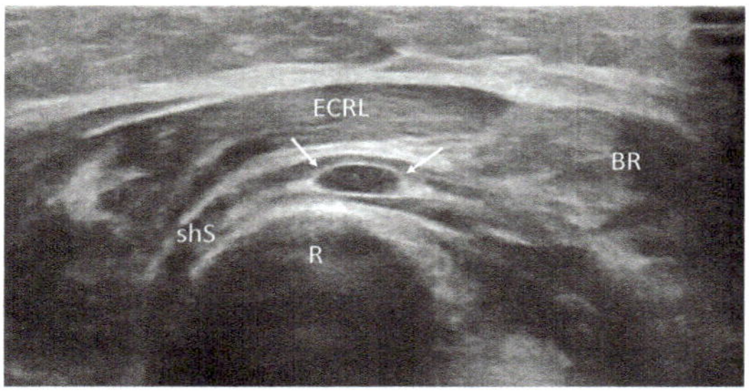

Fig. 23.10 Posterior interosseus nerve (PIN) injury. Transverse US image demonstrates a hypoechoic and swollen PIN (*arrows*) distally to the Fröhse's arcade after trauma. *ECRL* extensor carpi radialis longus, *BR* brachioradialis, *shS* superficial head of supinator muscle, *R* radius

To begin the US examination, it is useful to keep the elbow extended and the probe positioned immediately posterior to the medial epicondyle (identifiable by palpation). The ulnar nerve appears hypoechoic, surrounded by hyperechoic fat, and it can be ovoid or have a bilobed, bifid, or trifid appearance. The mean cross-sectional area of the ulnar nerve in the cubital tunnel was approximately 6.6 mm and slight enlargement of the nerve at the epicondyle compared to ulnar nerve area at the level of the upper arm proximally could be normal.

In the cubital tunnel syndrome, the ulnar nerve appears thickened and hypoechoic proximal to the tunnel and may flatten or remain thickened within it (Fig. 23.11a–c). It is useful to identify the causes of nerve compression, such as joint effusion, synovitis and osteophytes (Fig. 23.12). The presence of an anconeus-epitrochlearis muscle may represent another possible cause of ulnar nerve entrapment, which

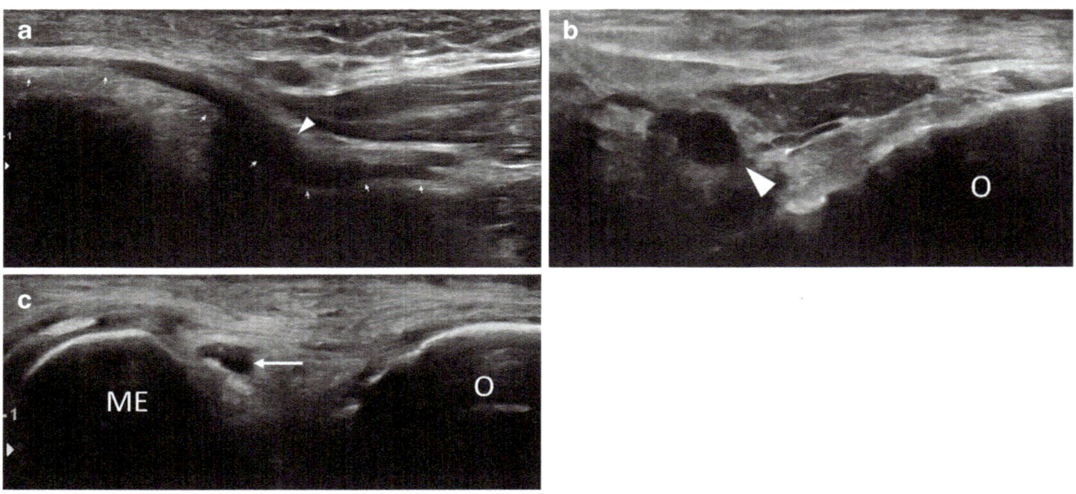

Fig. 23.11 (**a**–**c**) Cubital tunnel syndrome. Longitudinal (**a**) and transverse (**b**) US images just proximally and at the cubital tunnel level (**c**). The ulnar nerve (*arrows*) appears swollen and hypoechoic (*arrowheads* in **a** and **b**) just before entering the cubital tunnel. In the tunnel the nerve appears normal in dimension (*arrow* in **c**). *ME* medial epicondyle, *O* olecranon

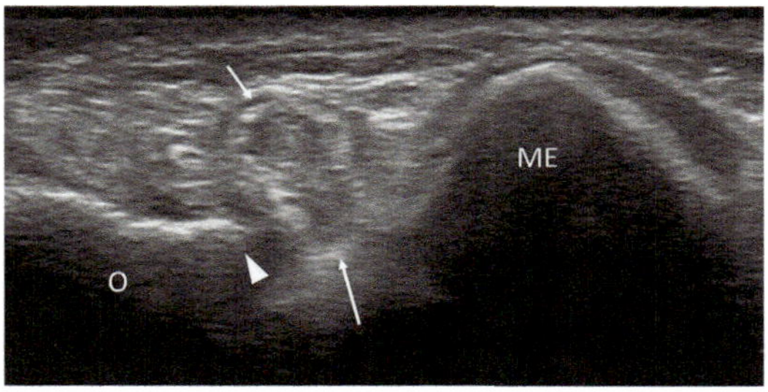

Fig. 23.12 Cubital tunnel syndrome. Transverse US image shows the ulnar nerve compressed by an olecranic spur (*arrowhead*). The ulnar nerve (*arrows*) appears pinched with hyperechoic and irregular margins. *ME* medial epicondyle, *O* olecranon

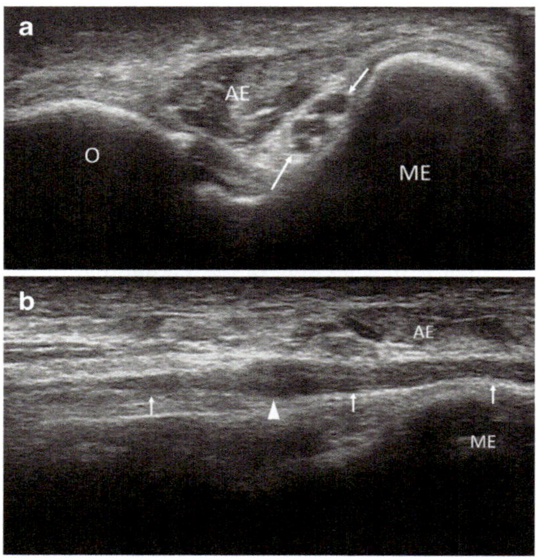

Fig. 23.13 (**a**, **b**) Transverse (**a**) and longitudinal (**b**) US images at the cubital tunnel level show the ulnar nerve (*arrows*) entrapped between an accessory muscle called anconeus epitrochlearis (AE) and the medial epicondyle humerus (ME). A focal nerve swelling (*arrowhead* in **b**) is noted just proximally to the compression site. *ME* medial epicondyle, *O* olecranon

occurs just proximal to the true cubital tunnel. It is visible with US as a muscle superficially to the ulnar nerve (Fig. 23.13a, b).

23.2.5.2 Guyon's Canal Syndrome

Guyon's canal represents an additional site of entrapment of the ulnar nerve, although this pathology is quite rare. Space-occupying lesions such as lipomas, cystic ganglia, ulnar artery pseudoaneurysms, or abnormal muscles are the main causes of this syndrome. Clinically it differs from that of the cubital tunnel because the sensitivity of the dorsum of the middle half of the fourth and fifth fingers is preserved.

23.2.6 Median Nerve

The median nerve originates from the medial and lateral cords of the brachial plexus, receiving innervation from C6, C7, C8, and T1. After its origin, the median nerve and brachial artery run along the medial aspect of the arm towards the elbow. The anterior interosseous nerve (AIN) emerges 5–8 cm distally to the lateral epicondyle on the posterior surface of the median nerve.

Rare entrapment sites of the median nerve are located near the elbow.

The *supracondylar process syndrome* is caused by the presence of the supracondylar process which is a beak-shaped bony process on the anteromedial aspect of the distal humerus. The ligament of Struthers' is a fibrous band usually extending from the tip of the process to the medial epicondyle.

The median nerve could be entrapped under the ligament of Struthers' or directly compressed by the bony process (Fig. 23.14).

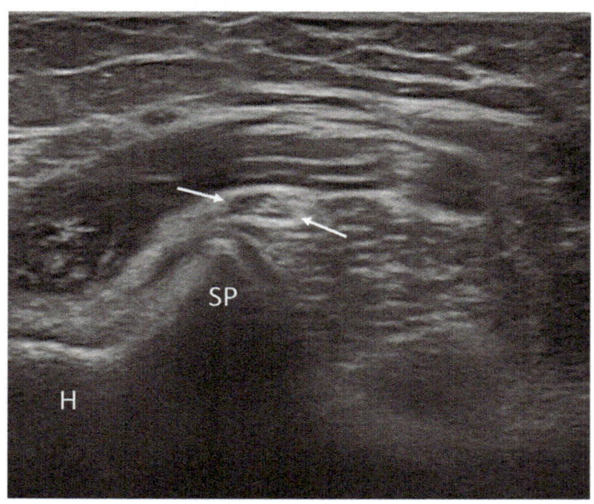

Fig. 23.14 Transverse US image of the anterior aspect of the middle third of the arm. Note the supracondylar process (SP) that dislocates the median nerve (*arrows*) deforming it. *H* humerus

In the *pronator syndrome* patients have pain and paresthesia in the volar aspect of the elbow and forearm and in the first, second, and third digits and radial half of the ring finger. US is very useful to detect the compression site. The *Kiloh-Nevin syndrome* is characterized by an extrinsic compression of the AIN that determines the difficulty in performing the OK sign with the affected hand.

Clinical and US detection of muscle atrophy often represents the first step in diagnosing these rare forms of entrapment.

23.2.6.1 Carpal Tunnel Syndrome

Carpal tunnel syndrome (CTS) is the most common entrapment neuropathy and consists of compression of the median nerve in the namesake tunnel. The median nerve in the carpal tunnel lies between the flexor retinaculum superiorly and the flexor tendons and carpal bones (scaphoid and trapezium) inferiorly. The CTS is characterized first by intermittent nocturnal paresthesia and pain. Subsequently there is a loss of sensation followed by motor symptoms such as weakness and thenar muscle atrophy.

Current recommendations by the American Academy of Orthopaedic Surgeons (AAOS) are to obtain a confirmatory test in patients for whom carpal tunnel surgery is being considered. Several authors today are in agreement to use US as a first-line test for confirmation of a clinical diagnosis of CTS to be a cost-effective strategy in the hands of a specialist.

The US diagnosis of STC includes several semiotic features. The most commonly used are median nerve thickening and evaluating the difference in cross-sectional area between the nerve in the carpal tunnel and proximally at the pronator quadratus muscle level in the distal forearm (Δ >2 mm^2 is pathologic). The severity grading is defined as mild when Δ is $\leq$6 mm^2, moderate when it is $\leq$9 mm^2, and severe when it is >9 mm^2. Distal flattening of the median nerve and palmar bulging of the flexor retinaculum (>2 mm beyond line joining the hamate-pisiform to the trapezium/scaphoid) are other important US features for the diagnosis of CTS. Power Doppler evaluation is also used by some authors in combination of nerve swelling measurements to increase the diagnostic accuracy of US in patients with clinically suspected CTS (Figs. 23.15a, b, and 23.16a, b).

Even if usually the CTS is congenital, US can assess the possible causes of compression: thickening of the flexor retinaculum, tenosynovitis, ganglion cysts, radiocarpal synovitis, or muscles' anatomic variants.

Anatomical variants of median nerve at wrist level include accessory branches proximal to the carpal tunnel; accessory branches in the distal carpal tunnel; thenar branch course variation; and high divisions of the median nerve (or bifid median nerve). The incidence of bifid median

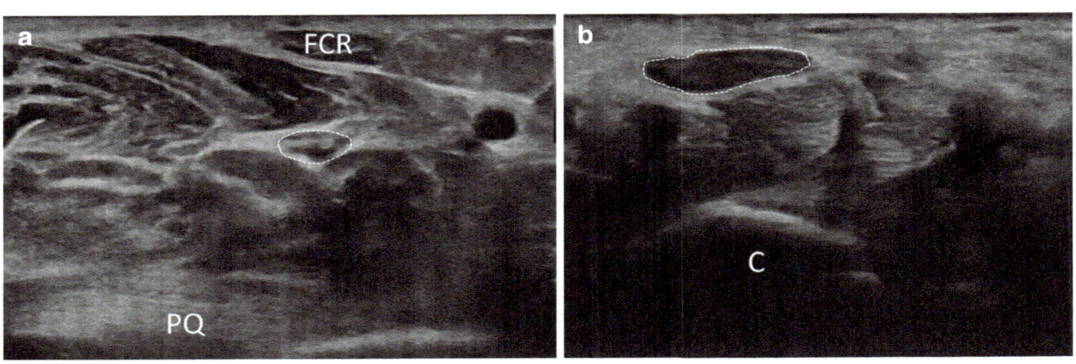

Fig. 23.15 (**a**, **b**) Carpal tunnel syndrome. Two transverse US images at the level of the distal third of pronator quadratus muscle (**a**) and at carpal tunnel level (**b**). The cross-sectional area of the median nerve (outlined) is 8 mm^2 in (**a**) and 14 mm^2 in (**b**) with a Δ of 6 mm^2, indicating high-grade carpal tunnel syndrome. *PQ* pronator quadratus muscle, *C* carpus, *FCR* flexor carpi radialis tendon

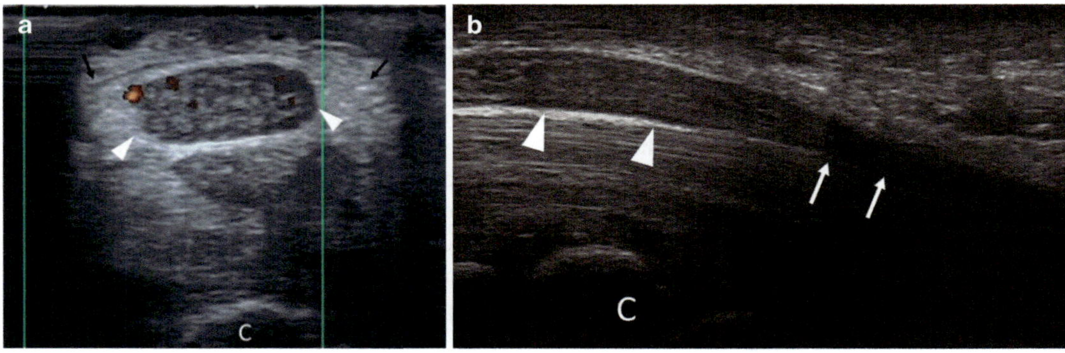

Fig. 23.16 (**a**, **b**) Carpal tunnel syndrome. Transverse (**a**) and longitudinal (**b**) US images at carpal tunnel level. The median nerve appears swollen and hypoechoic just proximally to the carpal tunnel (*arrowheads*) and flattening distally (*white arrows*). Note the palmar bowing of the flexor retinaculum (*black arrows*) and the increase of nerve vascularization at power Doppler

nerves was found to be 2.8% and it can be present with a persistent median artery (Fig. 23.17). Evaluation of the cross-sectional area implies summing the areas of the two branches of the median nerve with a new cutoff Δ value of 4 mm^2 instead of 2 mm^2.

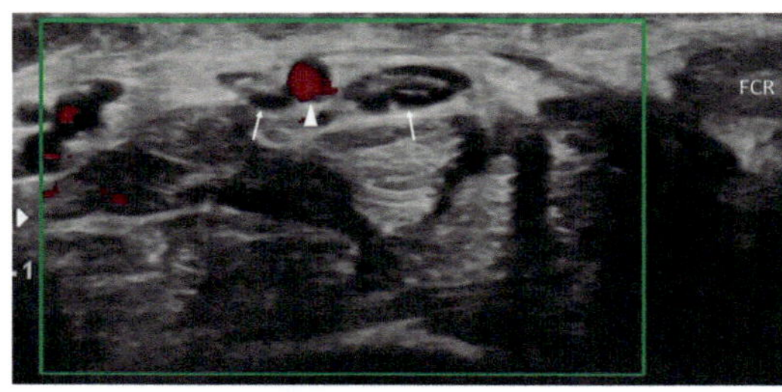

Fig. 23.17 Bifid median nerve. Transverse US image at carpal tunnel level shows a bifid median nerve (*arrows*) with a persistent median artery (*arrowhead*)

23.3 Entrapment Neuropathies of Lower Limb

23.3.1 Lateral Femoral Cutaneous Nerve Entrapment

The lateral femoral cutaneous nerve (LFCN) is a pure sensory nerve providing sensation to the anterolateral aspect of the thigh. The LFCN arises from the L2 and L3 nerve roots, courses lateral to the psoas muscle, crosses the iliacus muscle, and exits the pelvis running below or in a split of the lateral end of the inguinal ligament, medially to the anterior superior iliac spine (ASIS). Soon after crossing the ligament, the LFCN passes over or medially to the sartorius muscle into the thigh, where it divides into an anterior and a posterior branch, providing sensory innervation to the anterior and the lateral thigh, respectively.

Meralgia paresthetica is an entrapment neuropathy of the LFCN where it crosses the inguinal ligament with pain, numbness, paresthesia, or burning sensation in the anterolateral thigh. Causes of entrapment are abdominal bulging over the inguinal ligament in pregnancy and obesity with compression of the nerve at the lateral end of the inguinal ligament, ascites, tight clothing, seat belts, limb length discrepancy, avulsion fracture of the ASIS, proximal sartorius enthesopathy, and local soft-tissue masses. Recently, smartphone worn on the belt or tablet rested too frequently on a patient's lap has been found to cause LFCN entrapment.

The main US findings of LFCN neuropathy are nerve flattening under the inguinal ligament with hypoechoic nerve swelling proximal to the area of entrapment (Fig. 23.18a, b).

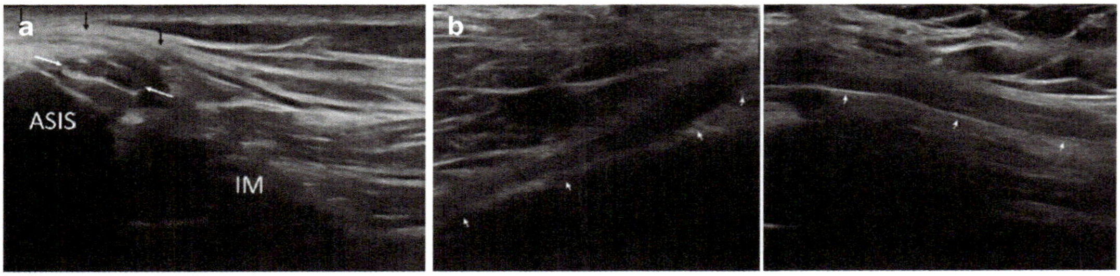

Fig. 23.18 (**a**, **b**) Meralgia paresthetica. Transverse (**a**) and longitudinal (**b**) US images show the entrapment of the lateral femoral cutaneous nerve between anterior superior iliac spine (ASIS) and inguinal ligament (*black arrows*). The nerve shows coalescence of fascicles and hyperechoic outer nerve sheath (*white arrows*). *IM* iliac muscle

23.3.2 Sciatic Nerve

The sciatic nerve (SN), the largest nerve in the body, originates from the L4 through S3 nerve roots, forming a single nerve within pelvis, and exits the pelvis posteriorly through the greater sciatic foramen inferior to the piriformis muscle. Distally to the piriformis muscle, SN is covered by gluteus maximus and runs halfway between the ischial tuberosity and the greater trochanter. After curving around the ischial spine, SN has a close relationship with hamstrings, descending lateral to their proximal origin and running behind them in the proximal thigh. SN provides motor fibers to the posterior thigh muscles and almost all sensory and motor functions below the knee.

23.3.2.1 Deep Gluteal Syndrome

This syndrome is caused by entrapment of SN occurring from gluteal region. The most common causes of SN entrapment are fibrovascular band, piriformis syndrome, ischiofemoral impingement, proximal hamstring tendon injury, femoral fracture, hip fracture dislocation, and total hip arthroplasty. In these cases US may reveal a focal increase in the nerve size, loss of the fascicular echotexture, and hypoechoic pattern of SN.

23.3.3 Common Peroneal Nerve

The common peroneal nerve (CPN), receiving contributions from the L4 through S2 nerve roots, takes off from SN at the apex of the popliteal fossa, coursing along the border of the biceps femoris muscle. CPN then travels superficially and wraps around the fibular head/neck, before entering the anterior compartment musculature of the leg through the peroneal tunnel, formed by the proximal fibula and peroneus longus muscle, where it divides into the superficial and deep peroneal nerves.

Compression neuropathy of CPN at fibular head is the most common neuropathy of the lower limb, presenting clinically with foot drop or motor weakness of ankle dorsiflexion. At the fibular head level the CPN is relatively fixed, located superficially and closely to the underlying bone of the fibula, making it particularly susceptible to injury. A remarkable predisposing factor for CPN neuropathies at fibular head is a recent weight loss, because it is associated with loss of subcutaneous fat, increasing the susceptibility of the nerve to compression at this level. Furthermore, anatomic variations of lateral gastrocnemius, distal biceps femoris tendon, and fibular head may predispose to compression of CPN.

Other causes of CPN neuropathy at fibular head/neck include space-occupying lesions, thickening of a surrounding fascia, traction- or contusion-nerve injuries during knee trauma (isolated or in association with fibular head fracture), and postsurgical scar tissue. Another less common cause is entrapment of the nerve by fabella, in close anatomical relation with CP (Fig. 23.19).

Compression of the deep peroneal nerve at the peroneal tunnel is less common.

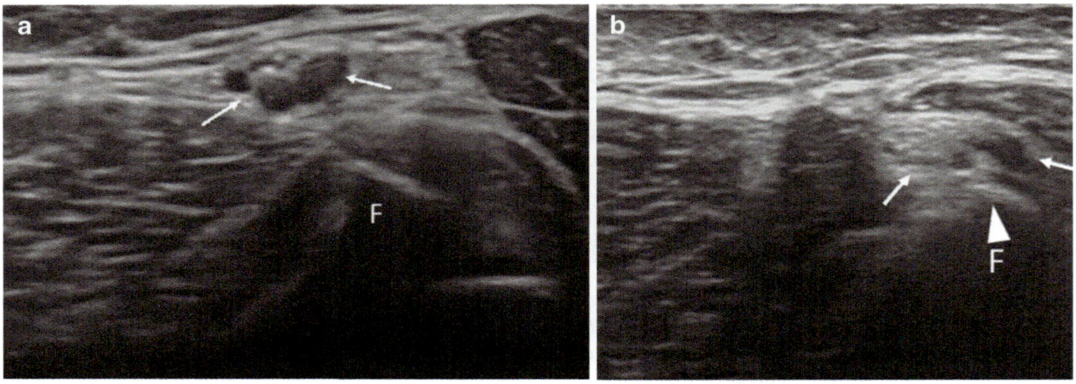

Fig. 23.19 (**a**, **b**) Common peroneal nerve impingement with fabella. Two transverse US images of common peroneal nerve (CPN) at lateral femoral condyle level, with extended knee in (**a**) and flexed knee with external rotation of the foot in (**b**). In (**a**) the CPN (*arrows*) appears thickened and hypoechoic; the fabella (F) is noted. In (**b**), with the knee in typical position of the legs crossed, the CPN (*arrows*) appears compressed and deformed by the fabella (F)

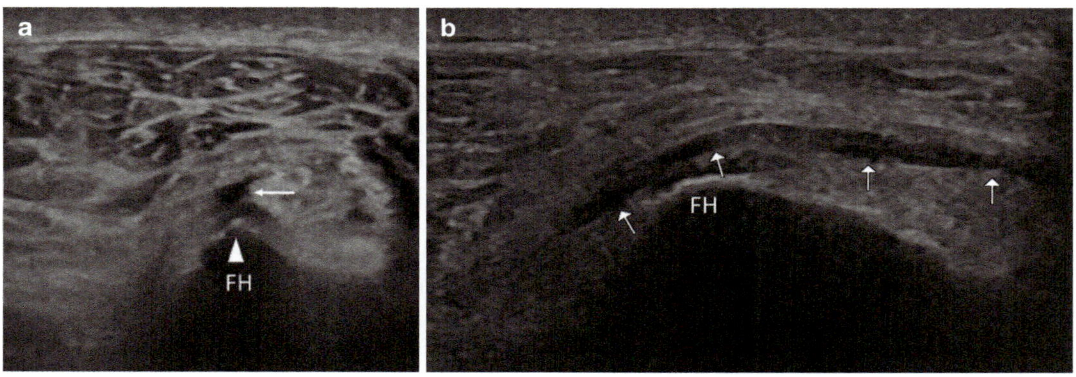

Fig. 23.20 (**a**, **b**) Common peroneal nerve entrapment. Transverse (**a**) and longitudinal (**b**) US images show the common peroneal nerve (*arrows*) compressed and dislocated by the below fibular head (FH).

The main US findings of CPN neuropathy are an evident fibular-CPN impingement, increased cross-sectional area (>11 mm^2), and flexion of its course at the fibular head, hypoechogenicity, loss of normal fascicular pattern, and sometimes hypervascularization on color or power Doppler (Fig. 23.20a, b). In cases of doubt on the direct ultrasound evaluation of the nerve, it may be useful to confirm the compromise of the only muscles innervated by the PCN to exclude other pathologies (Fig. 23.21).

23.3.4 Superficial Peroneal Nerve

After its origin from CPN in the peroneal tunnel, the superficial peroneal nerve (SPN) courses between the peroneus longus and extensor digitorum longus muscles. About 5 cm above the ankle joint SPN pierces the deep fascia, the most common site of mechanical entrapment, to enter the subcutaneous compartment, where it divides into its terminal sensory branches.

SPN provides motor innervation to the peroneus longus and brevis muscles and sensory

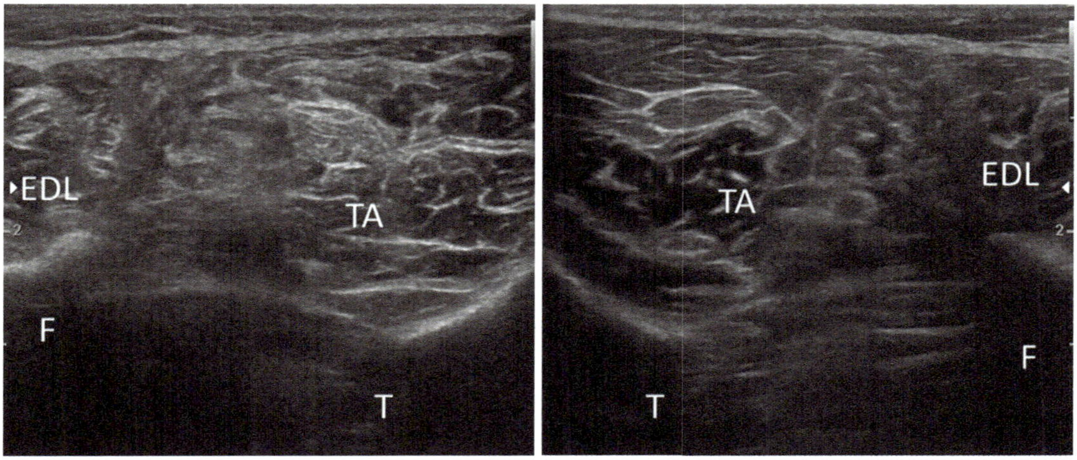

Fig. 23.21 Common peroneal nerve entrapment: Muscle atrophy. Transverse US images of anterior proximal third of the leg show the difference in echogenicity of the anterolateral muscles between the affected (on the left) and healthy side (on the right). On the left the tibialis anterior (TA) and the extensor digitorum longus (EDL) muscles appear hyperechoic due to the peroneal nerve entrapment

innervation to the lower two-thirds of the anterolateral leg and the dorsum of the foot.

The most common site of entrapment is the exit from the deep fascia and the generally reported symptoms are pain and sensory changes over the dorsum of the foot. Causes of SPN entrapment are repetitive plantar flexions and ankle inversions, scarring or fibrous bands, ganglion cyst, and muscle hernia through a fascial defect.

US is fundamental in assessing SPN, because, in addition to identifying the classic signs of entrapment neuropathy, it allows to detect any fascial defects and muscle hernias through a dynamic exam during muscle contraction.

23.3.5 Deep Peroneal Nerve

After its origin from CPN in the peroneal tunnel, the deep peroneal nerve (DPN), accompanied by the anterior tibial artery, courses distally along the anterior surface of interosseous membrane, providing motor innervation to extensor muscles of the foot and sensory innervation to tibiotalar joint. Impingement of the proximal course of the nerve within the proximal leg is uncommon.

23.3.5.1 Anterior Tarsal Tunnel Syndrome

At the ankle level the nerve becomes superficial and enters the anterior tarsal tunnel, containing the extensor tendons of the foot, dorsalis pedis artery and veins, and DPN. Just inferior or under the inferior extensor retinaculum, DPN divides into lateral and medial branches.

Entrapment of DPN and its branches may occur more commonly in three sites: deep to the inferior extensor retinaculum; deep to the extensor hallucis longus tendon at the level of the talo-navicular joint; and deep to the extensor hallucis brevis muscle at the first and second tarsal-metatarsal articulation levels (medial branch).

Generally, patients report sensory changes and pain across the top of the foot going into the space between the first and the second toe.

US may easily evaluate the nerve in its more superficial locations and detect entrapment causes.

Causes of DPN entrapment neuropathy are thickening or injury to the extensor retinaculum, synovitis, and osteophytosis at talo-navicular, navicular-cuneiform or tarso-metarsal joints (Fig. 23.22), os intermetatarseum, fractures, ice skate or ski boot wear, high-heeled or tight-fitting running shoes, ganglia originating from neigh-

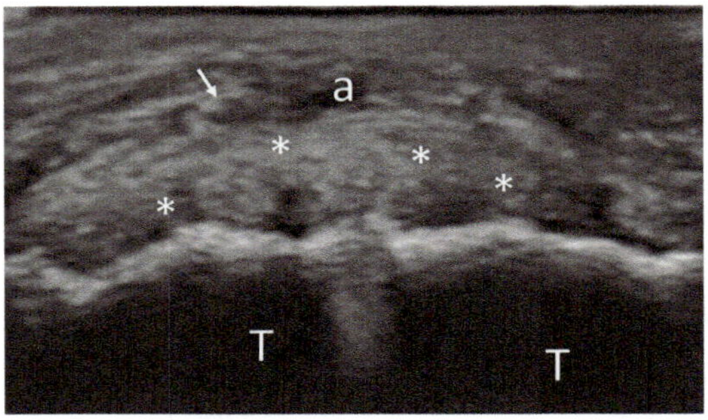

Fig. 23.22 Deep peroneal nerve. Transverse US images show synovitis (*asterisks*) of tarso-metatarsal joints with entrapment of superior deep peroneal nerve (*arrow*). *T* tarsus, *a* artery

boring joints, extensor tenosynovitis, anterior tibial or dorsalis pedis artery aneurysms, thrombosed dorsalis pedis vein, and prosthesis.

23.3.6 Tibial Nerve

The tibial nerve (TN) receives contributions from the L4 through S2 nerve roots. In the posterior knee TN takes off from SN at the apex of the popliteal fossa and runs through the popliteal fossa accompanied by popliteal artery and vein. This neurovascular bundle passes deep to the tendinous arch of the soleus muscle and, after yielding the peroneal artery, travels superficial to the tibialis posterior muscle to reach the tarsal tunnel.

At the ankle level, TN, now known as posterior tibial nerve (PTN), trifurcates into its terminal branches (medial plantar, lateral plantar, and medial calcaneal nerves) proximally, within or distally to the tarsal tunnel, the fibro-osseous tunnel in the posteromedial aspect of the ankle posterior to the medial malleolus, and deep to the flexor retinaculum.

The main compression neuropathies of TN and its branches include tarsal tunnel syndrome, jogger's foot, and Baxter neuropathy.

23.3.6.1 Tarsal Tunnel Syndrome (Posterior Tibial Nerve)

Tarsal tunnel syndrome is a compression neuropathy of PTN within the fibro-osseous tarsal tunnel on the posteromedial aspect of the ankle, containing PTN, posterior tibial artery and veins, posterior tibialis, and flexor tendons.

Excessive tension, compression, and entrapment of PTN in the tarsal tunnel may be due to valgus hindfoot, traumatic scar, talocalcaneal coalition, hypertrophic and accessory muscles, hypertrophic or inflamed tendons, and space-occupying lesions.

Symptoms of tarsal tunnel syndrome include pain and paresthesia along the plantar foot.

US of TN at the tarsal tunnel is very specific, being able to identify the causes of tarsal tunnel syndrome and direct findings of entrapment neuropathy, such as loss of nerve fascicular pattern, hypoechoic nerve enlargement proximal to the area of entrapment with flattening or disappearance of the nerve at the site of entrapment, and acute and pathologic angle changes in the path of the nerve or "kinking" (Fig. 23.23).

23.3.6.2 Jogger's Foot (Medial Plantar Nerve)

The medial plantar nerve (MPN) is the larger terminal branch of TN, providing motor innervation to the deep muscles of the plantar side of the foot and sensation from the respective side of the sole of the foot. MPN is most commonly entrapped between the abductor hallucis muscle and the "Henry's knot," that is, the crossing of the flexor digitorum longus tendon over the flexor hallucis longus tendon in the plantar aspect of the mid-

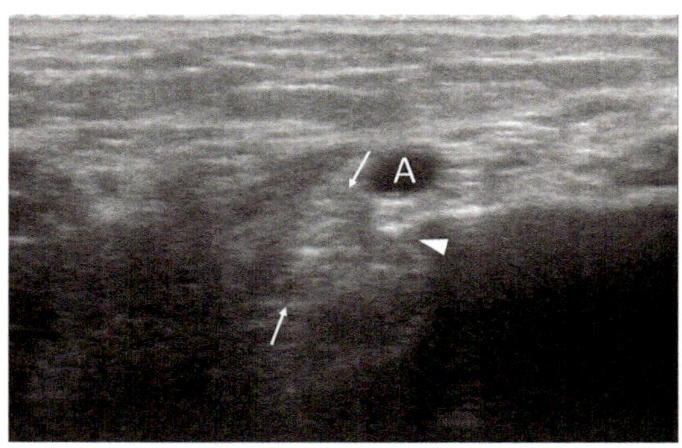

Fig. 23.23 Tarsal tunnel syndrome. Transverse US image of tarsal tunnel shows hypertrophy of the medial process of the talus. The bony spur (*arrowhead*) creating impingement with the tibial posterior nerve (*arrows*). *A* artery

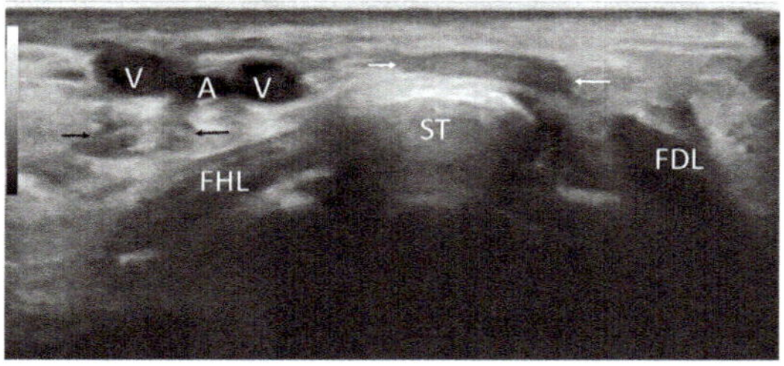

Fig. 23.24 Jogger's foot. Transverse US image of the posteromedial aspect of the ankle at calcaneal level shows hypertrophy of sustentaculum tali (ST) of calcaneus related to talocalcaneal coalition. The medial plantar nerve (*arrows*) results entrapped between the sustentaculum tali and superficial fascia. Note the lateral plantar nerve posteriorly (*black arrows*). *FHL* flexor hallucis longus, *FDL* flexor digitorum longus, *V* veins, *A* artery

foot, leading to pain on the medial plantar aspect of the foot. Tendinosis or tenosynovitis around "Henry's knot" may cause nerve irritation, particularly in regular runners; for this reason this condition is also called as "jogger's foot." Other less common causes of entrapment are plantar muscle hypertrophy, bony abnormalities and space occupying lesions (Fig. 23.24).

The "Henry's knot" is an excellent landmark to identify the nerve at US exam that is able to detect tendinosis or tenosynovitis around Henry's, space-occupying lesions, and direct findings of entrapment neuropathy.

23.3.6.3 Baxter Neuropathy (Inferior Calcaneal Nerves)

The inferior calcaneal nerve (ICN), or Baxter's nerve, is the first branch of the lateral plantar nerve, providing motor innervation to the abductor digiti minimi muscle and sensory innervation to the anterior aspect of the calcaneus.

Entrapment of ICN is also known as Baxter neuropathy. The entrapment sites are where ICN travels between the abductor hallucis and medial margin of the quadratus plantae muscles and where ICN runs between calcaneus and flexor digitorum brevis muscle-aponeurosis complex. Causes of entrapment are plantar calcaneal enthesopathy, plantar fasciitis, bone spurs, muscle hypertrophy, varicosities, and hyperpronation of the foot. The most common symptoms are heel pain, numbness along the lateral third of the sole of the foot, and weakness of the abductor digiti minimi. US is useful to assess the nerve and detect space-occupying lesions, other causes of external compression, as well as a denervation atrophy, but MRI appears to be more sensitive to identify the abductor digiti minimi muscle atrophy.

23.3.7 Interdigital Nerves

The interdigital nerves (IN) originate from the medial and lateral plantar nerves at the level of the metatarsal bases and course through a fibro-osseous tunnel formed by the metatarsal heads and intermetatarsal ligament, innervating the web spaces.

IN are typically involved in Morton's neuroma, which is not a true neuroma, but an entrapment neuropathy, characterized by perineural fibrosis of the interdigital nerve.

It is caused by repetitive compressive trauma of IN against the transverse intermetatarsal ligament resulting in local edema of the endoneurium, axonal degeneration, neovascularization, and perineural fibrosis. Sometimes it may be associated with intermetatarsal bursitis.

Morton's neuroma most commonly affects women, likely due to wearing narrow shoes inducing traction of IN. It is also observed in runners and dancers, typically caused by hyperextension of the metatarsophalangeal joints and repetitive trauma to the metatarsals.

The second and third intermetatarsal spaces are more commonly involved due to their smaller dimensions and the larger dimensions of the third IN, receiving contributions from both the medial and lateral plantar nerves.

Patients typically refer to burning or electric pain and paresthesia in the affected web space and may report sensation of walking on a lump or pebble.

US is a reliable tool in confirming the clinical diagnosis of Morton's neuroma. The best technique to visualize Morton's neuroma is to place the transducer on the plantar aspect of the web space of clinical interest applying a "Mulder's test" maneuver. At US the Morton's neuroma

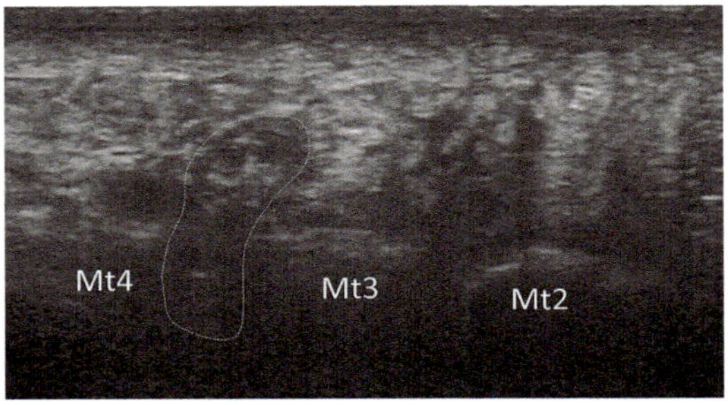

Fig. 23.25 Morton's neuroma Transverse US image of third intermetatarsal space during Mulder's test shows the so-called Morton's neuroma as hypo-isoechoic mass (outlined) between the third and fourth metatarsal heads (Mt)

appears as a rounded or ovoid, hypoechoic nodule in the intermetatarsal space. It is reported that the mean size of the measured neuromas on US was 4.9 ± 1.45 mm (range: 4–9 mm) (Fig. 23.25). The US Tinel sign, consisting of the evocation of pain with the pressure exerted by the transducer, may also be present and help in diagnosing Morton's neuroma.

23.3.8 Medial Proper Plantar Digital Nerve

The medial proper plantar digital nerve, also known as the medial hallucal digital nerve, is the most medial branch of the medial plantar nerve and is located at the medial plantar aspect of the hallux adjacent to the medial sesamoid bone, providing sensory innervation to the medial aspect of the hallux. Focal irritation of the nerve may result in the formation of a neuroma known as Joplin neuroma, which may be visualized at US as a small area of hypoechoic focal thickening.

Further Readings

Abreu E, Aubert S, Wavreille G, et al. Peripheral tumor and tumor-like neurogenic lesions. Eur J Radiol. 2013;82:38–50.

Allagui M, Maghrebi S, Touati B, et al. Posterior interosseous nerve syndrome due to intramuscular lipoma. Eur Orthop Traumatol. 2014;5:75–9.

Amin MF, Berst M, El-Khoury GY. An unusual cause of the quadrilateral space impingement syndrome by a bone spike. Skeletal Radiol. 2006;35:956–8.

Ay S, Bektas U, Yilmaz C, Diren B. An unusual supracondylar process syndrome. J Hand Surg Am. 2002;27:913–5.

Balalis K, Topalidou A, Balali C, et al. The treatment of Morton's neuroma, a significant cause of metatarsalgia for people who exercise. Int J Clin Med. 2013;4:19–24.

Bäumer P, Kele H, Xia A, et al. Posterior interosseous neuropathy: Supinator syndrome vs fascicular radial neuropathy. Neurology. 2016;87:1884–91.

Baxter DE, Thigpen CM. Heel pain—operative results. Foot Ankle. 1984;5:16–25.

Beltran LS, Bencardino J, Ghazikhanian V, Beltran J. Entrapment neuropathies III: lower limb. In: Seminars in musculoskeletal radiology. Semin Musculoskelet Radiol .Thieme Medical Publishers. 2010;14:501–11.

Bencardino J, Rosenberg ZS, Beltran J, et al. Morton's neuroma: is it always symptomatic? Am J Roentgenol. 2000;175:649–53.

Bianchi S, Martinoli C. Ultrasound of the musculoskeletal system. Switzerland: Springer Science & Business Media; 2007.

Bignotti B, Assini A, Signori A, et al. Ultrasound versus MRI in common fibular neuropathy. Muscle Nerve. 2017;55:849–57.

Bignotti B, Cadoni A, Assini A, et al. Fascicular involvement in common fibular neuropathy: evaluation with ultrasound. Muscle Nerve. 2016;53:532–7.

Bignotti B, Signori A, Sormani MP. Ultrasound versus magnetic resonance imaging for Morton neuroma: systematic review and meta-analysis. Eur Radiol. 2015;25(8):2254–62. https://doi.org/10.1007/s00330-015-3633-3.

Bodner G, Bernathova M, Galiano K, et al. Ultrasound of the lateral femoral cutaneous nerve: normal findings in a cadaver and in volunteers. Reg Anesth Pain Med. 2009;34:265–8.

Bodner G, Buchberger W, Schocke M, et al. Radial nerve palsy associated with humeral shaft fracture: evaluation with US—initial experience. Radiology. 2001;219:811–6.

Bowley MP. Entrapment neuropathies of the lower extremity. Med Clin North Am. 2018;103(2):371–82. https://doi.org/10.1016/j.mcna.2018.10.013.

Boykin RE, Friedman DJ, Higgins LD, Warner JJP. Suprascapular neuropathy. JBJS. 2010;92:2348–64.

Cahill BR, Palmer RE. Quadrilateral space syndrome. J Hand Surg Am. 1983;8:65–9.

Carro LP, Hernando MF, Cerezal L, et al. Deep gluteal space problems: piriformis syndrome, ischiofemoral impingement and sciatic nerve release. Muscles Ligaments Tendons J. 2016;6:384.

Chari B. Nerve entrapment in ankle and foot. Ultrasound Imag. 2018;22:354–63.

Chihlas CN, Ladocsi LT, Sholley MM, et al. Position of the fabella relative to the path of the common peroneal nerve across the lateral head of the gastrocnemius muscle. Clin Anat Off J Am Assoc Clin Anat Br Assoc Clin Anat. 1993;6:163–6.

Chipman JN, Mott RT, Stanton CA, Cartwright MS. Ultrasonographic tinel sign. Muscle Nerve Off J Am Assoc Electrodiagn Med. 2009;40:1033–5.

Cho D, Saetia K, Lee S, et al. Peroneal nerve injury associated with sports-related knee injury. Neurosurg Focus. 2011;31:E11.

Chundru U, Liebeskind A, Seidelmann F, et al. Plantar fasciitis and calcaneal spur formation are associated with abductor digiti minimi atrophy on MRI of the foot. Skeletal Radiol. 2008;37:505–10.

Claessen FMAP, Peters RM, Verbeek DO, et al. Factors associated with radial nerve palsy after operative treatment of diaphyseal humeral shaft fractures. J Shoulder Elb Surg. 2015;24:e307–11.

Cruz-Martinez A, Arpa J, Palau F. Peroneal neuropathy after weight loss. J Peripher Nerv Syst. 2000;5:101–5.

Damarey B, Demondion X, Boutry N, et al. Sonographic assessment of the lateral femoral cutaneous nerve. J Clin Ultrasound. 2009;37:89–95.

Davidson JJ, Bassett FH, Nunley JA. Musculocutaneous nerve entrapment revisited. J shoulder Elb Surg. 1998;7:250–5.

Duparc F, Coquerel D, Ozeel J, et al. Anatomical basis of the suprascapular nerve entrapment, and clinical relevance of the supraspinatus fascia. Surg Radiol Anat. 2010;32:277–84.

Felci GRS. Delayed radial nerve palsy due to entrapment of the nerve in the callus of a distal third humerus fracture. Turk Neurosurg. 2008;18:194–6.

Feng S-H, Hsiao M-Y, Wu C-H, Özçakar L. Ultrasound-guided diagnosis and management for quadrilateral space syndrome. Pain Med. 2017;18:184–6.

Ferkel E, Davis WH, Ellington JK. Entrapment neuropathies of the foot and ankle. Clin Sports Med. 2015;34:791–801. https://doi.org/10.1016/j.csm.2015.06.002.

Flynn LS, Wright TW, King JJ. Quadrilateral space syndrome: a review. J shoulder Elb Surg. 2018;27:950–6.

Foresti M, Foresti M. Superficial peroneal nerve compression due to peroneus brevis muscle herniation. J Radiol Case Rep. 2019;13:10–7. https://doi.org/10.3941/jcr.v13i11.3757.

Fowler JR, Maltenfort MG, Ilyas AM. Ultrasound as a first-line test in the diagnosis of carpal tunnel syndrome: a cost-effectiveness analysis. Clin Orthop Relat Res. 2013;471:932–7.

Gamil AM, Shalaby MH, Shehata KA, El Deeb AM. Value of grayscale and power doppler high-resolution ultrasound in assessment of patients with clinically suspected carpal tunnel syndrome. J Ultrasound Med. 2020;39:1155–62.

Garwood ER, Duarte A, Bencardino JT. MR imaging of entrapment neuropathies of the lower extremity. Radiol Clin NA. 2018;56:997–1012. https://doi.org/10.1016/j.rcl.2018.06.012.

Grant TH, Omar IM, Dumanian GA, et al. Sonographic evaluation of common peroneal neuropathy in patients with foot drop. J Ultrasound Med. 2015;34:705–11.

Hobson-webb LD, Juel VC. Common entrapment neuropathies. Continuum (Minneap Minn). 2017;23:487–511.

Hochman MG, Zilberfarb JL. Nerves in a pinch: imaging of nerve compression syndromes. Radiol Clin. 2004;42:221–45.

Hung C-Y, Chang K-V, Chen P-T, et al. Sonoelastography for the evaluation of an axillary schwannoma in a case of quadrilateral space syndrome. Clin Imaging. 2014;38:360–3.

Ikiz ZAA, Ucerler H, Uygur M. Dimensions of the anterior tarsal tunnel and features of the deep peroneal nerve in relation to clinical application. Surg Radiol Anat. 2007;29:527–30.

Jacobson JA, Fessell DP, Lobo LDG, Yang LJ-S. Entrapment neuropathies I: upper limb (carpal tunnel excluded). Semin Musculoskelet Radiol. © Thieme Medical Publishers. 2010;14:473–86.

Jacobson JA, Wilson TJ, Yang LJ. Sonography of common peripheral nerve disorders with clinical correlation. J Ultrasound Med. 2016;35:683–93.

Kang PB, Preston DC, Raynor EM. Involvement of superficial peroneal sensory nerve in common peroneal neuropathy. Muscle Nerve Off J Am Assoc Electrodiagn Med. 2005;31:725–9.

Karwa KA, Do DP, Tavee JO. Journal of the Neurological Sciences Smart device neuropathy. J Neurol Sci. 2016;370:132–3. https://doi.org/10.1016/j.jns.2016.09.040.

Katirji B. Peroneal neuropathy. Neurol Clin. 1999;17:567–91.

Kim Y, Ha DH, Lee SM. Ultrasonographic findings of posterior interosseous nerve syndrome. Ultrasonography. 2017;36:363.

Kim S-J, Hong SH, Jun WS, et al. MR imaging mapping of skeletal muscle denervation in entrapment and compressive neuropathies. Radiographics. 2011;31:319–32.

Klauser AS, Buzzegoli T, Taljanovic MS, et al. Nerve entrapment syndromes at the wrist and elbow by sonography. Semin Musculoskelet Radiol. 2018;22 Thieme Medical Publishers:344–53.

Klauser AS, Faschingbauer R, Jaschke WR. Is sonoelastography of value in assessing tendons? Semin Musculoskelet Radiol Thieme Medical Publishers. 2010;14:323–33.

Klauser AS, Halpern EJ, De Zordo T, et al. Carpal tunnel syndrome assessment with US: value of additional cross-sectional area measurements of the median nerve in patients versus healthy volunteers. Radiology. 2009;250:171–7.

Kotani H, Miki T, Senzoku F, et al. Posterior interosseous nerve paralysis with multiple constrictions. J Hand Surg Am. 1995;20:15–7.

Kroonen LT. Cubital tunnel syndrome. Orthop Clin. 2012;43:475–86.

La Rocca VR, Rosenberg ZS, Kiprovski K. MRI of the distal biceps femoris muscle: normal anatomy, variants, and association with common peroneal entrapment neuropathy. Am J Roentgenol. 2007;189:549–55.

Łabętowicz P, Synder M, Wojciechowski M, et al. Protective and predisposing morphological factors in suprascapular nerve entrapment syndrome:

a fundamental review based on recent observations. Biomed Res Int. 2017;2017:4659761.
Lau JTC, Daniels TR. Tarsal tunnel syndrome: a review of the literature. Foot Ankle Int. 1999;20:201–9.
Lee M, Kim S, Song H, et al. Morton neuroma: evaluated with ultrasonography and MR imaging. Korean J Radiol. 2007;8(2):148–55.
Lee S, Shin K, Gil Y, et al. Anatomy of the lateral femoral cutaneous nerve relevant to clinical findings in meralgia paresthetica. Muscle Nerve. 2017;55:646–50.
Lenchik L, Brigido MK, Shahabpour M, Marcelis S. Normal anatomy and compression areas of nerves of the foot and ankle: US and MR imaging with anatomic correlation. Radiographics. 2015;35:1469–82.
Letters C. Clinical letters. 2016–2018. 2017.
Lucchetta M, Briani C, Liotta GA, et al. Ultrasonographic Tinel sign: comment. Muscle Nerve Off J Am Assoc Electrodiagn Med. 2010;41:570–1.
Ma H, Van Heest A, Glisson C, Patel S. Musculocutaneous nerve entrapment: an unusual complication after biceps tenodesis. Am J Sports Med. 2009;37:2467–9.
Malek E, Salameh JS. Common entrapment neuropathies. Semin Neurol. 2020;39(5):549–59.
Marciniak C. Fibular (peroneal) neuropathy electrodiagnostic features and clinical correlates. Phys Med Rehabil Clin NA. 2013a;24:121–37. https://doi.org/10.1016/j.pmr.2012.08.016.
Marciniak C. Fibular (peroneal) neuropathy: electrodiagnostic features and clinical correlates. Phys Med Rehabil Clin. 2013b;24:121–37.
Martin HD, Shears SA, Johnson JC, et al. The endoscopic treatment of sciatic nerve entrapment/deep gluteal syndrome. Arthrosc J Arthrosc Relat Surg. 2011;27:172–81.
Martinoli C, Bianchi S, Pugliese F, et al. Sonography of entrapment neuropathies in the upper limb (wrist excluded). J Clin Ultrasound. 2004;32:438–50.
Martinoli C, Miguel-Perez M, Padua L, et al. Imaging of neuropathies about the hip. Eur J Radiol. 2013;82:17–26.
Masakado Y, Kawakami M, Suzuki K, et al. Clinical neurophysiology in the diagnosis of peroneal nerve palsy. Keio J Med. 2008;57:84–9.
Masear VR, Hill JJ Jr, Cohen SM. Ulnar compression neuropathy secondary to the anconeus epitrochlearis muscle. J Hand Surg Am. 1988;13:720–4.
McDonagh C, Alexander M, Kane D. The role of ultrasound in the diagnosis and management of carpal tunnel syndrome: a new paradigm. Rheumatology. 2015;54:9–19.
Melendez MM, Glickman LT, Dellon AL. Peroneal nerve compression in figure skaters. Clin Res Foot Ankle. 2013;1:102.
Miller SL, Gill J, Webb GR. The proximal origin of the hamstrings and surrounding anatomy encountered during repair: a cadaveric study. JBJS. 2007;89:44–8.
Miller MD, Thompson SR. DeLee & Drez's Orthopaedic Sports Medicine E-Book. Elsevier Health Sciences, Amsterdam; 2014.
Molina AEP, Bour C, Oberlin C, et al. The posterior interosseous nerve and the radial tunnel syndrome: an anatomical study. Int Orthop. 1998;22:102–6.
Musson RE, Sawhney JS, Lamb L, et al. Foot & Ankle International. Los Angeles, CA: Sage Publishing; 2014. https://doi.org/10.3113/FAI.2012.0196.
Nagano A. Spontaneous anterior interosseous nerve palsy. J Bone Joint Surg Br. 2003;85:313–8.
Nakasa T, Fukuhara K, Adachi N, Ochi M. Painful os intermetatarseum in athletes: report of four cases and review of the literature. Arch Orthop Trauma Surg. 2007;127:261–4.
Ng I, Vaghadia H, Choi PT, Helmy N. Ultrasound imaging accurately identifies the lateral femoral cutaneous nerve. Anesth Analg. 2008;107:1070–4.
Ozturk E, Sonmez G, Colak A, et al. Sonographic appearances of the normal ulnar nerve in the cubital tunnel. J Clin Ultrasound. 2008;36:325–9.
Padua L, Coraci D, Erra C, et al. Carpal tunnel syndrome: clinical features, diagnosis, and management. Lancet Neurol. 2016;15:1273–84.
Palmer BA, Hughes TB. Cubital tunnel syndrome. J Hand Surg Am. 2010;35:153–63.
Park BJ, Joeng ES, Choi JK, Kang S. Ultrasound-guided lateral femoral cutaneous nerve conduction study. Ann Rehabil Med. 2015;39:47–51.
Paul L, Lakshmi GV, Alex L. A cadaveric study of the Arcade of Frohse. Indian J Clin Anat Physiol. 2020;7:195–200.
Peters PG, Adams SB, Schon LC. Interdigital neuralgia. Foot Ankle Clin. 2011;16:305–15.
Pham M, Bäumer P, Meinck H-M, et al. Anterior interosseous nerve syndrome: fascicular motor lesions of median nerve trunk. Neurology. 2014;82:598–606.
Polguj M, Sibiński M, Grzegorzewski A, et al. Variation in morphology of suprascapular notch as a factor of suprascapular nerve entrapment. Int Orthop. 2013;37:2185–92.
Polguj M, Sibiński M, Grzegorzewski A, et al. Morphological and radiological study of ossified superior transverse scapular ligament as potential risk factor of suprascapular nerve entrapment. Biomed Res Int. 2014;2014:613601.
Pomeroy G, Wilton J, Anthony S. Entrapment neuropathy about the foot and ankle: an update. JAAOS. 2015;23:58–66.
Puig S, Turkof E, Sedivy R, et al. Sonographic diagnosis of recurrent ulnar nerve compression by ganglion cysts. J Ultrasound Med. 1999;18:433–6.
Safran MR. Nerve injury about the shoulder in athletes, part 1: suprascapular nerve and axillary nerve. Am J Sports Med. 2004;32:803–19.
Samarawickrama D, Therimadasamy AK, Chan YEEC, et al. Nerve ultrasound in electrophysiologically verified tarsal tunnel syndrome. Muscle Nerve. 2016;53(6):906–12. https://doi.org/10.1002/mus.24963.
Sanders TG, Tirman PFJ. Paralabral cyst: an unusual cause of quadrilateral space syndrome. Arthrosc J Arthrosc Relat Surg. 1999;15:632–7.

Shamrock AG, Das JM. Radial tunnel syndrome. In: StatPearls [Internet]. Treasure Island, FL: StatPearls Publishing; 2020.

Shon H-C, Park J-K, Kim D-S, et al. Supracondylar process syndrome: two cases of median nerve neuropathy due to compression by the ligament of Struthers. J Pain Res. 2018;11:803.

Sirico F, Castaldo C, Baioccato V, et al. Prevalence of musculocutaneous nerve variations: Systematic review and meta-analysis. Clin Anat. 2019;32:183–95.

Spinner RJ, Dellon AL, Rosson GD, et al. Tibial intraneural ganglia in the tarsal tunnel: is there a joint connection? J foot ankle Surg. 2007;46:27–31.

Still GP, Fowler MB. Joplin's neuroma or compression neuropathy of the plantar proper digital nerve to the hallux: clinicopathologic study of three cases. J Foot Ankle Surg. 1998;37:524–30.

Tagliafico AS, Bignotti B, Martinoli C. Elbow US: anatomy, variants, and scanning technique. Radiology. 2015;275:636–50.

Tagliafico AS, Michaud J, Marchetti A, et al. US imaging of the musculocutaneous nerve. Skeletal Radiol. 2011;40:609–16.

Tagliafico A, Serafini G, Lacelli F, et al. Ultrasound-guided treatment of meralgia paresthetica (lateral femoral cutaneous neuropathy) technical description and results of treatment in 20 consecutive patients. J Ultrasound Med. 2011;30:1341–6.

Takebe K, Hirohata K. Peroneal nerve palsy due to fabella. Arch Orthop Trauma Surg. 1981;99:91–5.

Tawfik EA, El Zohiery AK, Abouelela AAKH. Proposed sonographic criteria for the diagnosis of idiopathic tarsal tunnel syndrome. Arch Phys Med Rehabil. 2016;97(7):1093–9. https://doi.org/10.1016/j.apmr.2015.11.012.

Toms AF, Rushton LA, Kennedy NR. Muscle herniation of the peroneus longus muscle triggering superficial fibular nerve paresthesia. Sonography. 2018;5:36–40.

Torriani M, Kattapuram SV. Dynamic sonography of the forefoot: the sonographic Mulder sign. Am J Roentgenol. 2003;180:1121–3.

Visser LH, Hens V, Soethout M, et al. Diagnostic value of high-resolution sonography in common fibular neuropathy at the fibular head. Muscle Nerve. 2013;48:171–8.

Weiss C, Imhoff AB. Sonographic imaging of a spinoglenoid cyst. Ultraschall der Medizin. 2000;21:287–9.

Weng W-C, Wei Y-C, Huang W-Y, et al. Risk factor analysis for meralgia paresthetica: a hospital-based study in Taiwan. J Clin Neurosci. 2017;43:192–5.

Yates B, Merriman LM. Merriman's assessment of the lower limb. Amsterdam: Elsevier Health Sciences; 2009.

Yoshida N, Tsuchida Y. Posterior interosseous nerve palsy due to Bado type-III Monteggia fracture. Case Reports. 2018;2018:bcr2018226254.

Yücesoy C, Akkaya T, Özel Ö, et al. Ultrasonographic evaluation and morphometric measurements of the suprascapular notch. Surg Radiol Anat. 2009;31:409.

Part IV

Ultrasound in Healing Evaluation and in Therapy Monitoring

Bone Fracture Healing

24

Armanda De Marchi, Davide Orlandi,
Enzo Silvestri, Luca Cavagnaro,
and Alessandro Muda

Contents

24.1 Introduction

The reparative process after bone fracture depends on several conditions: mechanism of injury, site of lesions, kind of fracture, and methods of fracture treatment. The healing process has different steps involving nonosseous tissue components like cartilage and blood vessels until the complete repair.

Bone fracture repair is generally assessed using ionizing radiation-based imaging modalities such as plain films, fluoroscopy, and computed tomography (CT).

Signs of fracture healing using plain films and fluoroscopy are not normally evident until after 6–8 weeks of recovery when the callus has become sufficiently calcified to be visible on X-ray; in fact their main limitation is the low sensitivity for the healing process during the early phase. In addition, when dealing with fractures treated by metal hardware, radiographic evaluation is also limited by the presence of the latter.

CT is really useful for investigating cortical bone fractures and soft-tissue calcifications, due to the good contrast between tissues, and also for the evaluation of the healing process but is affected by some limitations such as the presence of metal hardware artifacts and a very poor sensitivity in the detection of trabecular bone involvement. In

A. De Marchi
Radiologia CIDIMU: Centro Italiano di Diagnostica Medica Ultrasonica, Torino, Italy

D. Orlandi (✉)
Department of Radiology, Ospedale Evangelico Internazionale, Genova, Italy

E. Silvestri
Radiology, Alliance Medical, Genova, Italy

L. Cavagnaro
Ortopedia e Traumatologia 2- Joint Replacement, Unit/Bone Infection Unit, Ospedale Santa Corona, Pietra Ligure (SV), Italy

A. Muda
Department of Radiology, IRCCS Policlinico San Martino-IST, Genova, Italy

F. Martino et al. (eds.), *Musculoskeletal Ultrasound in Orthopedic and Rheumatic disease in Adults*,
https://doi.org/10.1007/978-3-030-91202-4_24

this setting MRI could be considered the gold standard, being able to perform a detailed assessment of bone and soft-tissue involvement. Nowadays, thanks to metallic artifact reduction sequences (MARS) MRI could also be performed in patients treated by metal hardware or prosthesis.

24.2 Ultrasound Evaluation of Bone Fracture Healing

Ultrasound (US) provides a safe and noninvasive monitoring of the first steps of bone-healing process, improving the current subjective clinical fracture assessment [8, 9]. US represents an efficient diagnostic imaging modality to visualize and assess the first step of bone healing, which is the soft-tissue reparation stage. At this stage ultrasound is able to detect simultaneously the bony surface and the incoming soft callus before its transformation in a dense calcific callus. In this way US has been used successfully to evaluate also what is assumed to be callus production.

An animal study indicates that a direct correlation exists between this "presumed to be callus" tissue seen with US and actual fracture callus as determined by histological examination.

In a study where an external limb-lengthening distraction device (Ilizarov frame) was used, Young et al. studied the value of sonography in the evaluation of new bone production at the distraction site to determine whether it could be used to image the new bone before it became visible on plain radiography. In this study the sonographic evaluation with linear and/or sector transducers was used, depending on the skin accessibility within the Ilizarov frame, and was begun at either 7 or 15 days after surgery and at 4 and 6–8 weeks. The authors confirmed that new bone formation appears like some hyperechoic spots until the development of a dense hyperechoic line.

Such information may provide valuable prognostic information for the early assessment of fracture healing and the related need for secondary operative procedures.

It is possible also with ultrasound to predict the future repair process to identify healing complications as early as possible like hematoma and cyst, which can hinder the new bone production.

Compared to X-ray ultrasound could substantially improve the monitoring of fracture repair by allowing earlier detection of bridging callus, nonunion lesions, and complications.

US imaging is performed with linear or convex probes in the peripheral region of the fracture encompassing almost the total circumference of the long bone across the entire length of the fracture site. Instead of conventional 2D ultrasound, some authors have highlighted the use of 3D freehand ultrasound in complex fractures where 3D details of fracture site and bone fragment are important.

Bone growth depends on the rapid growth of new capillaries; conventional color Doppler modalities can obtain information about these vessels (Fig. 24.1).

Caruso et al. also used color Doppler ultrasonography in tibial fracture patients with delayed fracture healing, detecting the lack of blood flow signals and persistence of high resistance indices. 3D power Doppler ultrasound (PDU) used in

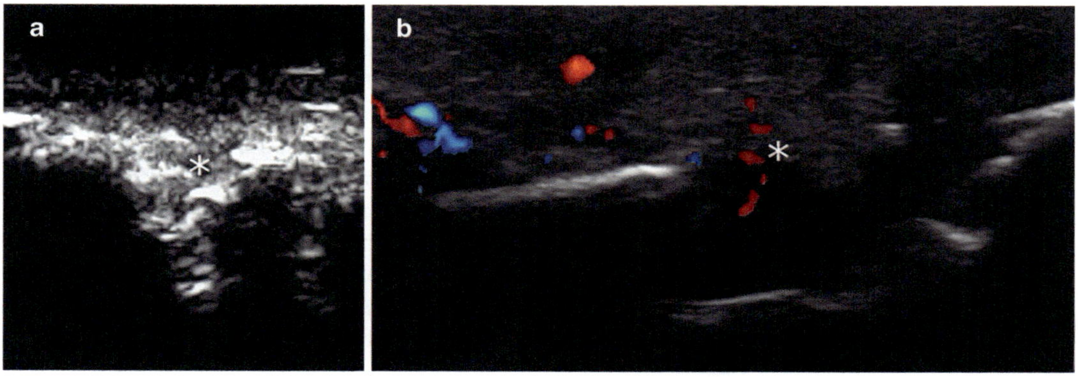

Fig. 24.1 Contrast-enhanced ultrasound evaluation (**a**) and color Doppler (**b**) performed during callus formation 4 weeks after fracture treatment showing few vessels in the gap of the fracture (*asterisks*)

another study on fracture healing in a rat model is not yet used for the clinical assessment of fracture cases. As a precondition of osteogenesis, neovascularization plays a crucial role in the whole process and directly affects bone activity. In this field contrast-enhanced ultrasound (CEUS) represents a noninvasive imaging modality, which is able to evaluate the angiogenesis at the site of bone fracture. The US contrast agents' property to remain within the vessels is very useful to detect a true microvascular pattern.

Regarding the use of CEUS in bone fracture healing evaluation literature highlights a lack of a standardized timing for US contrast medium procedure in this setting. In this pilot study for the early diagnosis of fracture, healing was at 6 and 9 weeks postoperatively. In recent papers CEUS examination was performed at a 12-week follow-up to capture the vascularization of soft callus formation, which begins after the initial inflammatory phase and slows down before the hard callus formation or remodeling phase in tibial nonunion fractures.

In another recent study CEUS was performed 15 days before the treatment and 7 days and 4 and 8 weeks after treatment in noninfected long bone nonunion fractures.

As evidenced in this recent literature, the neoangiogenesis in graft bone increased from the 3rd to 14th day and then gradually decreased by days 21–28.

The different operative and nonoperative treatments represent the cause for no standardized imaging procedure to early detect the bone formation.

CEUS is also a useful method in monitoring the healing process in long bone noninfected nonunion fractures. Krammer et al. reported that an early evaluation of success recovery after tibial nonunion can be realized with CEUS. In another recent paper authors showed that a combination of CEUS and peripheral cytokine expression analysis is a promising novel tool in the early prediction of the outcome of the nonunion therapy.

Recently, following the technological development of ultrasound machines, different brands have developed microvascular imaging techniques (e.g., SMI) able to display very-low-velocity blood flows, allowing imaging of microvessels without any contrast agent. However, in a recent paper some authors compared the performances of CEUS and SMI in the evaluation of bone healing, showing that SMI neovascularity detection sensitivity is lower than CEUS.

In conclusion, the monitoring of the fracture repair is crucial; therefore, a noninvasive diagnostic method such as US could help the traditional X-ray modalities to reveal the progress of the biologic processes during fracture healing.

Further Readings

Augat P, et al. Imaging techniques for the assessment of fracture repair. Injury. 2014;45(Suppl 2):S16–22.

Augat P, et al. Quantitative assessment of experimental fracture repair by peripheral computed tomography. Calcif Tissue Int. 1997;60(2):194–9.

Caruso G, et al. Monitoring of fracture callus with color Doppler sonography. J Clin Ultrasound. 2000;28(1):20–7.

De Marchi A, et al. Perfusion pattern and time of vascularization with CEUS increase accuracy of differentiating between benign and malignant tumours in 216 musculoskeletal soft tissue masses. Eur J Radiol. 2015;84:142–50.

De Marchi A, et al. Study of neurinomas with ultrasound contrast media: review of a case series to identify characteristics imaging patterns. Radiol Med. 2011;116:634–43.

Den Boer F. Quantification of fracture healing with three-dimensional computed tomography. Arch Orthop Trauma Surg. 1998;117:345–50.

Firoozabadi R, et al. Qualitative and quantitative assessment of bone fragility and fracture healing using conventional radiography and advanced imaging technologies – focus on wrist fracture. J Orthop Trauma. 2008;22(8 Suppl):S83–90.

Fischer C, et al. Dynamic contrast enhanced sonography and dynamic contrast-enhanced magnetic resonance imaging for preoperative diagnosis of infected nonunions. J Ultrasound Med. 2016;35:933–42.

Fleicher AC. Sonographic depiction of tumor vascularity and flow; from in vivo models to clinical applications. J Ultrasound Med. 2000;19(1):55–61.

Giannoudis PV, et al. The diamond concept—open questions. Injury. 2008;39(Suppl 2):S5–8.

Hamblen D, Simpson AH. Outline of fractures. 12th ed. London, UK: Churchill Livingstone; 2007.

Haubruck P, et al. A preliminary study of contrast-enhanced ultrasound (CEUS) and cytokine expression analysis (CEA) as early predictors for the outcome of tibial nonunion therapy. Diagnostics (Basel). 2018;8:55.

Hijazy A, et al. Quantitative monitoring of bone healing process using ultrasound. J Franklin Inst. 343(4–5):495–500. Proceedings of the First International Conference on Modeling, Simulation and Applied Optimization, Sharjah, U.A.E. 2005; February 1–3

Kang M-L, et al. Vascular endothelial growth factor transfected adipose-derived stromal cells enhance bone regeneration and neovascularization from bone marrow stromal cells. J Tissue Eng Regen Med. 2017;11:3337–48.

Krammer D, et al. Contrast enhanced ultrasound quantifies the perfusion within tibial non unions and predicts the outcome of revision surgery. Ultrasound Med Biol. 2018;44:1853–9.

Leunig M, et al. Quantitative assessment of angiogenesis and osteogenesis after transplantation of bone: comparison of isograft and allograft bone in mice. Acta Orthop Scand. 1999;70:374–80.

Jin L, et al. MD Studies of superb microvascular imaging and contrast-enhanced ultrasonography in the evaluation of vascularization in early bone regeneration. J Ultrasound Med. 2019;38:2963–71.

Moed BR, et al. Ultrasound for the early diagnosis of fracture healing after interlocking nailing of the tibia without reaming. Clin Orthop. 1995;310:137–44.

Moed BR, et al. Ultrasound for the early diagnosis of tibial fracture healing after static inter- locked nailing without reaming: clinical results. J Orthop Trauma. 1998;12(3):206–13.

Moed BR, et al. Ultrasound for the early diagnosis of tibial fracture healing after static interlocked nailing without reaming: histologic correlation using a canine model. J Orthop Trauma. 1998;12:200–5.

Müller S, et al. Assessment of bone microcirculation by contrast-enhanced ultrasound (CEUS) and positron emission tomography/computed tomography in free osseous and osseocutaneus flaps for mandibular reconstruction: preliminary results. Clin Hemorheol Microcirc. 2016;49:115–28.

Orlandi D, et al. Advances power Doppler technique increase synovial vascularity detection in patients with rheumatoid arthritis. Ultrasound Med Biol. 2017;43:1880–7.

Park AY, et al. An innovative ultrasound technique for evaluation of tumor vascularity in breast cancers: superbmicro-vascular imaging. J Breast Cancer. 2016;19:210–3.

Pozza S, et al. Technical and clinical feasibility of contrast-enhanced ultrasound evaluation of long bone non-infected nonunion healing. Radiol Med. 2018;123:703–9.

Colier R, Donarski R. "Non-invasive method of measuring the resonant frequency of a human tibia in vivo", part 1 & 2. J Biomed Eng. 1987;9:321–31.

Ross EF. 3D ultrasound for imaging components of musculoskeletal system. PhD thesis; 2009.

Sun MH, et al. Three-dimensional high frequency power Doppler ultrasonography for the assess-ment of microvasculature during fracture healing in a rat model. J Orthop Res. 2012;30(1):137–43.

Blokhuis T, et al. The reliability of plain radiography in experimental fracture healing. Skelet Radiol. 2001;30:151–6.

Tall M. Treatment of aseptic tibial shaft nonunion without bone defect. Orthop Traumatol Surg Res. 2018;104:S63–9.

Yung JW, et al. Sonographic evaluation of bone production at distraction site in Ilizarov limb-lengthening procedures. AJR Am J Roentgenol. 1990;154(1):125–8.

Tendon and Muscle Rupture Repair

25

Giovanni Rusconi, Giulio Pasta, Davide Orlandi, Enzo Silvestri, and Francesco Di Pietto

Contents

25.1 Introduction

The main objectives of ultrasound after a diagnosis of muscle injury are the control of the evolution of the lesion for a timely and safe return to play, the early recognition of possible complications, the prevention of recurrences, or the detection of those cases which deserve surgical therapy.

Ultrasound is a useful tool to evaluate the aspects of muscle healing and offers higher spatial resolution than magnetic resonance imaging. In addition to these features, the possibility of a color Doppler analysis and a dynamic study should be considered. Serial ultrasound evaluations of muscle injury may reduce the recurrence

G. Rusconi · F. Di Pietto
Dipartimento di Diagnostica per Immagini "Pineta Grande Hospital", Castel Volturno (CE), Italy

G. Pasta
Specialista in Radiologia e Diagnostica per Immagini, Studio Associato di Radiologia Dr. Pasta, Emilia-Romagna, Italy

D. Orlandi (✉)
Department of Radiology, Ospedale Evangelico Internazionale, Genova, Italy

E. Silvestri
Radiology, Alliance Medical, Genova, Italy

F. Martino et al. (eds.), *Musculoskeletal Ultrasound in Orthopedic and Rheumatic disease in Adults*, https://doi.org/10.1007/978-3-030-91202-4_25

rate of strains and allow for a standardized return-to-play criteria.

It has been suggested that between 2 and 48 h after injury is the ideal timing of examination. If the examination is performed too early post-injury then the hematoma may not have had adequate time to fully form and there may be a risk of false-negative examination, or underappreciation of the severity of the injury.

25.2 Healing After Muscle Injury

25.2.1 Skeletal Muscle Healing Process

The healing of a skeletal muscle after contusion, strain, or laceration injury is usually divided into a three-phase process:

1. Destruction phase, in which there is the rupture and necrosis of the myofibers, the consequent inflammatory reaction, and the formation of a hematoma between the ruptured muscle stumps.
2. Repair phase, characterized by the phagocytosis of the necrotized tissue, the regeneration of the myofibers, and the capillary ingrowth into the injured area, resulting in the production of a connective tissue scar.
3. Remodeling phase, during which the maturation of the regenerated myofibers, the contraction and reorganization of the scar tissue, and the recovery of the functional capacity of the muscle occur. Repair and remodeling phases are usually closely associated or overlapping.

25.2.2 Hematoma and Scar Tissue

Hematoma is a localized collection of blood that forms secondary to trauma or surgery but spontaneous formation is also not uncommon, especially in patients with coagulation disorders or on anticoagulant therapy.

The physical consistency of the collection varies according to its phase, from a hyperacute to a chronic stage. In the very first hours after the trauma, the hematoma can still be diffuse, not collected, with hyperechoic aspect at ultrasound examination. For these reasons it could be difficult to clearly identify it in a very early phase. In the subsequent phase (after 2–3 days), the clot dissolves and the collection becomes to appear as a cystic, purely liquid collection characterized by low echogenicity or complete anechogenicity at US (Fig. 25.1).

As healing progresses, after some days or weeks, the hematoma will begin to organize and

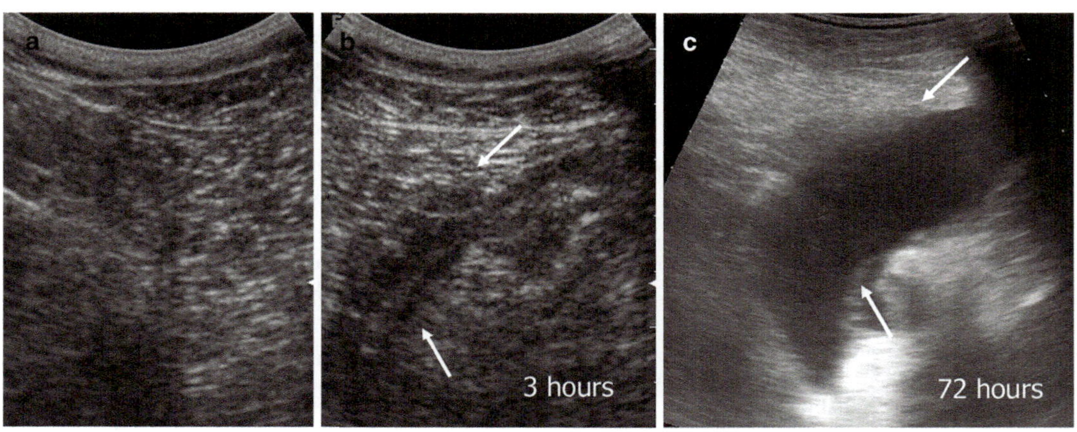

Fig. 25.1 Ultrasound examination performed at 3 h (**b**), reassessed at 72 h (**c**), after direct blunt trauma. At the 3-h evaluation the large hematoma of the muscle belly of the vastus intermedius has hyperechoic appearance. At 72-h evaluation the hematoma becomes hypo/anechoic. (**a**) Corresponding healthy contralateral side

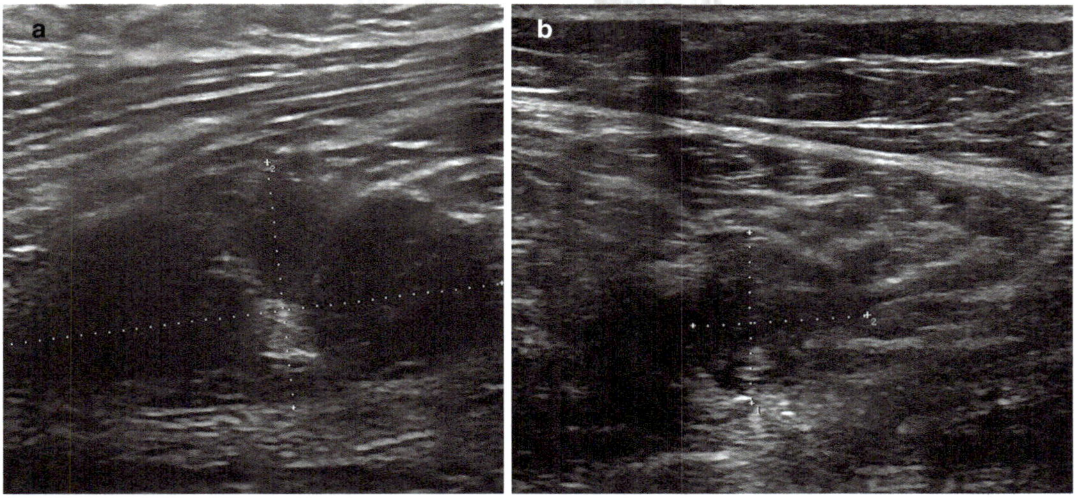

Fig. 25.2 Ultrasound examination 3 days after trauma (**a**) showing hypoechoic hematoma with full-thickness tear of the proximal myotendinous junction of the biceps femoris muscle. At 20 days (**b**) the hematoma is largely reabsorbed and becomes echoic due to organization and partial scarring of the fibers

in the chronic phase it could have a solid mass or a mixed cystic-solid appearance, characterized by septa formation and calcification, due to chronic hemoglobin degradation products (Fig. 25.2).

The presence and extent of hematoma should be assessed in both short and long axis imaging planes. As mentioned above, 48 h post-injury is the ideal time for initial examination; if it is performed prior to this time, consider to repeat examination within a few days to document any additional hematoma that may not have been optimally visualized at the initial examination. In many cases hematomas may decrease in dimension and resolve spontaneously, but US-guided percutaneous aspiration may be considered when there is a significant hematoma or in those cases in which chronic hematomas do not resolve in time, in order to drain the fluid collected and promote the healing process. Other possible indications to drainage are those patients with severe pain or elite athletes, to achieve an early return to play.

Power Doppler imaging can be a useful tool in the evaluation of a muscle injury because it can add information about neovascularization. In fact, it has been reported that there is new vessel formation until 8 weeks after injury, which gradually decreases at 12-week ultrasound follow-up after injury (Fig. 25.3).

While hematoma is mainly observed in the initial phases of injury, in the subsequent remodeling phase there is progressive scar formation. Fibrotic scars are hyperechoic linear zones within the muscle after a trauma and sometimes the healing process may lead to an excessive scar tissue formation, especially in larger lesions and when the return to play is too early (Fig. 25.4).

They cause few symptoms if the patient is well aware of their presence and warms his/her muscles adequately before a competition and stretches his/her muscles deeply after the competition. Usually, scar thickness is significantly larger at 8 and 12 weeks compared with 4 weeks and it has been reported that fibrous tissues remained at 1-year follow-up after injury (Fig. 25.5).

There is a risk of recurrent injury associated to the extent of residual fibrous scar tissue in the muscle belly. Dynamic ultrasound examination can help in its assessment by revealing the differences in muscle contraction in the scar areas through contralateral comparison.

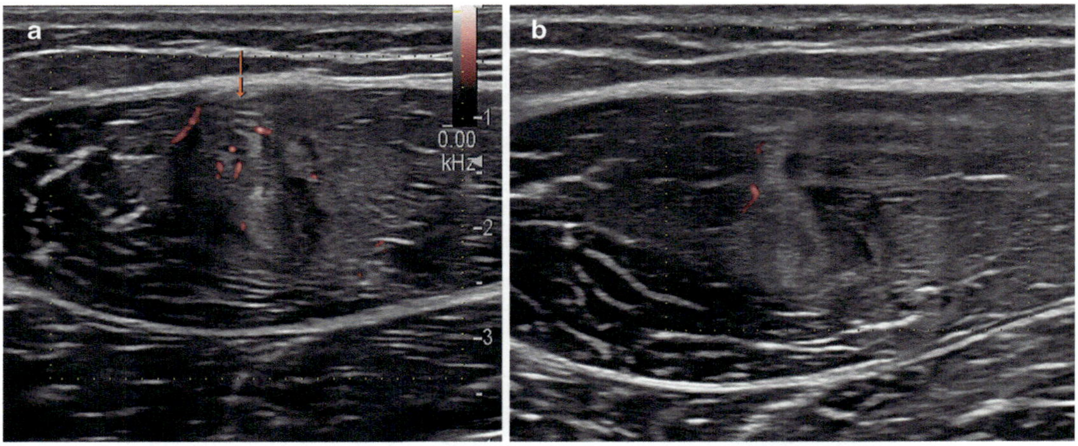

Fig. 25.3 Indirect strain injury (grade I) at the myotendinous junction of the indirect tendon of the rectus femoris. (**a**) US at 7 days shows peritendinous hyperemia at power Doppler analysis, expression of an ongoing repair process. (**b**) 1-month follow-up of the same patient. Reduction of peritendinous vascular signals at power Doppler analysis

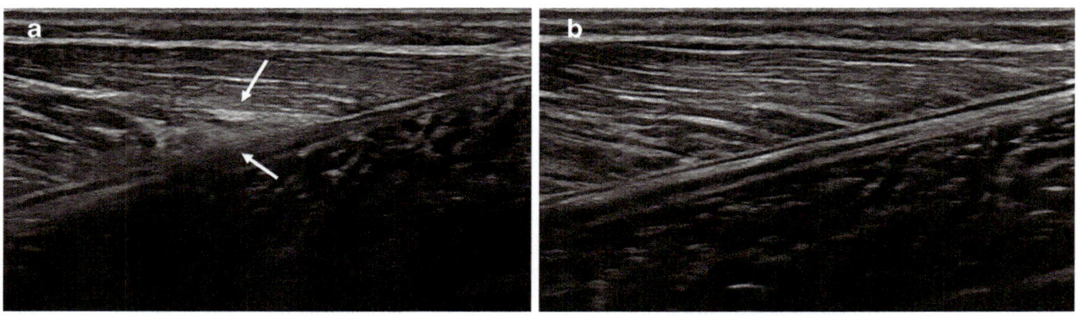

Fig. 25.4 Scar tissue at the site of a previous distal myofascial tear of the medial head of the gastrocnemius (*arrows*) (**a**). Corresponding healthy contralateral side (**b**)

25.3 Muscle Healing Process Complications

25.3.1 Cyst

Cysts result from an incomplete resorption of a hematoma after a muscle trauma and appear as well-defined lesions with anechoic content and consequent posterior acoustic enhancement. They may be intermuscular (Fig. 25.6) or intramuscular (Fig. 25.7) and the most common location is the calf. Biggest ones causing mass effect may need percutaneous needle evacuation.

25.3.2 Calcific Myonecrosis

Calcific myonecrosis refers to a rare disease occurring as a very late sequela after a closed fracture or trauma, often associated to compartment syndrome. The symptoms of calcific myonecrosis appear, on average, 37 years following the initial injury (range: 10–64 years).

It involves almost exclusively the lower limb and typically the anterior muscles of the leg, even if it has been occasionally reported at other sites.

It is a benign lesion, characterized by the formation of a dystrophic enlarging mass; in particular, the injured muscle is replaced by a complex mass consisting of a central cystic core containing necrotic muscle, fibrin, and cholesterol, with peripheral plaque-like amorphous calcifications.

US is often the first imaging method to evaluate the lesion and demonstrates extensive, shadowing, echogenic foci, consistent with calcifications, with a central complex hypoechoic area, but in many cases other imaging modalities are needed. The main differential diagnosis of calcific myonecrosis is the more common myositis ossificans (MO), but its aspect and its enlargement could mimic soft-tissue sarcomas. US may also help to guide the aspiration of the central fluid component to help the healing process, and to guide the biopsy for a histologic diagnosis.

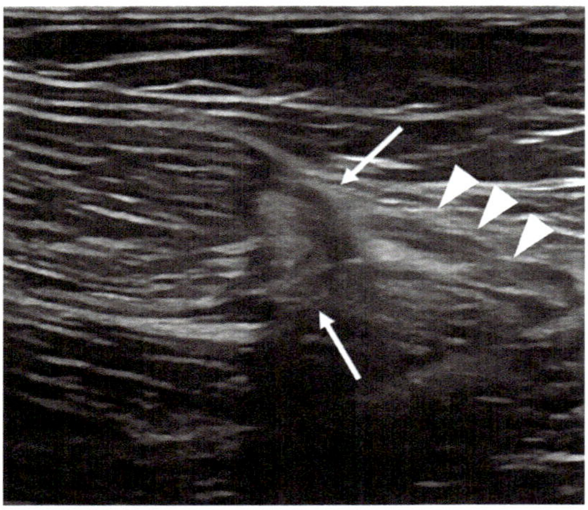

Fig. 25.5 Follow-up of a grade III injury of the adductor longus. Distal retraction of the muscle belly (*arrows*) with extensive scar tissue at the myotendinous junction (*arrowheads*)

25.3.3 Myositis Ossificans

Myositis ossificans (MO) is a benign process characterized by heterotopic ossification usually within large muscles, involving most commonly the extremities, the thigh, and the anterior side of the arm.

Despite the term "myositis", it is not an inflammatory condition and several hypotheses have been proposed about the pathophysiology. The lesion is thought to develop through inappropriate differentiation of fibroblasts into osteogenic cells after traumatic muscle injury, resulting in extraosseous bone formation.

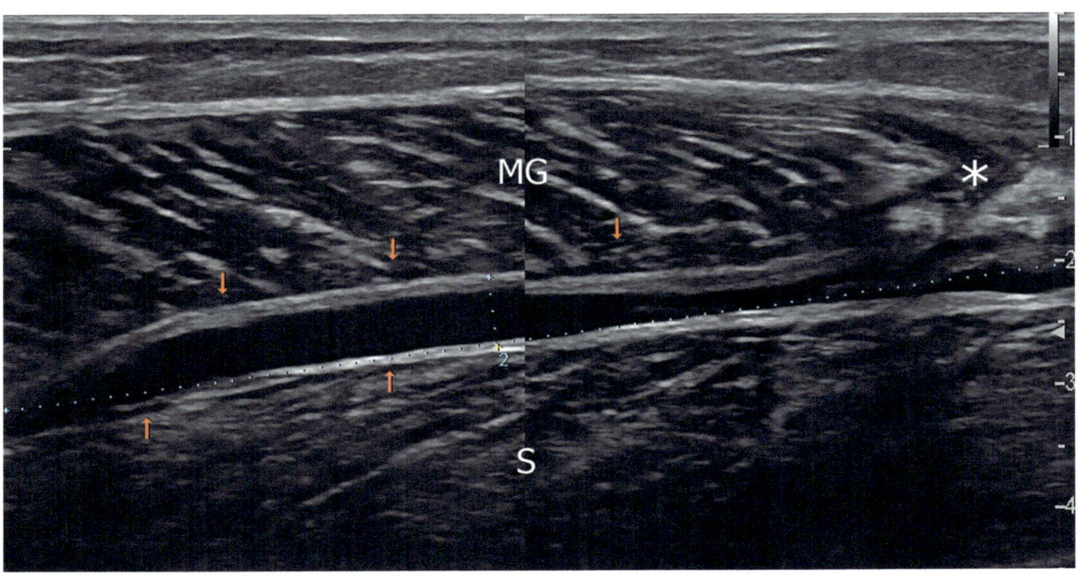

Fig. 25.6 Large cystic interfascial collection between medial head of the gastrocnemius (MG) and soleus (S) after a distal myofascial junction tear of the medial head of the gastrocnemius (*asterisk*)

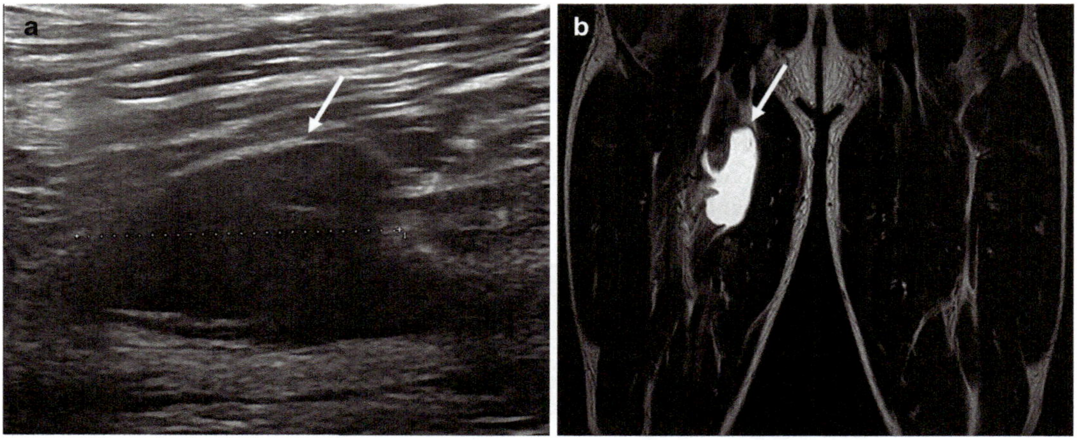

Fig. 25.7 Intramuscular cyst after a grade II injury of the semimembranosus (*white arrows*). (**a**) Long-axis ultrasound scan showing hypoechoic aspect of the cyst. (**b**) Coronal FSE T2 MRI of the same patient

As MO occurs as a result of a severe contusion trauma, the most affected population is young adults. Another group of patients especially prone to MO are paraplegics, in which recognized episodes of trauma are often absent, and the disease frequently occurs around knees and hips.

It is considered a skeletal so-called "don't touch lesion", which is important to recognize because it can mimic malignant lesions. For example, osteosarcoma has a histologically similar appearance, and this may lead to inappropriate management.

MO clinically presents as a painful, tender mass, and histologically is characterized by a zonal organization: a peripheral, well-organized mature lamellar bone zone, an intermediate osteoid region, and a proliferating fibroblast central zone, with granulation tissue and localized areas of hemorrhage.

MO also has a typical "maturation" pattern and imaging findings change according to an early, a subacute, and a mature phase. In particular, at US examination, early MO lesions are heterogeneous hypoechoic soft-tissue masses, with a focal hyperechoic central area. As the lesion matures, after 4 weeks, the center develops diffuse reflective areas and a peripheral lamellar calcification, leading to posterior acoustic shadowing. It is also possible to detect increased vascularity at color Doppler analysis. After about 2 months, mature calcified mass may present irregularity of the peripheral rim and may regress in size, disappearing spontaneously in approximately 30% of cases.

Peripheral calcification is a peculiar feature of myositis ossificans and makes this condition more easily diagnosed with X-ray, even if US can detect the ossification process approximately 2 weeks earlier than plain radiographs (Fig. 25.8).

25.3.4 Muscle Hernia

Muscle hernias represent a focal defect in the muscle fascia with protrusion of muscle through the defect. They are most commonly found in the lower extremities, typically the tibialis anterior muscle.

They are often asymptomatic, but can cause cramping sensations or pain during or after activity. They may also present as a palpable mass, and be referred for imaging with suspicion of neoplasia.

Ultrasound is the modality of choice in the evaluation of suspected muscle hernia, although MRI may be required if there are uncertain US findings. The hernia is often hypoechoic to the surrounding muscle and may assume a mushroom shape as it protrudes through the fascial defect (Fig. 25.9).

The mass may not be palpable when the patient is relaxed, which is a clinical clue to the diagnosis; therefore a dynamic US evaluation is

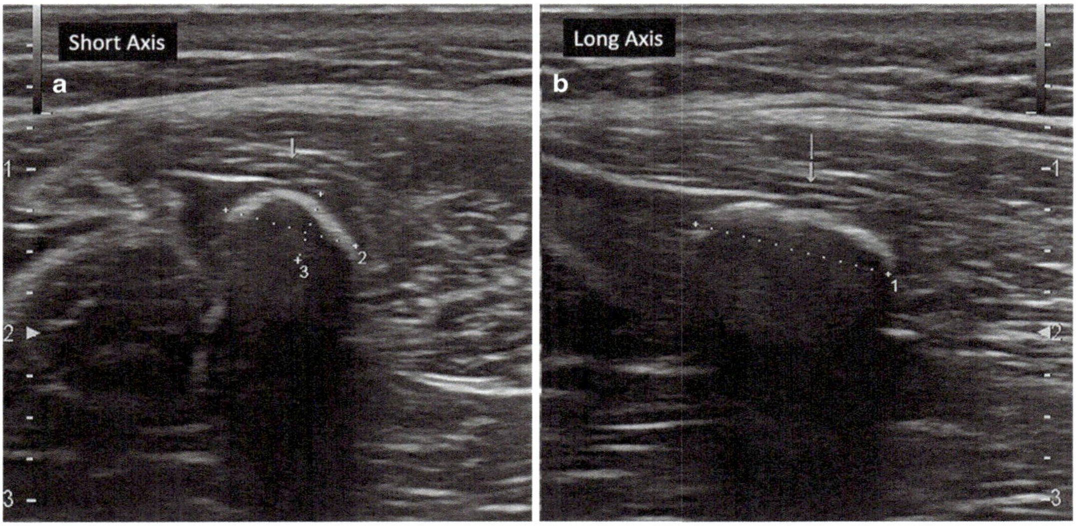

Fig. 25.8 US short (**a**) and long (**b**) axis scan of myositis ossificans. Macroscopic shell calcification with posterior acoustic shadowing after traumatic injury at the level of the proximal third of the muscle belly of the semimembranosus

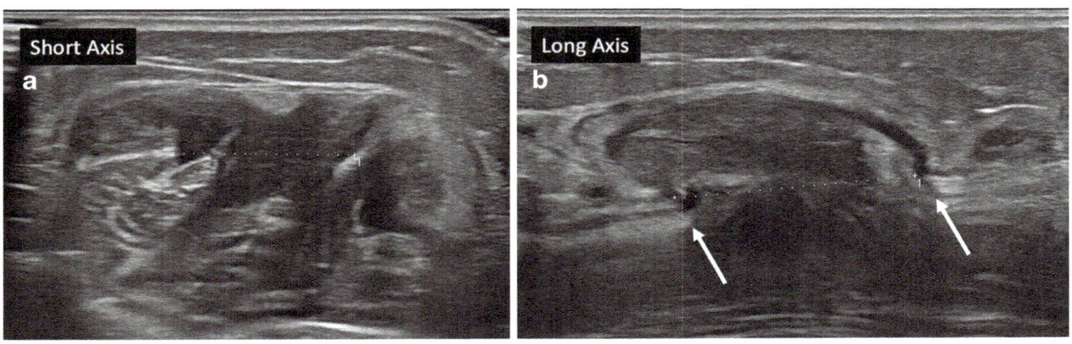

Fig. 25.9 Wide defect in the superficial fascia of the muscle belly of the tibialis anterior with secondary herniation of its fibers. (**a**) Short-axis scan. (**b**) Long-axis scan. Margins of the muscle hernia (*arrows*) are clearly identified

recommended to properly depict the hernia, asking the patient to contract the muscle. When the hernia is not clinically evident, it is also important to decrease the pressure on the probe in order to avoid the accidental reduction of the hernia.

25.3.5 Morel-Lavallée Lesion

Morel-Lavallée lesions are closed degloving injuries associated with severe trauma.

This lesion typically occurs when the skin and subcutaneous fatty tissue traumatically and abruptly separate from the underlying fascia as a result of shearing forces acting on the subcutaneous tissues.

The potential space created superficial to the fascia is filled by various types of fluid, ranging from serous fluid to frank blood, due to the rupture of the vessels perforating the fascia layers and consequent bleeding. It classically occurs in the thigh and the most frequent site is over the greater tro-

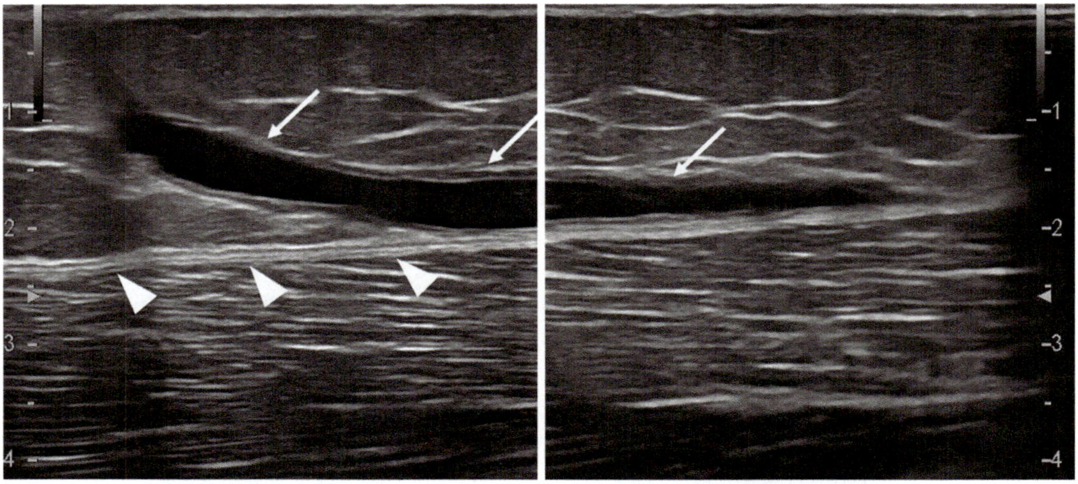

Fig. 25.10 Morel-Lavallée lesion. Post-contusive anechoic collection (*arrows*), with serohematic content and well-defined margins, located superficially to the iliotibial band (*arrowheads*) in the lateral region of the thigh

chanter of the femur, although it can be seen in the lumbar region, over the scapula, or over the knee.

At US examination, acute lesions may appear as thin heterogeneous hyperechoic collections due to debris such as necrotic fat lobules. Then, the collection may spontaneously resolve or become persistent.

In a chronic phase, the collection becomes fusiform, the fluid tends to become more homogeneous and anechoic, and local inflammatory reaction promotes the development of a fibrous pseudocapsule (Fig. 25.10).

However, it is difficult to establish the age of the lesion, as rebleeding of a chronic lesion may confer a persistent heterogeneous hyperechoic appearance.

25.4 Ultrasound After Tendon Surgery Repair

While injured muscle fibers have the ability to heal, even though with the formation of a scar tissue, tendons usually require a surgical repair. The sonographic appearance of the postoperative tendon is very variable, ranging from hyperechoic to hypoechoic appearance. Moreover, the normal fibrillar echotexture may be present or completely absent and the tendon thickness may also be increased or decreased. This could be a problem because the US criteria to diagnose a tendon tear include abnormal hypoechogenicity, loss of the normal fibrillar echotexture, and reduction of the tendon thickness.

Generally, normal operated tendons are larger than native ones. Progressive thickening starts between 3 and 6 months after the intervention and is irreversible. Some intratendinous Doppler signals can be identified and can even increase between the first and third months after surgery. It usually decreases after 6 months. At US follow-up beyond 6 months after surgery, detection of tendon thinning, a liquid collection in or around the tendon, and persistent intratendinous Doppler signals suggest inadequate healing or rerupture. The diagnosis of a recurrent full-thickness tendon tear after surgery also takes advantage of dynamic US imaging, by evaluating active and passive tendon motion.

Some of the most involved tendons that undergo surgery repair are rotator cuff, distal biceps brachii, peroneal and Achilles tendons. Their peculiar postoperative aspects and more frequent complications after surgery will be discussed hereafter.

Rotator cuff: Common indications for rotator cuff repair include a full-thickness tear or a high-grade partial-thickness tear for which conserva-

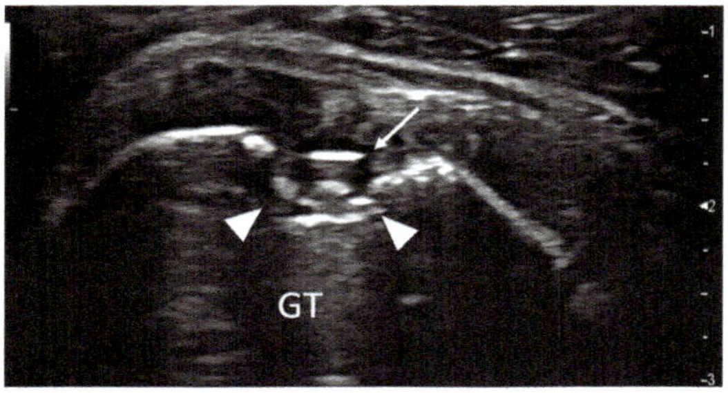

Fig. 25.11 US follow-up after surgical reinsertion of the supraspinatus tendon. At the level of the greater tuberosity (GT), a depression of the cortical contour (*arrowheads*) produced by the orthopedic surgeon in the anchor implant site (*white arrow*) is visible

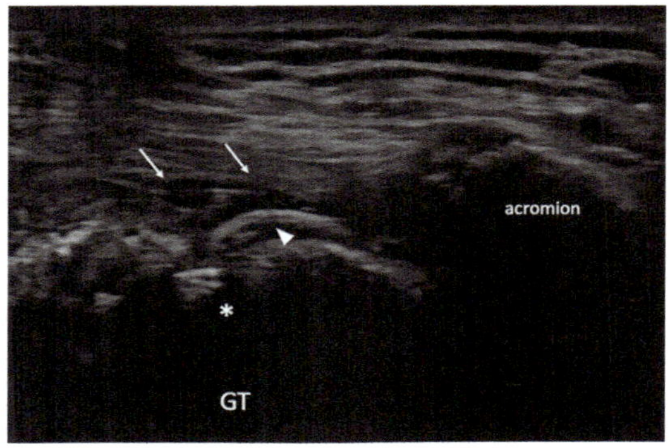

Fig. 25.12 Ultrasound examination after surgical reinsertion of the supraspinatus tendon, which has inhomogeneous echostructure, due to a hyperechoic linear streak referable to the suture thread (*arrowhead*) attached to the greater tuberosity (GT) by means of an anchor (*)

tive management has failed. Although symptomatic smaller partial-thickness tears may be treated with just debridement, higher grade partial-thickness (>50% tendon thickness) and full-thickness tears are commonly repaired by attaching the torn tendon fibers onto the osseous footprint of the humeral greater tuberosity. At US, hyperechoic suture material within the tendon substance and hyperechoic anchors at the bone cortex may be observed (Fig. 25.11). They both may produce posterior acoustic shadowing and they can also displace in subdeltoid bursa.

Postoperative rotator cuff tendons can have a highly variable imaging appearance, with a heterogeneous echotexture at US exam which lasts for years after surgery (Fig. 25.12).

Initially, the tendon may have a thick or thin aspect and is hypoechoic with loss of the normal fibrillar architecture; it becomes more echogenic with time. Peribursal soft tissues may demonstrate persistent inhomogeneous echogenicity, and fluid in the subacromial bursa is also a normal finding in a postoperative setting.

An irregularity of the tendon surface is not so important in the postoperative patient, as it is a common finding in asymptomatic patients in the follow-up after surgery; however careful clinical correlation is always needed.

With regard to the recurrent rotator cuff tears, many of them are massive, with resultant complete absence of the tendons in the physiological location. Furthermore, at dynamic US, lack of tendon translation across the repair site with associated tendon retraction is diagnostic for a full-thickness tendon tear.

Distal biceps brachii tendon (DBBT): In most individuals, the DBBT is composed of two separate components. The first derives from the long head of the biceps muscle, originating at the supraglenoid tuberosity, whereas the second is issued from the short head, originating at the coracoid process. Although partial tears are usually treated conservatively, complete tears require surgical repair, with a high satisfaction rate reported. Hyperechoic fibrillar structure becomes heterogeneous because of small hypoechoic areas around the suture material or small calcareous deposits (Fig. 25.13). Decreased mobility and elasticity of the tendon may also be observed within the first few months.

Most frequent postoperative complications related to DBBT repair are heterotopic ossification, nerve injury, and tendon re-rupture, occurring in 15–40% of patients.

Heterotopic ossification may develop within several weeks after surgery and US can identify it earlier than does radiography, showing hyperechoic nodules or streaks with posterior acoustic attenuation within muscles. Nerve lesions and tendon re-rupture are considered major complications and should be diagnosed as soon as possible. Dynamic US evaluation of nerves'

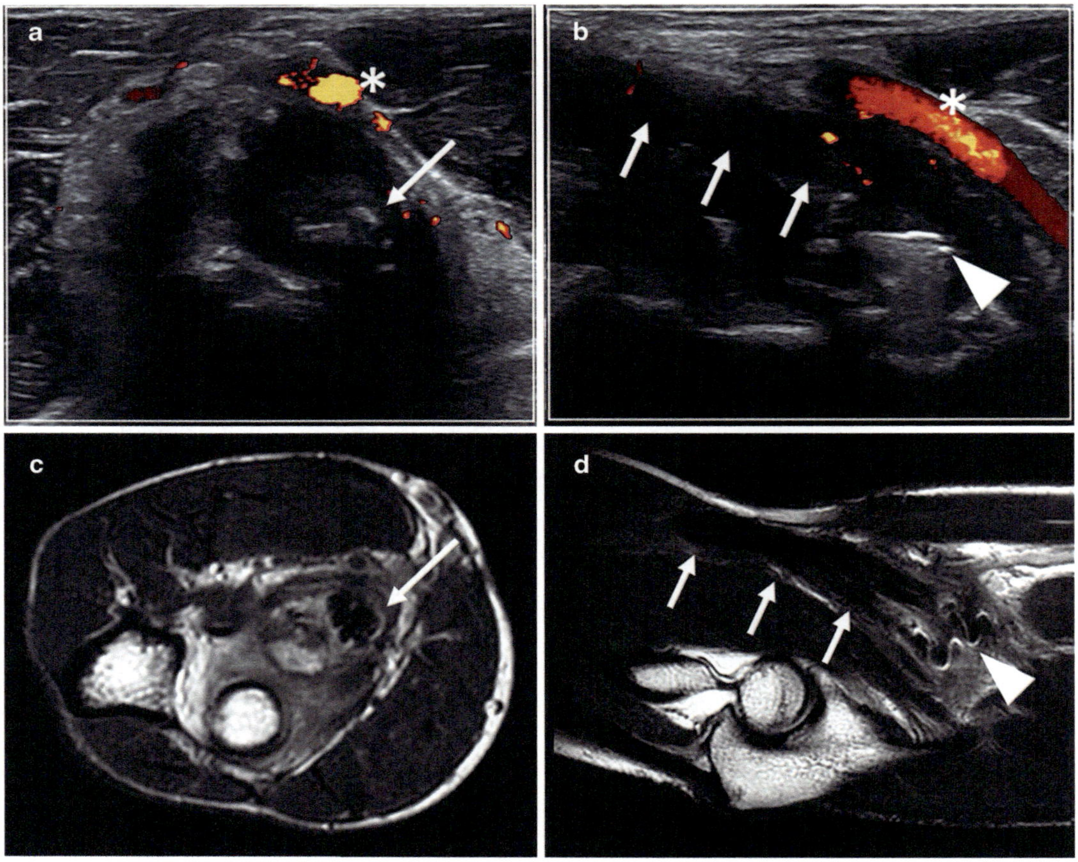

Fig. 25.13 US examination after surgical reinsertion of the distal biceps brachii tendon. (**a**) Short-axis US scan, (**b**) long-axis US scan. The reinserted tendon (*white arrows*) is thickened and inhomogeneous with some intratendinous vascular signals at power Doppler, suggesting ongoing reparation process. The asterisk indicates the brachial artery. The arrowhead indicates the hyperechoic metal anchor characterized by posterior acoustic reverberation artifact. (**c**) Axial FSE PD MRI and (**d**) FSE T2 MRI examination of the same patient. Note the magnetic susceptibility artifact caused by the metal anchor (*arrowhead*) in MRI

relationship with orthopedic material is helpful in determining a nerve abnormal structure or possible conflict.

Re-rupture usually occurs within 3 weeks after surgery and is typically the result of too early or excessive rehabilitation. MR imaging is also very sensitive for diagnosing complete tears after surgery, but it is less sensitive in detecting partial tears. Moreover, MRI is complicated by the patient difficulty in achieving correct positioning of the elbow after surgery or by the presence of metal orthopedic material.

Peroneal Tendon Tears: The peroneal tendons (PT) are part of the peroneal tendon complex, which is composed of the peroneus brevis (PB) and peroneus longus (PL) muscles and tendons, PT sheaths, and superior and inferior peroneal retinacula. First approach for peroneal tenosynovitis, tendinopathy, and partial tears is classically a conservative management, including pharmacological therapy, physiotherapy, and immobilization, with relief expected in 4–6 weeks.

Operative intervention may be indicated when conservative treatments fail or in tendon dislocation/subluxation and high-grade symptomatic and full-thickness tendon tear, especially in patients with high functional demands. Peroneal

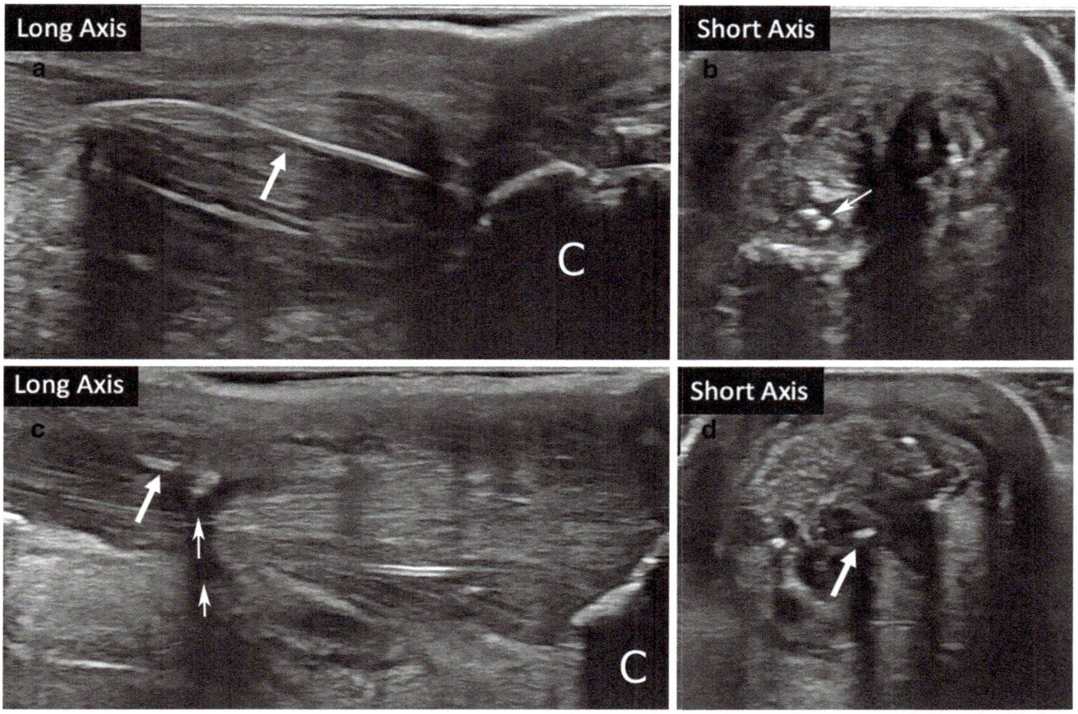

Fig. 25.14 Distal (**a, b**) and proximal (**c, d**) US scan of surgical suture repair of the Achilles tendon. The tendon appears thickened and inhomogeneous, characterized by intratendinous hyperechoic strikes with posterior acoustic shadowing, referable to the suture threads (*white arrows*)

tendon tears are characteristically longitudinal (split lesions) rather than transverse, and peroneus brevis tears are much more common than those of the peroneus longus. When evaluating tendon injuries, it is important to investigate for frequently associated damage of the anterolateral ligament complex of the ankle. Most important postoperative findings to report after surgery are the viability of the remaining tendon, any recurrent or residual tear of one or both peroneal tendons, underlying tendinopathy, and extent of changes within the tendon.

At US examination, the echogenicity for repaired tendons varies from hyperechoic to hypoechoic, with changes of the normal fibrillar pattern due to varying degrees of granulation tissue or scar remodeling. Hypoechoic defects and Doppler spots of vascularization within a tendon repair site caused by the granulation tissue may persist for several years and mimic recurrent tear.

There are immediate and late complications of peroneal tendon surgery. Immediate complications include intratendinous and/or peritendinous hematoma and infections. Late complications include recurrent degeneration or tears, dislocations, and peritendinous adhesions. Patients with postoperative hematoma and infection usually have pain and swelling with complex collection detected at US imaging. Presence of fluid associated with retracted tendon ends or nonvisualization of the tendon, dislodged suture anchor, and broken suture are signs of tendon recurrent tear. A dynamic ultrasound study to evaluate tendon movement by moving the extremity can be used to confirm a tendon tear. Complications of peroneal tendon groove refashioning include redislocation, decreased range of motion, sural nerve injury, and friction of the tendon after repair leading to recurrent tendinosis and tear. Calcifications and suture granuloma are other possible but uncommon complications.

Achilles tendon: The Achilles tendon is the most commonly injured of all the ankle tendons. Predisposing factors include overuse injury, diabetes, peripheral vascular disease, inflammatory and degenerative changes, and obesity. Some drugs are also associated to an increased risk of tendinopathy and tear (glucocorticoids, oral contraceptives). The middle third of the tendon is the most prone to rupture because it is known to be the less vascularized zone of the tendon.

Different surgery techniques can be performed according to the degree of lesion. If tendon ends are still closely approximated, primary end-to-end repair is usually feasible. When severe retraction is present and the gap is too large to reattach the tendon ends, then either a tendon graft or a synthetic augmentation can be used. Grafts from the plantaris, flexor hallucis longus, and peroneal tendons are commonly used to add mechanical strength to the repair.

The repaired tendon is normally larger and/or wider than normal and maintains the increased thickness for at least 2 years after surgery. At US examination, heterogeneous echotexture with loss of the internal fibrillary structure and presence of surgical material within the tendon are considered as normal aspects after surgery (Fig. 25.14). Fluid collections, irregular contours, and extensive intratendinous calcifications should be considered pathologic aspects.

At Doppler imaging there might be a subtle increase during the initial healing process that regresses as the scar matures, but increased vascularity signals at 2 years after surgery may suggest tendinopathy or reinjury.

Variations of peritendinous vascularization are considered less important than intratendinous one.

Dynamic US evaluation shows a physiologic reduction of the tendon's mobility in the first few months after surgery.

Post-traumatic re-rupture is the main complication after surgical treatment of the Achilles tendon rupture. Although clinical symptoms could be clear, sonographic diagnosis may not be obvious, due to the altered echostructure of both the tendon and the peritendinous soft tissues. A dynamic US evaluation during dorsiflexion and plantar flexion movements is necessary to reveal discontinuity of the tendon. It should also be considered that sometimes the gliding of the tendon is prevented by the scar tissue around the repair site. In fact, although initial formation of scars provides continuity at the repair site, an excessive production has to be considered pathological. In this case, at US it may be difficult distinguishing the margins of the tendon from the surrounding tissue and there are hypoechoic areas around the repaired tendon. Other possible complications include infection, calcifications, and suture granuloma, as may happen after surgical repair of other tendons.

Further Readings

Amin NH, Volpi A, Lynch TS, et al. Complications of distal biceps tendon repair: a meta-analysis of single-incision versus double-incision surgical technique. Orthop J Sports Med. 2016;4(10):2325967116668137.

Batz R, Sofka CM, Adler RS, et al. Dermatomyositis and calcific myonecrosis in the leg: ultrasound as an aid in management. Skelet Radiol. 2006;35(2):113–6.

Beltran LS, Bencardino JT, Steinbach LS. Postoperative MRI of the shoulder. J Magn Reson Imaging. 2014;40(6):1280–97.

Brodsky J, Toppins A. Postsurgical imaging of the peroneal tendons. Semin Musculoskelet Radiol. 2012;16(03):233–40.

Chun KA, Cho KH. Postoperative ultrasonography of the musculoskeletal system. Ultrasonography. 2015;34(3):195–205.

Cohen MJ. US imaging in operated tendons. Ultrasound. 2012;15(1):69–75.

Counsel P, Breidahl W. Muscle injuries of the lower leg. Semin Musculoskelet Radiol. 2010;14(2):162–75.

Creteur V, Madani A, Sattari A, et al. Ultrasonography of complications in surgical repair of the distal biceps Brachii tendon. J Ultrasound Med. 2019;38(2):499–512.

Devilbiss Z, Hess M, Ho GWK. Myositis Ossificans in sport: a review. Curr Sports Med Rep. 2018 Sep;17(9):290–5.

Di Pietto F, Chianca V, Zappia M, et al. Articular and peri-articular hip lesions in soccer players. The importance of imaging in deciding which lesions will need surgery and which can be treated conservatively? Eur J Radiol. 2018;105:227–38.

Drakonaki EE, Sudoł-Szopińska I, Sinopidis C, et al. High resolution ultrasound for imaging complications of muscle injury: is there an additional role for elastography? J Ultrason. 2019;19(77):137–44.

Garon MT, Greenberg JA. Complications of biceps distal repair. Orthop Clin N Am. 2016;47:435–44.

Gilat R, Atoun E, Cohen O, et al. Recurrent rotator cuff tear: is ultrasound imaging reliable? J Shoulder Elb Surg. 2018;27(7):1263–7.

Gitto S, Draghi AG, Bortolotto C, et al. Sonography of the Achilles tendon after complete rupture repair: what the radiologist should know. J Ultrasound Med. 2016;35(12):2529–36.

Grasset W, Mercier N, Chaussard C, et al. The surgical treatment of peroneal tendinopathy (excluding subluxations): a series of 17 patients. J Foot Ankle Surg. 2012;51:13–9.

Guermazi A, Roemer FW, Robinson P, et al. Imaging of muscle injuries in sports medicine. Radiology. 2017;

Hall MM. Return to play after thigh muscle injury: utility of serial ultrasound in guiding clinical progression. Curr Sports Med Rep. 2018 Sep;17(9):296–301.

Hollawell S, Baione W. Chronic Achilles tendon rupture reconstructed with Achilles tendon allograft and xenograft combination. J Foot Ankle Surg. 2015;54(6):1146–50.

Jacobson JA, Lax MJ. Musculoskeletal sonography of the postoperative orthopedic patient. Semin Musculoskelet Radiol. 2002;6(1):67–77. Review

Kumar Y, Farmazalian A, Shivani A, et al. Peroneal tendon pathology: pre- and post-operative high resolution US and MR imaging. Eur J Radiol. 2017;92:132–44.

Kwee RM, Kwee TC. Calcified or ossified benign soft tissue lesions that may simulate malignancy. Skelet Radiol. 2019;48(12):1875–90.

LiMarzi GM, Scherer KF, Richardson ML, et al. CT and MR imaging of the postoperative ankle and foot. Radiographics. 2016;36(6):1828–48. Review

Lungu E, Michaud J, Bureau NJ. US assessment of sports-related hip injuries. Radiographics. 2018;38(3):867–89.

Möller M, Kälebo P, Tidebrant G, et al. The ultrasonographic appearance of the ruptured Achilles tendon during healing: a longitudinal evaluation of surgical and nonsurgical treatment, with comparisons to MRI appearance. Knee Surg Sports Traumatol Arthrosc. 2002;10:49–56.

Orlandi D, Corazza A, Arcidiacono A. Ultrasound-guided procedures to treat sport-related muscle injuries. Br J Radiol. 2016;89(1057):20150484.

Peetrons P. Ultrasound of muscles. Eur Radiol. 2002;12:35–43.

Pierce JL, Nacey NC, Jones S, et al. Postoperative shoulder imaging: rotator cuff. Labrum and Biceps Tendon Radiographics. 2016;36:1648–71.

Tyler P, Saifuddin A. The imaging of myositis Ossificans. Semin Musculoskelet Radiol. 2010;14(2):201–16.

Yoshida K, Itoigawa Y, Maruyama Y. Healing process of gastrocnemius muscle injury on ultrasonography using B-mode imaging, power Doppler imaging, and shear wave Elastography. J Ultrasound Med. 2019;38(12):3239–46.

Therapy Efficacy Evaluation in Synovitis

26

Marina Carotti, Emilio Filippucci, Fausto Salaffi, and Fabio Martino

Contents

26.1 Introduction

In chronic inflammatory joint diseases, synovial tissue is the major site of inflammation. Latest reports indicate that ultrasonography may be an important imaging technique to determine the degree of synovitis in inflamed joints of patients with chronic inflammatory arthritis. Furthermore, the use of power Doppler technique with high-frequency probes allows for a sensitive detection of synovial proliferation with abnormal blood flow, especially in the small joints of the hands and feet.

Power Doppler technique analyzes Doppler changes induced by the moving red blood cells

M. Carotti
Clinica di Radiologia, Dipartimento di Scienze Radiologiche – Azienda Ospedali Riuniti di Ancona Universita' Politecnica delle Marche, Ancona, Italy

E. Filippucci · F. Salaffi
Clinica Reumatologica, Dipartimento di Scienze Cliniche e Molecolari, Università Politecnica delle Marche, Jesi (Ancona), Italy

F. Martino (✉)
Radiology, Sant'Agata Diagnostic Center, Bari, Italy

F. Martino et al. (eds.), *Musculoskeletal Ultrasound in Orthopedic and Rheumatic disease in Adults*,
https://doi.org/10.1007/978-3-030-91202-4_26

and is particularly helpful for the quantification of low blood flows at synovial tissue level. Contrast-enhanced ultrasound (CEUS) may be a promising tool to evaluate inflammatory arthritis, because of its ability to provide dynamic imaging, and high sensitivity for angiogenesis. Angiogenesis is emerging as a key player in the pathogenesis of many chronic inflammatory arthritis. A number of scoring systems, improving reliability and consequently the responsiveness of US in clinical trials, have been proposed. However, there is still a lack of an expert-derived consensus, especially on the core set of joints to scan. We have attempted to summarize the emerging B-mode ultrasound, color/power Doppler ultrasound, and CEUS imaging techniques and their applications in quantifying synovial inflammation.

26.2 Musculoskeletal Ultrasound Scoring Methods

In patients with rheumatoid arthritis, sonographic findings of synovial inflammation were found predictive for irreversible joint damage (i.e., bone erosions), and they can be significantly changed by disease-modifying antirheumatic drugs. Color and power Doppler techniques have shown to be of diagnostic value in the detection of vascularity in intra-articular synovial tissue and provide a measure of neovascularization within the synovial lining of tendons and within tendons themselves. The ultrasound quantification of synovial inflammation is essential for at least three reasons: (i) for diagnosing active synovitis, (ii) for therapy monitoring, and (iii) as a predictive factor for relapse in patients in remission.

26.2.1 Ultrasound Scoring Systems

Several semiquantitative scoring systems using grayscale findings and power Doppler signals have been proposed (Table 26.1). In most of the published studies, grayscale and Doppler findings have been graded independently and each elementary component had its dedicated scoring system.

Recently, the EULAR-OMERACT (*European League Against Rheumatism-Outcome Measures in Rheumatology*) group for musculoskeletal ultrasound has agreed on the use of a four-grade semiquantitative scoring system for both B-mode-detected and Doppler-detected synovitis, which have demonstrated good multi-examiner intra-observer and inter-observer reliability in RA patients.

In 2003, Szkudlarek et al. developed a four-step semiquantitative US grading system for joint effusion, synovial thickening, and power Doppler signal at synovium level in five preselected small joints of patients with RA: second and third metacarpophalangeal joints, second proximal interphalangeal joint, and first and second metatarsophalangeal joints. Joint effusion was defined as a compressible anechoic intracapsular area and the amount of fluid semiquantitatively scored as follows: grade 0: no effusion; grade 1: minimal amount; grade 2: moderate amount (without distension of the joint capsule); and grade 3: extensive amount (with distension of the joint capsule). Synovial thickening was defined as a non-compressible hypoechoic intracapsular area scored as follows: grade 0: none; grade 1: minimal synovial thickening filling the angle between the periarticular bones, without bulging over the line linking tops of the bones; grade 2: synovial thickening bulging over the line linking tops of the periarticular bones without extension along the bone diaphysis; and grade 3: synovial thickening bulging over the line linking tops of the periarticular bones with extension to at least one of the bone diaphysis. Semiquantitative grading of the PD signal in the synovium was described as follows: grade 0: no flow; grade 1: single-vessel signals; grade 2: confluent vessel signals in less than half of the area of the synovium; and grade 3: vessel signals in more than half of the area of the synovium (Figs. 26.1 and 26.2).

In 2000, Wakefield et al. described the first semiquantitative scoring system for the assessment of bone erosions. A bone erosion was defined as an interruption of the bony cortex with an irregular floor documented in longitudinal and transverse planes. The size of the definite bone erosion was measured using its maximal diame-

Table 26.1 Main ultrasound scoring systems for synovitis listed in chronological order

Author	Year	Pathologies	No. of patients	Grade	Examined joints	Joint region
Wakefield et al.	2000	Bone erosion	100	0–3	Unilateral MCP II-V	Ulnar, radial, palmar, and dorsal
Szkudlarek et al.	2003	Joint effusion, synovial thickening, PD activity	30	0–3	Unilateral MCP II, III, PIP II, MPT I and II	Dorsal
Scheel et al.	2005	Effusion/synovial hypertrophy	46	0–3	Unilateral MCP II–V, PIP II–V, assessment	Palmar, dorsal
Naredo et al.	2005	Joint effusion, synovial thickening, PD activity	49	0–3 sum of bilateral 60-, 18-, 16-, 12-, 10-, and 6-joint score	Dorsal	
Backhaus et al.	2009	Synovitis, tenosynovitis, paratendonitis, PD activity, bone erosions	120	0–3; 0–1 for tenosynovitis and erosion	Unilateral wrist, MCP II, III PIP II, III, MPT II, V	Dorsal, palmar, lateral
Ellegaard et al.	2010	PD activity	109	0–3	Unilateral wrist	Dorsal
Dougados et al.	2010	Synovitis	76	0–3; 0–1 for tenosynovitis	Bilateral 28 joints vs. 38 joints (28 + MTPs) vs. 20 joints (20 MCPs + 20 MTPs)	Dorsal, plantar
Hammer et al.	2011	Synovitis, tenosynovitis PD activity, bursitis	20	0–3	Bilateral 78 joints vs. 44 joints, 28 joints, 12 joints, and 7 joints	Dorsal
Kawashini et al.	2011	Synovitis, bursitis	24	0–3	Bilateral elbows, wrists, knees, and ankles	Dorsal, palmar
Bachkaus et al.	2012	Synovitis, tenosynovitis, paratendonitis, bone erosions	432	0–3	Sum of wrist, MTP II-V, MCP/PIP II and III	Dorsal, plantar
Ohmdorf et al.	2012	Synovitis, tenosynovitis, paratendonitis, bone erosions	6	0–3	Dominant wrist, MCP II and III, PIP II–V, MPT II and V	Dorsal, radial, and plantar
Harlung et al.	2012	Synovitis, tenosynovitis PD activity	199	0–3	Shoulder, elbow, hip, and knee	Dorsal, ventral, and lateral
Yoshimi et al.	2014	PD activity	234	0–3	Wrists, knees, MCP I-V, PIP II and III	Dorsal, palmar
Aga et al.	2015	GSUS and PDUS scores	439	0–3	7-joint/2 tendon (MCP, PIP, MTP), radiocarpal, elbow, tibialis	Dorsal, palmar, plantar
Luz et al.	2016	Synovitis, tenosynovitis PD activity, bone erosions	48	0–3; 0–1 for tenosynovitis	Wrist, MCP II and III, PIP II and III	Dorsal, palmar
Janta et al.	2016	Synovitis, tenosynovitis, PD activity	47	0–3	12-joint (wrist, hand, ankle, MTP); B-mode, PD, tenosynovitis	Dorsal, palmar
Sun et al.	2017	Synovitis, PD activity	235	0–3	Bilateral wrists, MCP I-V, PIP I-V	Dorsal

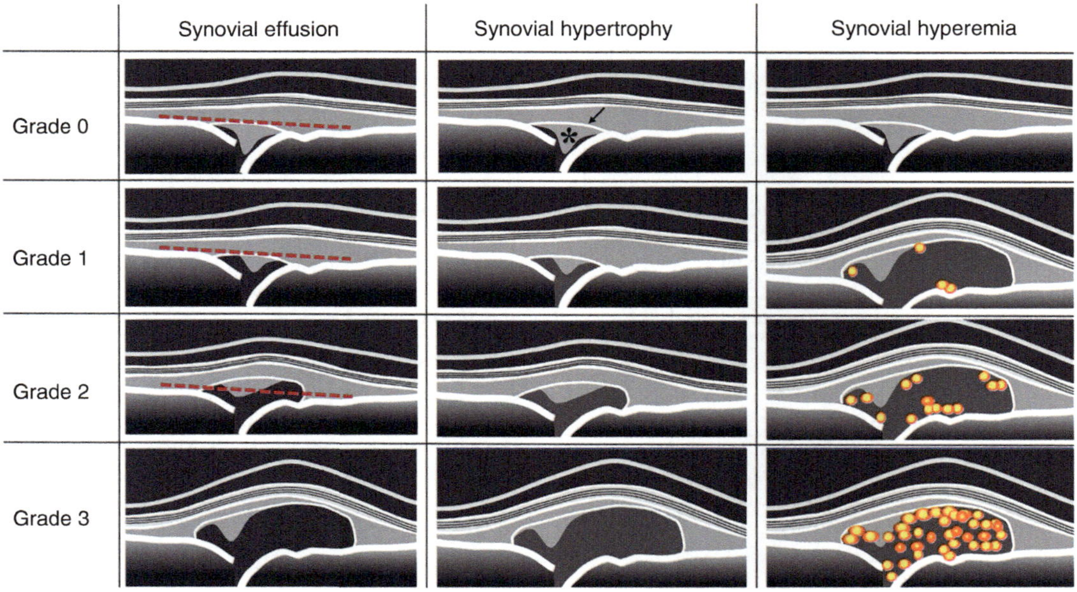

Fig. 26.1 Ultrasound semiquantitative scoring scheme of synovial effusion, synovial hypertrophy, and synovial hyperemia assessing synovitis grade at MCP joint using dorsal longitudinal scan. Red dotted line = tangent line to tops of joint bones; asterisk = dorsal plate; arrow = capsule profile

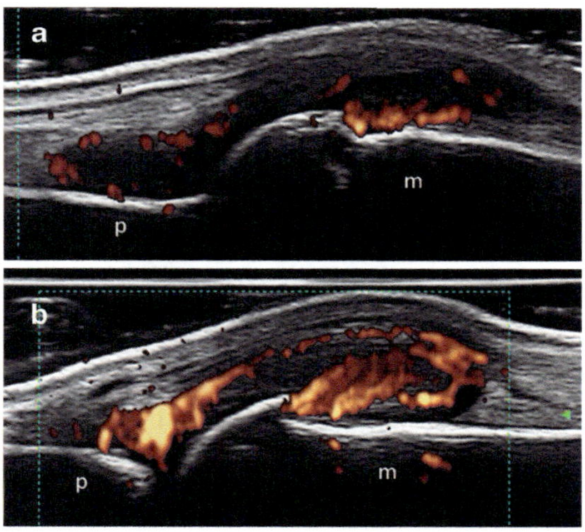

Fig. 26.2 Rheumatoid arthritis. Active synovitis detected using a longitudinal dorsal scan at metacarpophalangeal joint level. Both images (**a**) and (**b**) show representative examples of synovitis grade 3 using grayscale scoring system. Using power Doppler assessment grade 2 and grade 3 can be assigned, respectively, to (**a**) and (**b**). p proximal phalanx, m metacarpal bone

ter and the following scoring system was proposed: small erosion: <2 mm; moderate erosion: 2–4 mm; and large erosion: >4 mm (Fig. 26.3).

In a recent study by Hurnakova J et al., cartilage damage of the metacarpal head was assessed in patients with rheumatoid arthritis and in patients with osteoarthritis using a very-high-frequency probe (up to 22 MHz) and the following five-grade semiquantitative scoring system: 0 = normal hyaline cartilage; 1 = loss of the sharpness of the cartilage superficial margin; 2 = partial-thickness defect of the cartilage layer; 3 = full-thickness defect of the cartilage layer with normal subchondral bone profile; and 4 = complete loss of the cartilage layer and subchondral bone damage (Fig. 26.4).

For tenosynovitis and tendon damage a taskforce of the OMERACT US group agreed on a four-grade semiquantitative scoring system (i.e., grade 0, normal; grade 1, minimal; grade 2, moderate; grade 3, severe). Both longitudinal and transverse planes should be used to assess both inflammatory findings and tendon ruptures.

The data acquired by all scoring systems depend on both acquisition and interpretation processes and the following practical tips are fundamental to consider, especially when a comparison between a previous or future ultrasound

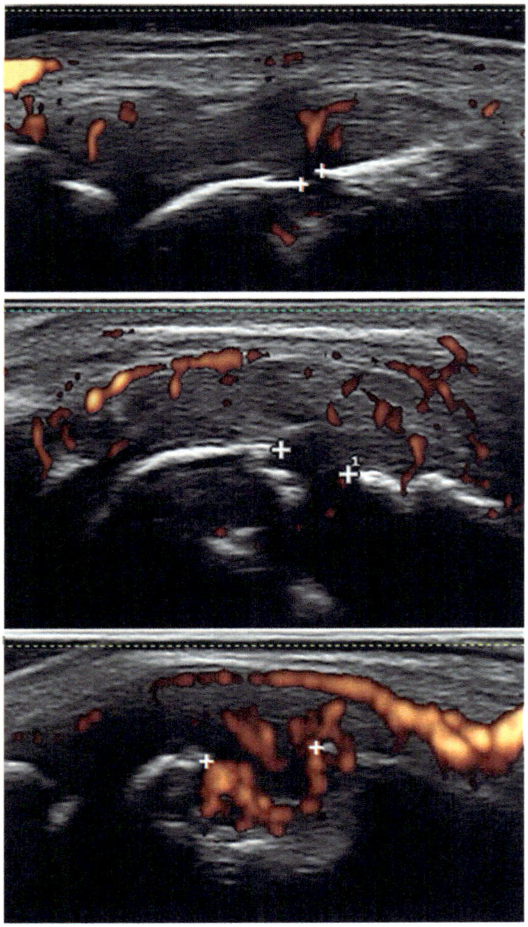

Fig. 26.3 Rheumatoid arthritis. Second metacarpophalangeal joint on longitudinal radial scan. Representative examples showing bone erosions with different sizes. p proximal phalanx; m metacarpal bone

examination is, respectively, requested or planned.

As regards the acquisition process, it may be based on anatomic or pathologic references: in other words, the sonographer may save the images using standard scanning planes described using fixed anatomic landmarks, or according to the maximal expression of synovitis.

The images acquired using standard scans are easily compared, but they may underestimate or completely miss synovitis; conversely the method based on pathologic findings may lead to the acquisition of images with different anatomic backgrounds, but they display the outcome measure which is essential for therapy monitoring. Thus, ultrasound examination should not be limited to placing the probe in a selected number of scanning planes, but it should entail the movement of the probe from one side of the anatomic site under examination to the other side, to look for the maximal expression of synovial inflammation.

Interpretation of ultrasound findings indicative of synovitis for therapy monitoring must consider the following main issues: intra- and inter-observer reliability and sensitivity to change. In fact, interpretation based only on presence/absence is likely to provide a higher degree of intra- and inter-observer agreement, but it may miss early improvements due to treatment; conversely adopting a semiquantitative scoring system allows for a more sensitive-to-change method which distinguishes different grades of synovitis. In other words, presence/absence approach misses the benefit obtained by a treatment inducing a change from synovitis grade 3 at baseline to grade 1 at follow-up examination, because it requires the complete disappearance of the ultrasound findings indicative of synovial inflammation to record an improvement.

26.2.2 Examined Joints

Several core sets of joints have been proposed to assess rheumatoid arthritis activity with ultrasound; however, to date, there is no clear consensus on the optimal joint count to use in daily clinical practice. To include ultrasound in the clinical routine, it is of major importance to scan the lowest number of joints and tendons that is able to give relevant information on the inflammatory process at patient level.

Hammer et al. published a study, in which a comprehensive US score including 78 joints was compared with reduced joint counts (7-, 12-, 28-, and 44-joint scores) at different time points, during biologic agent treatment. They found high correlation between the reduced joint scores and the 78-joint score at all examination time points for power Doppler ultrasound.

In the development of scoring system, Scheel et al. examined semiquantitatively (0–3) and quan-

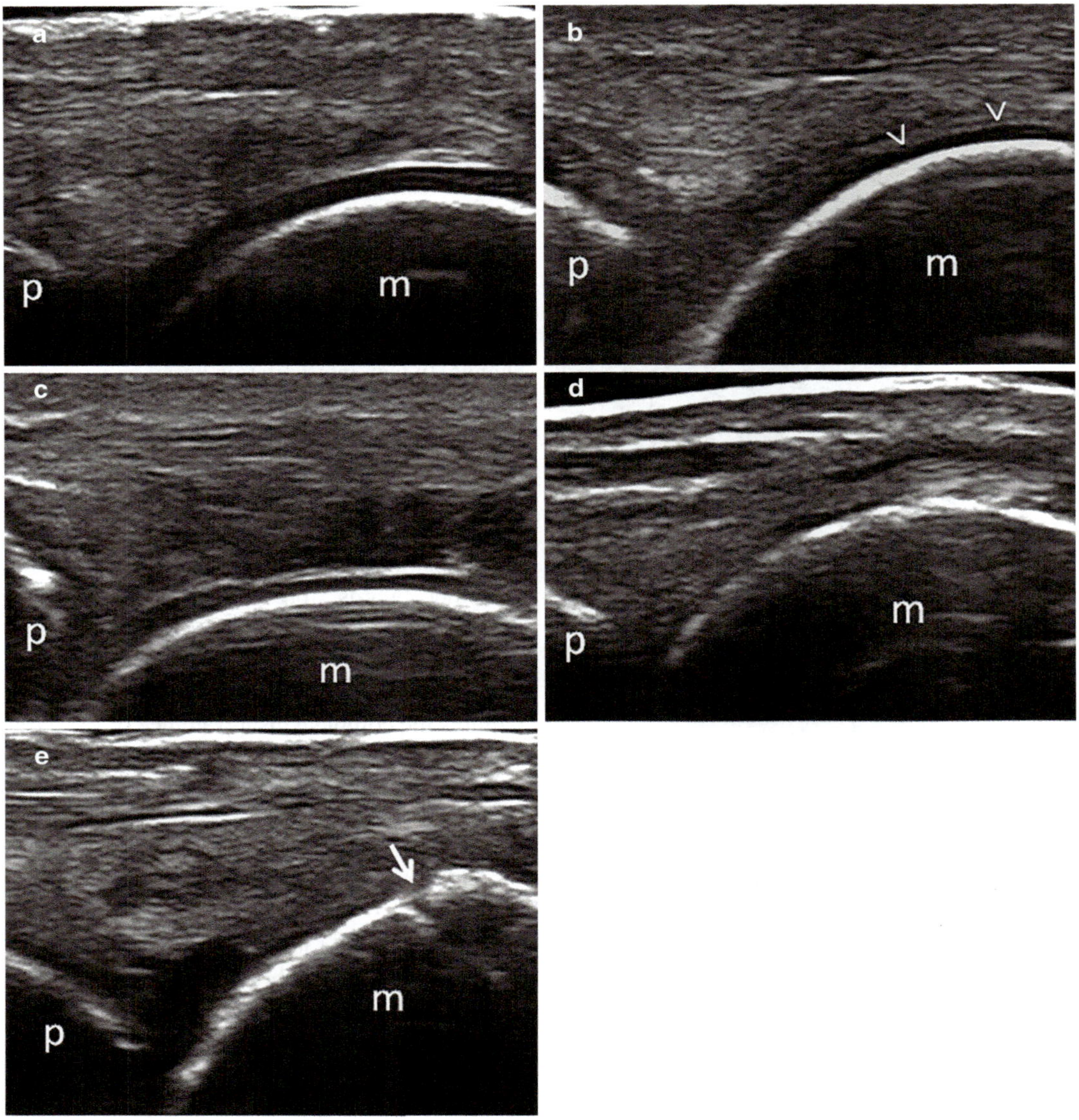

Fig. 26.4 Rheumatoid arthritis. Metacarpal head on longitudinal dorsal scan. Representative examples of different grades of cartilage damage. (**a**) Normal hyaline cartilage. (**b**) Loss of the sharpness of the cartilage superficial margin. (**c**) Partial-thickness defect of the cartilage layer. (**d**) Full-thickness defect of the cartilage layer with normal subchondral bone profile. (**e**) Complete loss of the cartilage layer and subchondral bone damage. p proximal phalanx; m metacarpal bone

titatively synovitis in the clinically most affected metacarpophalangeal and proximal interphalangeal joints of the hands of rheumatoid patients. They found no significant differences between semiquantitative scores and quantitative measurements and concluded that the examination of a reduced number of joints is preferable, in view of the shorter examination time required.

Naredo et al. investigated the validity of reduced joint counts including large and small joints on both sides. A 12-joint score including bilateral wrist, metacarpophalangeal and proximal interphalangeal joints of the second and third fingers, and knees was used to determine effusion, synovitis, and PD activity. Such a scoring system correlated highly with a corresponding 60-joint score. In fact, 12-joint score reflected the overall joint inflammation in patients with RA and is therefore useful for monitoring treatment.

Luz et al. proposed a novel ultrasound scoring system for hand and wrist joints for evaluation of patients with early RA. Such a scoring system involved the assessment of the wrist and second and third metacarpophalangeal and proximal interphalangeal joints. The score consisted of inflammation parameters (synovial proliferation, power Doppler signal, and tenosynovitis) and joint damage parameters (bone erosion and cartilage damage). The method proved to be a useful tool for monitoring inflammation and joint damage in patients with early RA, demonstrating significant correlations with longitudinal changes in disease activity and functional status.

More recently, 705 patients with definite RA were investigated and a selection of eight joints (bilateral wrist and metacarpophalangeal joints of second, third, and fifth fingers) was found simple and efficient to detect synovitis in daily practice.

In 2009, Backhaus et al. proposed a seven-joint US composite scoring system, including wrist, metacarpophalangeal and proximal interphalangeal joint of the second and third fingers, and metatarsophalangeal joint of the second and fifth toes. The joints were examined by B-mode and power Doppler ultrasound for synovitis, tenosynovitis/paratendonitis, and erosions (Table 26.2).

B-mode ultrasound synovitis was scored semiquantitatively according to Scheel et al., while the power Doppler signal was assessed using the scoring system of Szkudlarek et al. Tenosynovitis/paratendonitis and bone erosions in B-mode ultrasound were recorded on a binary basis (presence/absence). The authors concluded that the use of this score would provide a fast overview of disease activity in daily clinical practice and would be helpful in monitoring treatment.

To date the seven-joint US composite scoring system proposed by Backhaus et al. represents the most comprehensive (not only joints are included but also tendons; not only inflammatory findings are evaluated, but also bone erosions) and validated (not only in cross-sectional studies in comparison with clinical and other imaging data, but also in longitudinal studies testing its responsiveness) approach for assessing patients with rheumatoid arthritis. This accounts for its being the most used score in rheumatological clinical practice. From a practical point of view, its main limitation lies on the fact that it is based on a fixed set of anatomic structures to scan (Table 26.2). Since the anatomic structures are frequently affected joints in rheumatoid arthritis, this score works very well when assessing a cohort of patients with rheumatoid arthritis. However, in a specific single patient it may miss the most clinically involved joints. Thus, a possible solution in daily clinical practice could be to scan the seven joints indicated by Backhaus et al. together with the most clinically inflamed joint at the time of the visit.

26.2.3 Color and/or Power Doppler Ultrasound Methods

Color and/or power Doppler ultrasound techniques have gained importance because of their ability to assess abnormal blood flow at synovial tissue level, a key feature of the inflammatory process in patients with chronic arthritis. Apart from the outcome measure for monitoring disease activity during treatment (Fig. 26.5), Doppler findings have been proposed as predictors for relapse in patients in clinical remission and have been found able to predict erosive progression both in patients with early RA and in patients with low disease activity or remission.

Color and/or power Doppler ultrasound techniques are operator- and machine-dependent techniques. The following practical aspects should be considered during a Doppler examination of joint and periarticular structures. First, the patient must find a comfortable position during the scanning to avoid an increase of pressure at the anatomic site

Table 26.2 B-mode ultrasound (US) and power Doppler (PD) US assessing synovitis, tenosynovitis/paratendonitis, and bone erosions from the dorsal, palmar, and ulnar aspects of the wrist, metacarpophalangeal (MCP), proximal interphalangeal (PIP), and metatarsophalangeal (MTP) joints

	Wrist	Fingers	Toes	
Synovitis	Dorsal + PD Palmar + PD Ulnar + DP	**MCP II, III** Palmar + PD Dorsal-only PD **PIP II, III** Palmar + PD Dorsal-only PD	**MPT II, V** Dorsal + PD	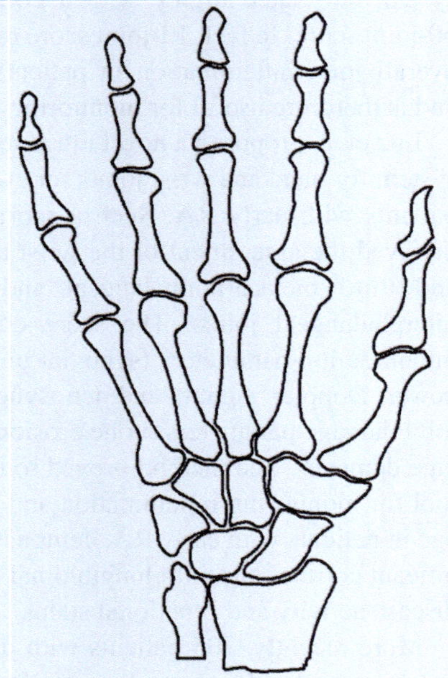
Paratendonitis/ tenosynovitis	Dorsal + PD Palmar + PD Ulnar + PD	**MCP II,** **III**Dorsal + PD Palmar + PD		
Bone erosions		**MCP II, III** Dorsal, palmar **MCP II** Radial **PIP II, III** Dorsal, palmar	**MTP II, V** Dorsal, plantar **MTP V** Lateral	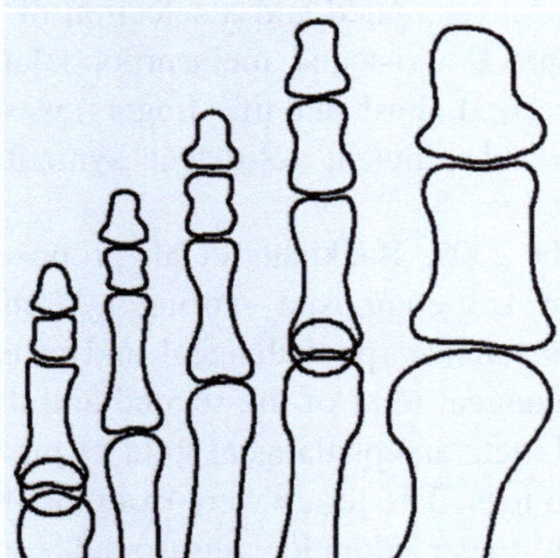
	1 joint	4 joints	2 joints	7 joints

under examination and consequent false-negative findings. Second, the sonographer should reduce as much as possible the compression on the tissues with the probe. Third, the Doppler parameters should be set to obtain the maximal sensitivity for the detection of synovial blood flow. Although they may vary using different ultrasound systems, the mean values of the main Doppler parameters can be the following:

- Doppler frequency: 6 MHz for large joints, i.e., knee; 9 MHz for smaller joints, i.e., wrist; and 11 MHz for very small joints and superficial structures, i.e., distal interphalangeal joints and tendons of the fingers and toes.
- Pulse repetition frequency (PRF): ranging from 750 Hz to 1.3 KHz.
- Doppler gain: the highest value not generating random noise artifacts.

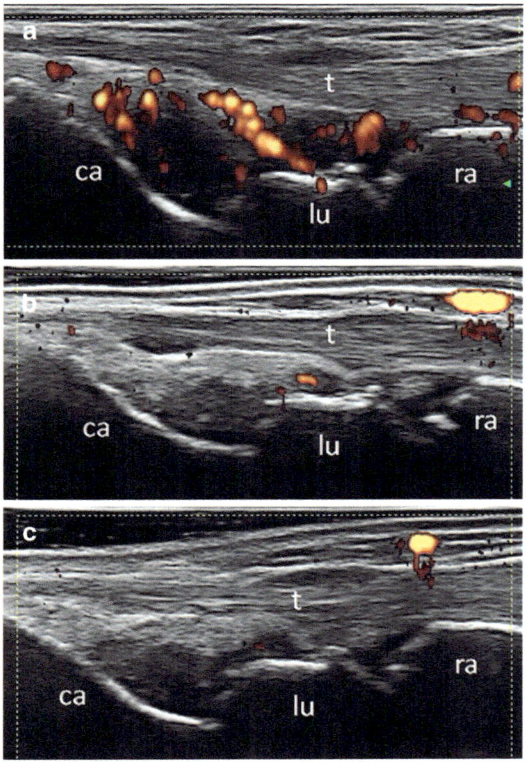

Fig. 26.5 Rheumatoid arthritis. Wrist synovitis. Ultrasound changes induced by intra-articular steroid injection assessed using a dorsal longitudinal view. (**a**) Baseline assessment showing active wrist synovitis. (**b**) Two weeks after the injection the same view allows the detection of the disappearance of ultrasound signs of synovitis. (**c**) One month after the injection, the image shows the persistent absence of ultrasound signs of synovitis. ca capitate bone, lu lunate bone, ra radius, t common extensor tendons of the fingers

26.2.4 Doppler Quantitative Assessment of Synovial Blood Flow

Using different machines, Doppler modalities, and settings may have a considerable influence on the quantification of inflammation by ultrasound in patients with chronic arthritis, and this must be taken into account when a follow-up examination is performed. Semi- or fully automated software tools for quantitative assessment of active synovitis may help reducing the interobserver variability. Quantitative Doppler scoring systems include the count of color pixels or the color pixel intensity, in a region of interest (ROI), outlined by the sonographer, in synovial tissue, inside the joint capsule, using dedicated post-processing software and spectral Doppler analysis with measurement of the resistive index (RI) (Fig. 26.6).

Spectral Doppler analysis can be used to obtain a quantitative estimation of the grade of the synovial perfusion. The normal flow at the level of soft tissues is characterized by high resistance (i.e., high values of RI), because the diastolic velocity has been considered to be zero. Conversely, the inflammatory process is characterized by an increased perfusion and permeability of vessels together with neovascularization, and consequently an increase of the diastolic velocity and low values of RI indicate an inflammation process.

Thus, RI value allows quantitative measurements of the synovial blood flow providing an estimation of the synovial activity in patients with chronic arthritis: the lower the value of RI, the higher the grade of synovitis.

26.3 Role of CEUS in the Assessment of Inflammatory Arthritis

Contrast-enhanced US (CEUS) consists of a suspension of stabilized gas-filled spheres, which once introduced into the bloodstream, intravenously, generate high-intensity signals which can be detected by the transducer. These tiny microbubbles are smaller than red blood cells, which thereby can be introduced into the vascular system, and keep stable during the whole process of examination. CEUS microbubbles are "blood pool" contrast agents because once injected inside the vessels, they remain inside the lumen and do not diffuse in the extra-arterial tissue or in the cells, showing the exact vascular patterns and neoangiogenesis in the inflamed synovium. This is important because angiogenesis is reported to be the earliest sign of rheumatoid arthritis and other inflammatory rheumatic diseases.

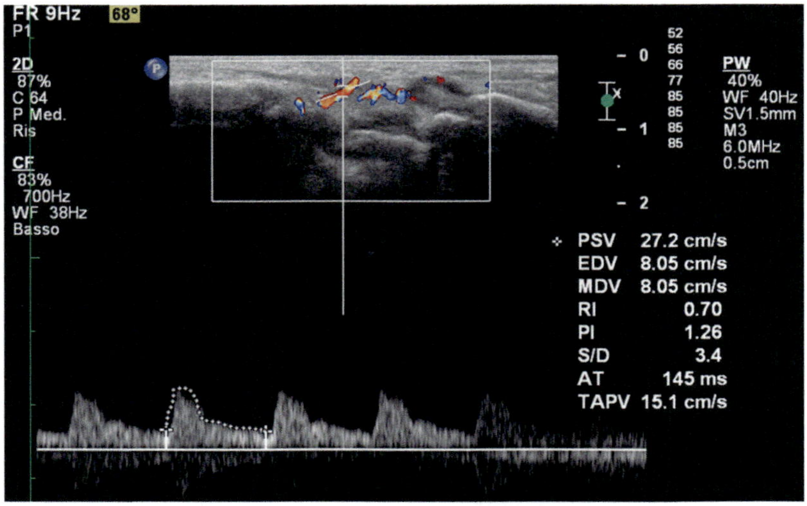

Fig. 26.6 Spectral Doppler analysis, with automatic calculation of the resistive index (RI). Abnormal vascularization, with decreased value of RI, due to persistent flow during the diastole, can be observed at the level of inflamed synovial tissue of the wrist in a patient with RA

The more recent type of US contrast agents consists of stabilized microbubbles of a sulfur hexafluoride gas (SonoVue®, Bracco, Milan, Italy). The use of CEUS improves the sensitivity of CDUS and PDUS in the identification of abnormal vascularization in joint inflammation, allowing a more exact measurement of the synovitis and a better characterization of the pannus, in terms of differentiation between hypervascularity, hypovascularity, and avascularity. This method has been shown to correlate with the histopathological quantitative and morphologic estimation of microvascular proliferation in synovial tissue.

26.3.1 Quantitative Analysis of CEUS

After an intravenous injection of the contrast microbubbles, a time-intensity curve (TIC) in the region of interest (ROI) is displayed by the software, showing an S-shaped wash-in and a nearly exponential washout (Fig. 26.7). The enhancement curves can be compared to those built with gadolinium DTPA in magnetic resonance studies. After the bolus injection, the slope of the ascending and descending curve, the time to peak, the maximum intensity, and the area under the TIC curve are the most common parameters calculated by the software, representative of the perfusion kinetics, and therefore they allow a detailed evaluation and quantification of synovial inflammation. Another approach of quantitative CEUS analysis of the vascular perfusion of synovium is pixel-based level and in a study a linear relationship was discovered between the parameters of quantitative CEUS and the frequencies of some interleukins in patients with psoriatic arthritis.

26.3.2 Applications of Quantitative Analysis of CEUS in Inflammatory Arthritis

Many studies have demonstrated that CEUS may be an excellent tool in the early diagnosis in inflammatory diseases, such as rheumatoid arthritis, psoriatic arthritis, and ankylosing spondylitis, as well as in degenerative disorders. Most of these studies have been performed in patients with rheumatoid arthritis. The capacity of CEUS compared to that of B-mode and power Doppler ultrasound for detection of vascularity in joints of rheumatoid patients was evaluated by the International Arthritis Contrast Ultrasound (IACUS) study group in a multicenter trial of five European centers. CEUS has been found more sensitive than color and power Doppler ultra-

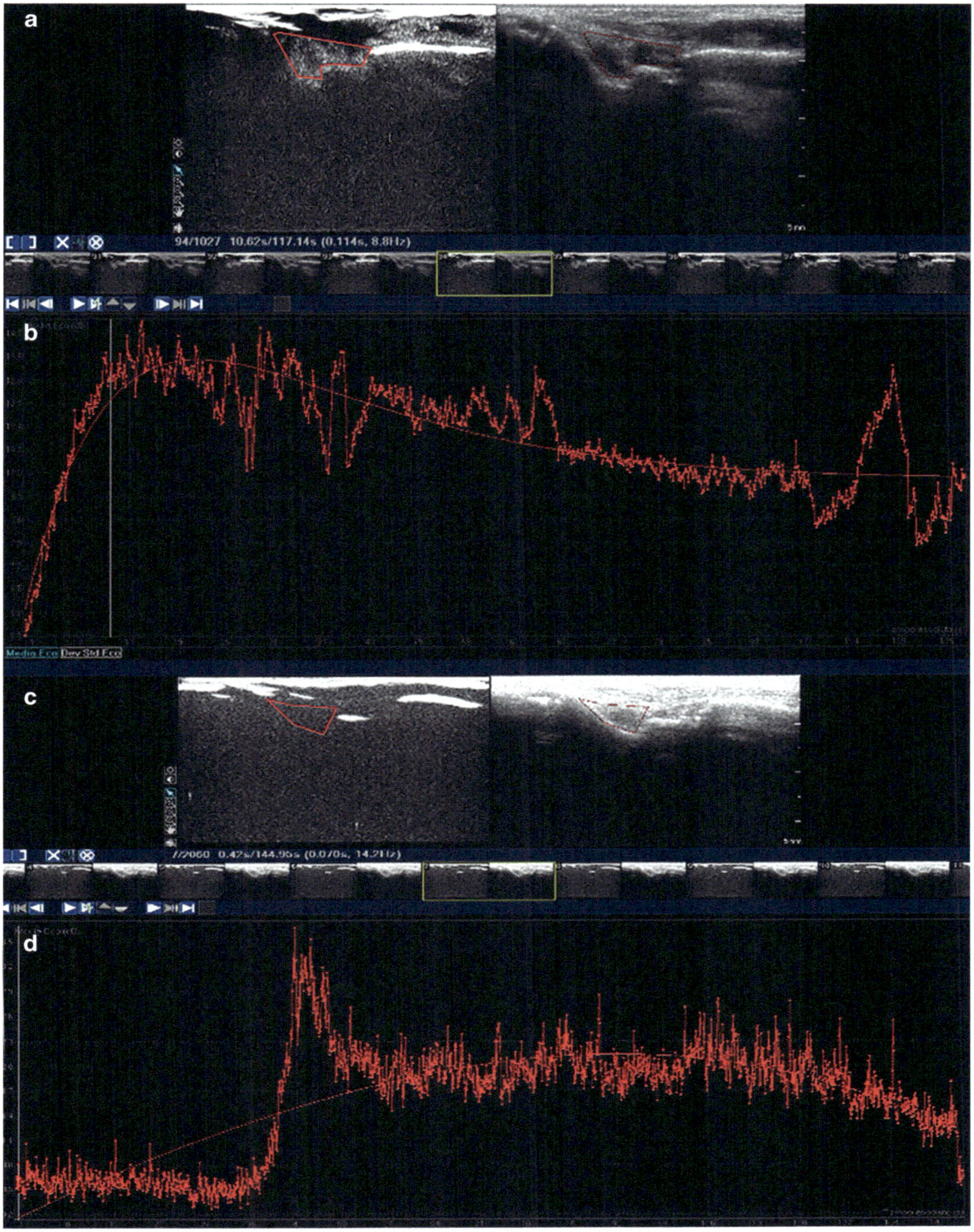

Fig. 26.7 Example of the time-intensity curve in patients with RA at baseline (**a**, **b**) and after 3 months of treatment with biologic agents (**c**, **d**)

sound in the differentiation between active and inactive synovitis. CEUS significantly improves the detection of synovial vascularization at the knee in rheumatoid patients and the area under the curve correlates with the clinical and laboratory findings of disease activity and with the degree of knee inflammation, being significantly higher in patients with clinically active synovitis compared with those with inactive synovitis. Apart from synovitis, CEUS was found to be useful in the detection of pathologic intra- and peritendinous vascularity associated with tenosynovitis; in the evaluation of vascularized erosive lesions, which are a sign of progressive active disease; and in the demonstration of vascularized synovial lining of the inflamed bursa. Similar results have been found in patients with spondylarthritis. It has been demonstrated that the perfusion kinetics of CEUS, such as refilling time, peak intensity, regional blood flow, and slope, are associated with vascular synovial pattern in patients with psoriatic arthritis. There is also evidence confirming that the hypervascularity can be shown in the inflamed sacroiliac joints with spondylarthritis.

26.3.3 Clinical Application of CEUS in Therapeutic Monitoring in Inflammatory Arthritis

The quantification of synovitis is a key aspect to support therapy decisions in daily practice in patients with inflammatory arthritis and imaging findings contribute to estimating synovial inflammation activity. In the EFSUMB (*European Federation of Societies for Ultrasound in Medicine and Biology*) guidelines, CEUS is described as a method whose findings may change as a result of adequate treatment. A number of studies confirmed that CEUS can play a role in the therapeutic monitoring in inflammatory arthritis and in the evaluation of true remission (Table 26.3). CEUS has been shown to be able to detect changes in synovial perfusion after intra-articular steroid injection in patients with RA and in patients treated with tumor necrosis factor alpha (TNFα) inhibitors. In these patients, CEUS was found to be useful in the short-term follow-up, as it seems to provide an indication of the presence or absence of residual disease activity.

26.3.4 Limitations

Apart from the advantages, some drawbacks must be considered when using CEUS to assess synovitis for therapy monitoring in clinical practice. In fact, CEUS imaging allows the assessment of only one joint per each dose of contrast medium administered intravenously which limits the examination to one or very few target districts. Moreover, the contrast agent administration involves an increase in the running costs, and carries a risk, albeit minimal, of side effects.

Table 26.3 Main studies focusing on the role of CEUS in therapeutic monitoring in inflammatory arthritis listed in t3.1 chronological order

Author	Year	Disease	Therapy	Quantification method	Results
Carotti et al.	2002	RA	Intra-articular injection of glucocorticosteroids	Time-intensity curve parameters	The mean values of the underlying time-intensity curves differed between patients with active and those with inactive synovitis
Salaffi et al.	2005	RA	Intra-articular injection of triamcinolone hexacetonide	Median values of the area underlying time-intensity curves	Synovitis activity was highly associated with changes of the value of the area underlying time-intensity curves. The values are also correlated with CRP and index score of synovitis activity
Klauser et al.	2005	RA	Conventional synthetic drugs	Enhancement and semiquantitative assessment	CEUS improved the differentiation of active versus inactive synovitis
Song et al.	2008	RA and SpA	Intra-articular injection of glucocorticosteroids	The slope values by time-intensity analysis	A significant improvement of clinical and CEUS parameters in patient 1, and elevated parameters in patient 2
Klauser et al.	2010	Tenosynovitis in RA, still disease, SSc, SpA	Not done	Extent of vascularity on semiquantitative assessment	CEUS was significantly more sensitive in the detection of vascularization, compared to power Doppler ultrasound
Ohmdorf et al.	2011	RA	Anti-TNF-alpha agents	Enhancement slope and semiquantitative assessment	CEUS showed the best sensitivity in detecting the changes after the treatment with anti-TNF-alpha among all the imaging techniques applied in the study
Stramare et al.	2013	RA	Anti-TNF-alpha agents	Enhancement and semiquantitative assessment	CEUS might be useful in the short-term follow-up of patients with RA
Mouterde et al.	2014 SpA	Nonsteroidal anti-inflammatory drugs	The slope values by time-intensity analysis	CEUS improved the detection of enthesitis in SpA patients	
Bonifati et al.	2014 PsA	Anti-TNF-alpha agents	The count of swollen (ACR 66), tender (ACR 68), and active inflamed joints	A significant reduction of all clinical variables, including CEUS	
Cozzi et al.	2015	PsA	Mud-bath treatment, anti-TNF-alpha agents	The count of swollen (ACR 66, tender (ACR 68), and active inflamed joints	A significant appearance delay and faster washout were observed in the therapeutic group
Tamas et al.	2015	Early arthritis	Conventional synthetic drugs	Peak, slope, area underlying time-intensity	Peak and area underlying time-intensity curve significantly decreased during the treatment with the remission of the symptoms

CEUS contrast-enhanced ultrasound, PsA psoriatic arthritis, RA rheumatoid arthritis, SpA spondylarthritis, SSc systemic sclerosis

Further Readings

Albrecht K, Grob K, Lange U, Müller-Ladner U, Strunk J. Reliability of different Doppler ultrasound quantification methods and devices in the assessment of therapeutic response in arthritis. Rheumatology (Oxford). 2008;47(10):1521–6.

Ammitzbøll-Danielsen M, Janta I, Torp-Pedersen S, Naredo E, Østergaard M, Terslev L. Three-dimensional Doppler ultrasound findings in healthy wrist and finger tendon sheaths - can feeding vessels lead to misinterpretation in Doppler-detected tenosynovitis? Arthritis Res Ther. 2016;18:70.

Backhaus M, Ohrndorf S, Kellner H, Strunk J, Backhaus TM, Hartung W, Sattler H, Albrecht K, Kaufmann J, Becker K, Sörensen H, Meier L, Burmester GR, Schmidt WA. Evaluation of a novel 7-joint ultrasound score in daily rheumatologic practice: a pilot project. Arthritis Rheum. 2009;61(9):1194–201. https://doi.org/10.1002/art.24646.

Brown AK, Conaghan PG, Karim Z, Quinn MA, Ikeda K, Peterfy CG, et al. An explanation for the apparent dissociation between clinical remission and continued structural deterioration in rheumatoid arthritis. Arthritis Rheum. 2008;58:2958–67.

Brown AK, Quinn MA, Karim Z, Conaghan PG, Peterfy CG, Hensor E, Wakefield RJ, O'Connor PJ, Emery P. Presence of significant synovitis in rheumatoid arthritis patients with disease-modifying antirheumatic drug-induced clinical remission: evidence from an imaging study may explain structural progression. Arthritis Rheum. 2006;54:3761–73.

Bruyn GA, Iagnocco A, Naredo E, Balint PV, Gutierrez M, Hammer HB, Collado P, Filippou G, Schmidt WA, Jousse-Joulin S, Mandl P, Conaghan PG, Wakefield RJ, Keen HI, Terslev L, D'Agostino MA, OMERACT Ultrasound Working Group. OMERACT definitions for Ultrasonographic pathologies and elementary lesions of rheumatic disorders 15 years on. J Rheumatol. 2019;46:1388–93.

Bruyn GAW, Hanova P, Iagnocco A, et al. Ultrasound definition of tendon damage in patients with rheumatoid arthritis. Results of a OMERACT consensus-based ultrasound score focusing on the diagnostic reliability. Ann Rheum Dis. 2014;73:1929–34.

Carotti M, Galeazzi V, Catucci F, Zappia M, Arrigoni F, Barile A, Giovagnoni A. Clinical utility of eco-color-power Doppler ultrasonography and contrast enhanced magnetic resonance imaging for interpretation and quantification of joint synovitis: a review. Acta Biomed. 2018;89(1-S):48–77.

Carotti M, Salaffi F, Manganelli P, Salera D, Simonetti B, Grassi W. Power Doppler sonography in the assessment of synovial tissue of the knee joint in rheumatoid arthritis: a preliminary experience. Ann Rheum Dis. 2002;61:877–82.

Carotti M, Salaffi F, Morbiducci J, Ciapetti A, Bartolucci L, Gasparini S, et al. Colour Doppler ultrasonography evaluation of vascularization in the wrist and finger joints in rheumatoid arthritis patients and healthy subjects. Eur J Radiol. 2012;81:1834–8.

D'Agostino MA, Terslev L, Aegerter P, Backhaus M, Balint P, Bruyn GA, Filippucci E, Grassi W, Iagnocco A, Jousse-Joulin S, Kane D, Naredo E, Schmidt W, Szkudlarek M, Conaghan PG, Wakefield RJ. Scoring ultrasound synovitis in rheumatoid arthritis: a EULAR-OMERACT ultrasound taskforce-part 1: definition and development of a standardised, consensus-based scoring system. RMD Open. 2017;3(1):e000428. https://doi.org/10.1136/rmdopen-2016-000428. eCollection

Filippucci E, Cipolletta E, Mashadi Mirza R, Carotti M, Giovagnoni A, Salaffi F, Tardella M, Di Matteo A, Di Carlo M. Ultrasound imaging in rheumatoid arthritis. Radiol Med. 2019;124:1087–100.

Filippucci E, Di Geso L, Grassi W. Progress in imaging in rheumatology. Nat Rev. Rheumatol. 2014;10:628–34.

Filippucci E, Salaffi F, Carotti M, Grassi W. Doppler ultrasound imaging techniques for assessment of synovial inflammation. Rep Med Imaging. 2013;6:83–91. https://doi.org/10.2147/RMI.S32950.

Fiocco U, Cozzi L, Chieco-Bianchi F, Rigon C, Vezzù M, Favero E, et al. Vascular changes in psoriatic knee joint synovitis. J Rheumatol. 2001;28:2480–6.

Fiocco U, Stramare R, Coran A, Grisan E, Scagliori E, Caso F, Costa L, Lunardi F, Oliviero F, Bianchi FC, Scanu A, Martini V, Boso D, Beltrame V, Vezzù M, Cozzi L, Scarpa R, Sacerdoti D, Punzi L, Doria A, Calabrese F, Rubaltelli L. Vascular perfusion kinetics by contrast-enhanced ultrasound are related to synovial microvascularity in the joints of psoriatic arthritis. Clin Rheumatol. 2015;34:1903–12.

Fiocco U, Stramare R, Martini V, Coran A, Caso F, Costa L, et al. Quantitative imaging by pixel-based contrast-enhanced ultrasound reveals a linear relationship between synovial vascular perfusion and the recruitment of pathogenic IL-17A-F IL-23+ CD161 + CD4+ T helper cells in psoriatic arthritis joints. Clin Rheumatol. 2017;36:391–9.

Foltz V, Gandjbakhch F, Etchepare F, Rosenberg C, Tanguy ML, Rozenberg S, et al. Power Doppler ultrasound, but not low-field magnetic resonance imaging, predicts relapse and radiographic disease progression in rheumatoid arthritis patients with low levels of disease activity. Arthritis Rheum. 2012;64:67–76.

Freeston JE, Wakefield RJ, Conaghan PG, Hensor EM, Stewart SP, Emery P. A diagnostic algorithm for persistence of very early inflammatory arthritis: the utility of power Doppler ultrasound when added to conventional assessment tools. Ann Rheum Dis. 2010;69:417–9.

Hammer HB, Kvien TK. Comparisons of 7- to 78-joint ultrasonography scores: all different joint combinations show equal response to adalimumab treatment in patients with rheumatoid arthritis. Arthritis Res Ther. 2011;13:R78.

Hurnakova J, Filippucci E, Cipolletta E, Di Matteo A, Salaffi F, Carotti M, Draghessi A, Di Donato E, Di Carlo M, Lato V, Horvath R, Komarc M, Pavelka K,

Grassi W. Prevalence and distribution of cartilage damage at the metacarpal head level in rheumatoid arthritis and osteoarthritis: an ultrasound study. Rheumatology (Oxford). 2019;58(7):1206–13. https://doi.org/10.1093/rheumatology/key443.

Kaiser MJ, Hauzeur JP, Blacher S, Foidart JM, Deprez M, Rossknecht A, Malaise MG. Contrast-enhanced coded phase-inversion harmonic sonography of knee synovitis correlates with histological vessel density: 2 automated digital quantifications. J Rheumatol. 2009;36:391–400.

Klauser A, Demharter J, De Marchi A, et al. The IACUS study group. Contrast enhanced gray-scale sonography in assessment of joint vascularity in rheumatoid arthritis: results from the IACUS study group. Euro Radial. 2005;15(12):2404–10.

Klauser A, Halpern EJ, Frauscher F, Gvozdic D, Duftner C, Springer P, Schirmer M. Inflammatory low back pain: high negative predictive value of contrast-enhanced color Doppler ultrasound in the detection of inflamed sacroiliac joints. Arthritis Rheum. 2005;53:440–4.

Löffler C, Sattler H, Uppenkamp M, Bergner R. Contrast-enhanced ultrasound in coxitis. Joint Bone Spine. 2016;83:669–74. https://doi.org/10.1016/j.jbspin.2015.10.012.

Luz KR, Pinheiro MM, Petterle GS, Dos Santos MF, Fernandes AR, Natour J, Furtado RN. A new musculoskeletal ultrasound scoring system (US10) of the hands and wrist joints for evaluation of early rheumatoid arthritis patients. Rev Bras Rheumatol Engl Ed. 2016;56(5):421–31.

Mouterde G, Aegerter P, Correas JM, Breban M, D'Agostino MA. Value of contrast-enhanced ultrasonography for the detection and quantification of enthesitis vascularization in patients with spondyloarthritis. Arthritis Care Res (Hoboken). 2014;66:131–8.

Mouterde G, Carotti M, D'Agostino MA. Contrast-enhanced ultrasound in musculoskeletal diseases. J Radiol. 2009;90(1 Pt 2):148–55.

Naredo E, D'Agostino MA, Wakefield RJ, Möller I, Balint PV, Filippucci E, Iagnocco A, Karim Z, Terslev L, Bong DA, Garrido J, Martínez-Hernández D, Bruyn GA, OMERACT Ultrasound Task Force*. Reliability of a consensus-based ultrasound score for tenosynovitis in rheumatoid arthritis. Ann Rheum Dis. 2013;72(8):1328–34. https://doi.org/10.1136/annrheumdis-2012-202092. Epub 2012 Sep 14

Naredo E, Gamero F, Bonilla G, et al. Ultrasonographic assessment of inflammatory activity in rheumatoid arthritis: comparison of extended versus reduced joint evaluation. Clin Exp Rheumatol. 2005;23:881–4.

Naredo E, Monteagudo I. Applications of Doppler techniques in rheumatology. Clin Exp Rheumatol. 2014;32(Suppl. 80):S12–9.

Ohrndorf S, Hensch A, Naumann L, Hermann KG, Scheurig-Münkler C, Meier S, Burmester GR, Backhaus M. Contrast-enhanced ultrasonography is more sensitive than grayscale and power Doppler ultrasonography compared to MRI in therapy monitoring of rheumatoid arthritis patients. Ultraschall Med. 2011;32(Suppl 2):E38–44.

Piscaglia F, Nolsøe C, Dietrich CF, Cosgrove DO, Gilja OH, Bachmann Nielsen M, Albrecht T, Barozzi L, Bertolotto M, Catalano O, Claudon M, Clevert DA, Correas JM, D'Onofrio M, Drudi FM, Eyding J, Giovannini M, Hocke M, Ignee A, Jung EM, Klauser AS, Lassau N, Leen E, Mathis G, Saftoiu A, Seidel G, Sidhu PS, ter Haar G, Timmerman D, Weskott HP. The EFSUMB guidelines and recommendations on the clinical practice of contrast enhanced ultrasound (CEUS): update 2011 on non-hepatic applications. Ultraschall Med. 2012;33(1):33–59.

Reece RJ, Canete JD, Parsons WJ, Emery P, Veale DJ. Distinct vascular patterns of early synovitis in psoriatic, reactive, and rheumatoid arthritis. Arthritis Rheum. 1999;42:1481–4.

Ribbens C, Andre B, Marcelis S, et al. Rheumatoid hand joint synovitis: gray-scale and power Doppler US quantifications following anti-tumor necrosis factor-a treatment: pilot study. Radiology. 2003;229:562–9.

Salaffi F, Carotti M, Manganelli P, Filippucci E, Giuseppetti GM, Grassi W. Contrast-enhanced power Doppler sonography of knee synovitis in rheumatoid arthritis: assessment of therapeutic response. Clin Rheumatol. 2004;23:285–90.

Salaffi F, Ciapetti A, Gasparini S, Carotti M, Filippucci E, Grassi W. A clinical prediction rule combining routine assessment and power Doppler ultrasonography for predicting progression to rheumatoid arthritis from early-onset undifferentiated arthritis. Clin Exp Rheumatol. 2010;28(5):686–94.

Sarzi-Puttini P, Filippucci E, Adami S, et al. Clinical, ultrasound, and predictability outcomes following Certolizumab Pegol treatment (with methotrexate) in patients with moderate-to-severe rheumatoid arthritis: 52-week results from the CZP-SPEED study. Adv Ther. 2018;35:1153–68.

Scheel AK, Hermann KG, Kahler E, et al. A novel ultrasonographic synovitis scoring system suitable for analyzing finger joint inflammation in rheumatoid arthritis. Arthritis Rheum. 2005;52:733–43.

Simpson E, Hock E, Stevenson M, Wong R, Dracup N, Wailoo A, Conaghan P, Estrach C, Edwards C, Wakefield R. What is the added value of ultrasound joint examination for monitoring synovitis in rheumatoid arthritis and can it be used to guide treatment decisions? A systematic review and cost-effectiveness analysis. Health Technol Assess. 2018;22:1–258.

Stramare R, Coran A, Faccinetto A, Costantini G, Bernardi L, Botsios C, Perissinotto E, Grisan E, Beltrame V, Raffeiner B. MR and CEUS monitoring of patients with severe rheumatoid arthritis treated with biological agents: a preliminary study. Radiol Med. 2014;119:422–31.

Sun X, Deng X, Geng Y, Ji L, Xie W, Zhang X, Zhang Z. A simplified and validated ultrasound scoring system to evaluate synovitis of bilateral wrists and hands in patients with rheumatoid arthritis. Clin Rheumatol. 2018;37(1):185–91.

Szkudlarek M, Court-Payen M, Jacobsen S, et al. Interobserver agreement in ultrasonography of the finger and toe joints in rheumatoid arthritis. Arthritis Rheum. 2003;48:955–62.

Taylor PC, Steuer A, Gruber J, Cosgrove DO, Blomley MJ, Marsters PA, et al. Comparison of ultrasonographic assessment of synovitis and joint vascularity with radiographic evaluation in a randomized, placebo-controlled study of infliximab therapy in early rheumatoid arthritis. Arthritis Rheum. 2004;50:1107–16.

Terslev L, Naredo E, Aegerter P, Wakefield RJ, Backhaus M, Balint P, Bruyn GAW, Iagnocco A, Jousse-Joulin S, Schmidt WA, Szkudlarek M, Conaghan PG, Filippucci E, D'Agostino MA. Scoring ultrasound synovitis in rheumatoid arthritis: a EULAR-OMERACT ultrasound taskforce-part 2: reliability and application to multiple joints of a standardised consensus-based scoring system. RMD Open. 2017;3(1):e000427. https://doi.org/10.1136/rmdopen-2016-000427. eCollection 2017

Torp-Pedersen S, et al. Power and color Doppler ultrasound settings for inflammatory flow. Impact on scoring of disease activity in patients with rheumatoid arthritis. Arthritis Rheumatol. 2015;67(2):386–95.

Torp-Pedersen ST, Terslev L. Settings and artefacts relevant in colour/power Doppler ultrasound in rheumatology. Ann Rheum Dis. 2008;67(2):143–9.

Wakefield RJ, Gibbon WW, Conaghan PG, et al. The value of sonography in the detection of bone erosions in patients with rheumatoid arthritis: a comparison with conventional radiography. Arthritis Rheum. 2000;43:2762–70.

Zhao CY, Jiang YX, Li JC, Xu ZH, Zhang Q, Su N, Yang M. Role of contrast-enhanced ultrasound in the evaluation of inflammatory arthritis. Chin Med J. 2017;130:1722–30.

Part V

Generalities in Ultrasound-guided Procedures

Introduction

27

Carlo Faletti, Davide Orlandi, and Enzo Silvestri

Contents

27.1 Introduction

One of the most important issues of medicine is, having established the location and the possible cause of a pathology, to identify its treatment with less discomfort for the patient.

Certainly, in the modern progression of therapeutic possibilities, taking advantage of what technology is able to provide, the need and willingness are to treat the greatest number of pathologies through the less invasive technical approach. In this setting, among the musculoskeletal and orthopedic panorama, we mention interventional procedures such as injections, arthrocentesis, and biopsies.

All of these procedures cannot be performed safely and effectively without the precise identification of the affected area and constant control of the procedural path. Nowadays, diagnostic imaging and especially ultrasound have proven to be excellent tools for a precise guidance of needles within soft tissues and joints, for use in a wide range of procedures. Moreover ultrasound is also able to perform dynamic evaluations of soft tissues related to the musculoskeletal system, and without patient exposure to ionizing radiation, allowing the clinician's technological and professional skills to play a fundamental role both in diagnostic and therapeutic terms.

This chapter describes, in a complete and timely manner, the various ultrasound-guided interventional procedures with prevalent reference to the musculoskeletal system and peripheral nerves.

C. Faletti
Direttore tecnico Radiodiagnostica Centro Diagnostico Cernaia, Asti Direttore scientifico Master MSK di II livello, Università degli studi di Torino, Turin, Italy

D. Orlandi (✉)
Department of Radiology, Ospedale Evangelico Internazionale, Genova, Italy

E. Silvestri
Radiology, Alliance Medical, Genova, Italy

F. Martino et al. (eds.), *Musculoskeletal Ultrasound in Orthopedic and Rheumatic disease in Adults*,
https://doi.org/10.1007/978-3-030-91202-4_27

Further Readings

Obradov M, Gielen L. Image-guided Intra- and Extra-articular musculoskeletal interventions. Switzerland AG: Springer Nature; 2018.

Sconfienza LM, Adriaensen M, Albano D, et al. Clinical indications for image-guided interventional procedures in the musculoskeletal system: a Delphi-based consensus paper from the European Society of Musculoskeletal Radiology (ESSR)-part I, shoulder. Eur Radiol. 2020;30(2):903–13.

Sconfienza LM, Adriaensen M, Albano D, et al. Clinical indications for image guided interventional procedures in the musculoskeletal system: a Delphi-based consensus paper from the European Society of Musculoskeletal Radiology (ESSR)-part III, nerves of the upper limb. Eur Radiol. 2020;30(3):1498–506.

Sconfienza LM, Adriaensen M, Albano D, et al. Clinical indications for image-guided interventional procedures in the musculoskeletal system: a Delphi-based consensus paper from the European Society of Musculoskeletal Radiology (ESSR)-Part II, elbow and wrist. Eur Radiol. 2020 Apr;30(4):2220–30.

Sconfienza LM, Serafini G, Silvestri E. Ultrasound-guided musculoskeletal procedures. The upper limb. Springer Verlag: Milan; 2012.

Silvestri E, Martino F, Puntillo F. Ultrasound-Guided Peripheral Nerve Blocks. Switzerland AG: Springer Nature; 2018.

Enzo S, Sconfienza LM, Orlandi D. Ultrasound-guided musculoskeletal procedures. The lower limb. Milan: Springer Verlag; 2015.

Joint and Bursal Infiltration 28

Marina Carotti, Emilio Filippucci, Fausto Salaffi,
Fabio Martino, Enzo Silvestri,
and Davide Orlandi

Contents

M. Carotti
Clinica di Radiologia,
Dipartimento di Scienze Radiologiche – Azienda Ospedali Riuniti di Ancona
Università Politecnica delle Marche,
Ancona, Italy

E. Filippucci · F. Salaffi
Clinica Reumatologica,
Dipartimento di Scienze Cliniche e Molecolari,
Università Politecnica delle Marche, Jesi (Ancona), Italy

F. Martino (✉)
Radiology, Sant'Agata Diagnostic Center,
Bari, Italy

E. Silvestri
Radiology, Alliance Medical, Genova, Italy

D. Orlandi
Department of Radiology, Ospedale Evangelico Internazionale, Genova, Italy

28.1 Generalities in Ultrasound-Guided Procedures in Rheumatology

Synovial fluid aspiration and intra- and periarticular injection treatment are part of the standard diagnostic and therapeutic armamentarium in rheumatological clinical practice.

The obtainment of synovial fluid sample allows its analysis which provides several diagnostic information including the definition of its inflammatory nature, the detection of crystals, and the identification of bacteria. Moreover, in case of acutely and significantly swollen joint due to a variable, but usually important, amount of synovial fluid, its aspiration can highly contribute to joint pain relief.

Steroid or hyaluronic acid injection represents an alternative or adjunctive therapeutic option to the systemic treatment in many rheumatic disorders (Table 28.1).

In Finland the intra-articular steroid injection is a recognized important part of the treatment

F. Martino et al. (eds.), *Musculoskeletal Ultrasound in Orthopedic and Rheumatic disease in Adults*,
https://doi.org/10.1007/978-3-030-91202-4_28

Table 28.1 The most commonly injected anatomic structures in rheumatological daily practice

Anatomic site	Anatomic target	Rheumatic disorder
Shoulder	Glenohumeral joint	Chronic inflammatory arthritis
	Acromion-clavicular joint	Polymyalgia rheumatica
	Subdeltoid bursa	CPPD
	Long head of the biceps tendon synovial sheath	Regional pain syndrome
Elbow	Elbow joint	Chronic inflammatory arthritis
	Olecranon bursa	Gout
	Cubital bursa	Lateral and medial epicondylitis
Wrist	Radio-carpal joint	Chronic inflammatory arthritis
	Inter-carpal joint	Carpal tunnel syndrome
	Distal radioulnar joint	CPPD
	Trapeziometacarpal joint	Thumb carpometacarpal joint OA
	Compartments of the extensor tendons on the dorsal aspects of the radius	
	Common finger flexor tendon synovial sheath	
	Flexor carpi radialis tendon synovial sheath	
Hand	Metacarpophalangeal joint	Chronic inflammatory arthritis
	Proximal interphalangeal joint	
	Distal interphalangeal joint	
	Digital synovial sheath of the finger flexor tendons	
Hip	Hip joint	Chronic inflammatory arthritis
	Iliopsoas bursa	Hip OA
	Trochanteric bursa	Polymyalgia rheumatica
Knee	Knee joint	Chronic inflammatory arthritis
	Prepatellar bursa	Knee OA
	Infrapatellar deep bursa	CPPD
		Gout
Ankle	Tibiotalar joint	Chronic inflammatory arthritis
	Subtalar joint	
	Tibialis posterior tendon synovial sheath	
	Peroneal tendon synovial sheath	
Foot	Metatarsophalangeal joint	Chronic inflammatory arthritis
	Plantar fascia	Gout

OA osteoarthritis, *CPPD* calcium pyrophosphate dihydrate crystal deposition disease

scheme in rheumatoid arthritis (RA) patients, and traditionally rheumatologists inject all swollen joints in patients with early RA unless in the presence of contraindications. Moreover, the results of a recent study indicate that neglecting intra-articular glucocorticoid injections is associated with lower remission rates, higher disease activity, and lower quality of life in RA patients with early stages of the disease. On the other end injecting small joints of the hands and wrists with persistent synovitis was found effective for up to 12 weeks after the US-guided steroid injection in RA patients who did not change their treatment during the observation period. Furthermore, in patients with early RA, US resulted to be useful in the identification of the joints which would obtain the maximal clinical benefit from a steroid injection, with moderate Doppler activity being the best predictor of treatment success in both swollen and not-swollen joints.

According to the latest Osteoarthritis Research Society International (OARSI) guidelines for the nonsurgical management of knee, hip, and polyarticular osteoarthritis, both intra-articular steroid and hyaluronic acid injections are recommended for patients with knee osteoarthritis (OA).

These procedures are normally carried out using anatomical landmarks with a variable successful rate mainly depending on both the degree of anatomical complexity and the size of the target area.

In particular the traditional non-imaging-guided approach may result to be inadequate when the target area is far from the skin and/or small in size or when a dry joint has to be injected.

In fact, both efficacy and side effects of an injection largely depend on the correct placement of the tip of the needle at the target area avoiding direct contact with nerves, tendons, articular cartilage, and blood vessels.

There is evidence revealing that conventional joint injections are often inaccurate. In fact, based on the experience of Jones et al. (1993), injections performed in different anatomic sites using a mixture of steroid and radiographic contrast medium were judged accurately by conventional radiography in only 56 (52%) out of 108 rheumatic patients. The percentage of successful placement reduces to 37% at shoulder level due to the inherent anatomical complexity.

It is now well established that steroid injections guided by US were significantly more accurate than those guided by clinical examination in patients with inflammatory arthritis. Difference in the number of joints accurately injected is particularly higher at shoulder, hip, elbow, and ankle level, suggesting that US may be especially helpful in guiding injections in joints with complex anatomy.

While there is still very little evidence supporting the superior clinical benefit of US-guided versus palpation-guided steroid injection, especially to treat tenosynovitis, accurate placement of the tip of the needle is obviously fundamental for the efficacy of the hyaluronic acid joint injection.

Although the use of ultrasound (US) to guide synovial fluid aspiration and injections reduces the number of incorrect placements of the tip of the needle, this imaging technique is still not systematically integrated into rheumatological practice. According to a survey of experts and scientific societies conducted in 2012, in most of the European countries less than 10% of the rheumatologists routinely use US to guide arthrocentesis and joint injection in their clinical practice.

US-guided injections can be carried out using two main methods.

In the first method the sonographer uses US imaging to obtain the relevant information to place the tip of the needle at the target area: detection of the target area, identification of the entrance point at skin level, and measurement of the distance between them.

In the second method the needle progression from the skin surface to the target area is directly visualized under real-time US scanning. In particular, this method includes the following steps:

1. Preliminary US examination aimed at detecting the target area and confirming the clinical indication to perform the injection therapy.
2. Identification of the US scanning plan to visualize the needle progression from the skin to the target area.
3. Disinfection of the skin area defined as point of entrance of the needle and covering of the probe using a glove or a condom.
4. Placement of a thin amount of sterile gel on the skin surface where to put the probe.
5. Real-time visualization of the needle progression through the soft tissues until the tip of the needle reaches the target area.
6. Visual confirmation of the synovial fluid aspiration if present and of the drug spreading into the target area during the injection (Fig. 28.1).

As well as for conventional approach, US-guided procedures should be performed after obtaining a patient informed consent and both patient and operator should gain a comfortable position during all the procedure.

The best US visualization of the needle requires a perpendicular insonation angle. Once the patient position and the needle progression pathway are defined, such an angle value is obtained with manual (i.e., moving the probe) and/or electronic (i.e., beam steering, virtual convex) changing of the US beam direction. Under perpendicular insonation the needle appears as a

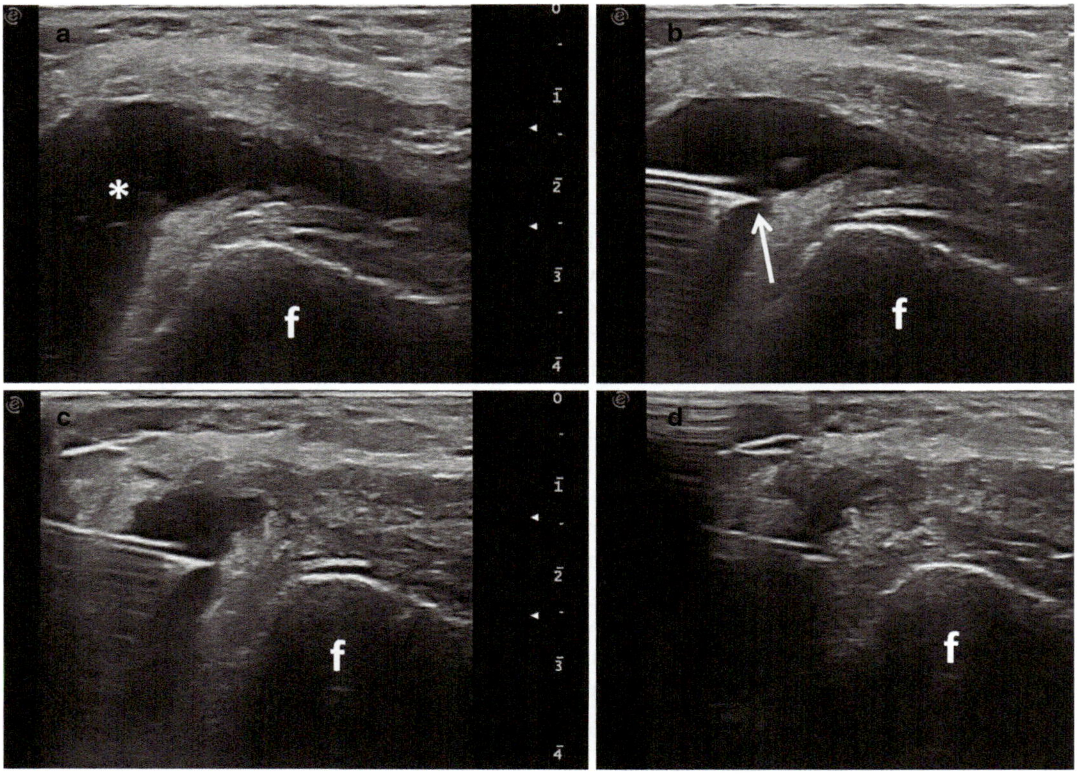

Fig. 28.1 Rheumatoid arthritis. Knee exudative synovitis. Anterior transverse suprapatellar view. (**a**) Identification of the target area. (**b**) Placement of the tip of the needle (*arrow*) at the target area. (**c**) Aspiration of the synovial fluid. (**d**) Injection of the steroid, appearing as an echoic material spreading into the suprapatellar pouch. * synovial fluid, *f* femur

sharply defined hyperechoic band with strong posterior reverberations on longitudinal view and as a small hyperechoic round spot on transverse view.

The longitudinal view allows the in-plane needle US imaging. This technique allows the real-time visualization of the needle tip and shaft while proceeding from the superficial level at one of the two upper corners of the screen to the target area in the deeper central part of the US field (Figs. 28.2 and 28.3). The in-plane US imaging is the one used in the great majority of the cases in rheumatology.

The out-of-plane needle US visualization uses the transverse view. Such an approach requires advanced scanning skills to ascertain the position of the tip of the needle during the procedure and shortens the needle pathway to reach the target area which results to be particularly helpful to reach deep targets.

Confirmation of the needle's correct placement can be obtained visualizing the spreading of steroid (appearing echoic), hyaluronic acid (appearing anechoic or hypoechoic), or air (appearing hyperechoic) within the target area or under color or power Doppler control (while injected the compound is visualized as a colored spot).

Peri-tendinous intrasynovial injection therapy with steroid has a well-established role in patients with chronic arthritis and tenosynovitis. A successful technique requires a correct positioning of the tip of the needle inside the tendon sheath avoiding the contact between the needle and the tendon.

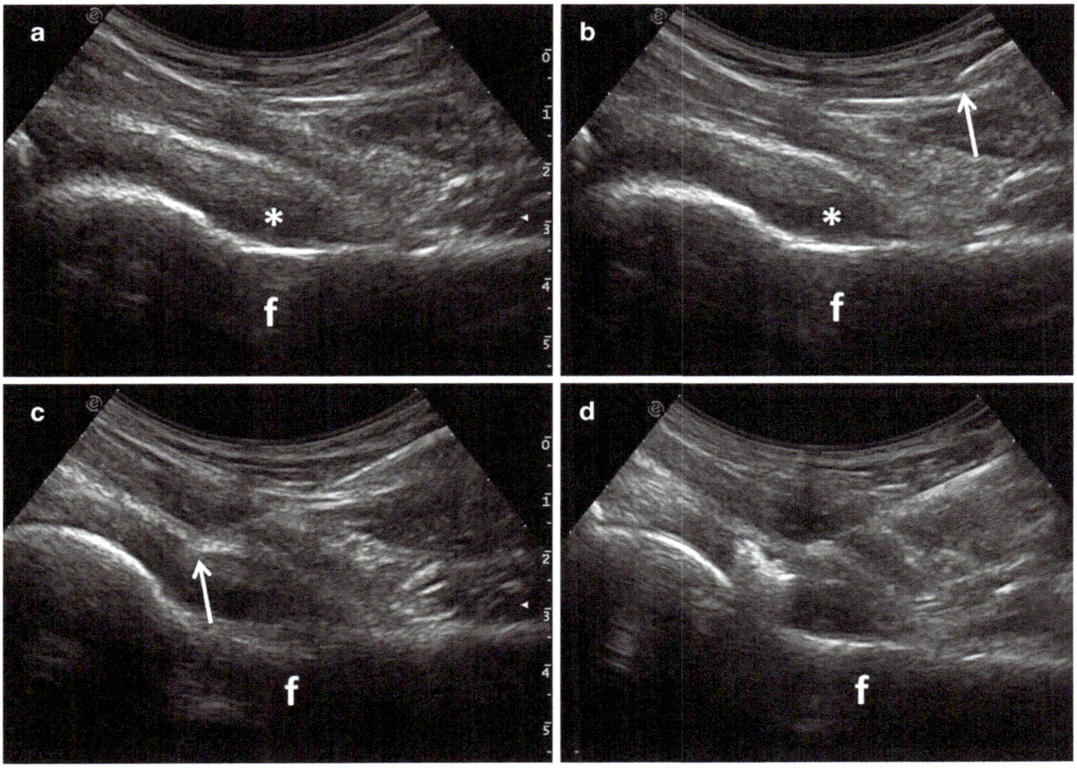

Fig. 28.2 Psoriatic arthritis. Hip exudative synovitis. Anterior longitudinal view. (**a**) Identification of the target area. (**b**) The tip of the needle appears at the upper right corner of the screen and is directed to the target area in the deeper central part of the ultrasound field. (**c**) The tip of the needle (*arrow*) is passing through the hip joint cavity. (**d**) Injection of sterile air, appearing as a hyperechoic material spreading inside the joint cavity, just before the steroid. * synovial fluid, *f* femur

The steroid injection within a widened synovial tendon sheath under US control appears to be very effective in minimizing the risk of damaging the tendon. The progression of the needle can be steadily monitored until the tip of the needle is properly placed within the tendon sheath and the steroid accurately injected into the peritendinous synovial space (Fig. 28.4).

Bursitis is a very common condition in rheumatological practice. Steroid injection is an effective and safe treatment in patient nonresponders to other conservative therapeutic options, including rest, local application of ice, and anti-inflammatory medication. In patients with clinical suspicion of bursitis, US approach allows confirmation of the diagnosis and needle guidance to aspirate synovial fluid and inject steroid.

US is very useful for the detection of popliteal cysts and for detailed visualization of their content.

Inner structure of the cyst is important to guide needle aspiration of the synovial fluid. Moreover, US control is critical to avoid puncture wounds of nerves and/or blood vessels and to ensure the correct position of the tip of the needle especially in patients with loculated cysts (Fig. 28.5).

In conclusion, the US guidance should be considered under the following main conditions:

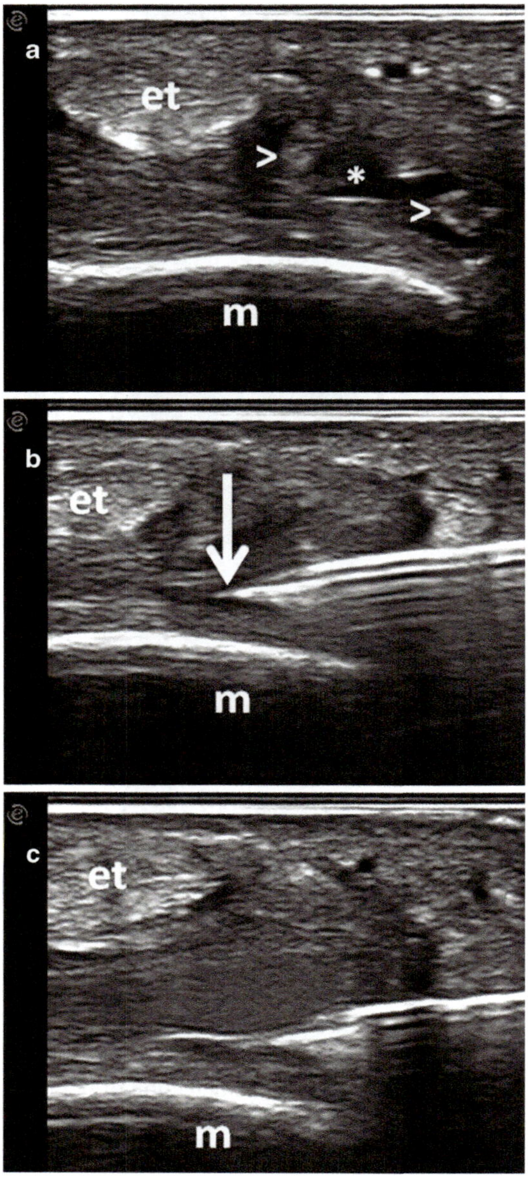

Fig. 28.3 Rheumatoid arthritis. Third metacarpophalangeal joint. Proliferative synovitis. Dorsal transverse view. (**a**) Identification of the target area: the joint cavity. (**b**) Placement of the tip of the needle (*arrow*) at the target area. (**c**) Injection of the steroid, appearing as an echoic material spreading into the joint cavity. * synovial fluid, *arrowhead* synovial hypertrophy, *et* finger extensor tendon, *m* metacarpal head

- To inject sites with a complex anatomy that are at risk to be injected inaccurately using the conventional approach (i.e., shoulder and ankle).
- If the anatomy is distorted by pathology or the anatomic landmarks are less accessible due to obesity or pathology.
- When hyaluronic acid is injected to provide visual feedback of its intra-articular spreading.
- In patients with previous failure of palpation-guided injection.

28.2 Viscosupplementation: Technique and Indications

Conservative treatment of OA includes weight loss, physical therapy, oral anti-inflammatory and analgesic medications, and intra-articular injections of steroids. Viscosupplementation, consisting of intra-articular injection of hyaluronic acid (HA) derivatives, is the main local treatment of mild or moderate OA.

The administration of hyaluronic acid with ultrasound-guided intra-articular injection has been demonstrated to be effective in moderate and severe osteoarthritis treatment. The aim of such a procedure is to reduce patients' disability and pain restoring the physiological properties of synovial fluid and improving articular function and recovery of working and social activity.

The intra-articular administration of hyaluronic acid has a role not only to restore the viscoelastic properties of synovial fluid (pure mechanical effect), but also to stimulate the endogenous production of hyaluronic acid by articular chondrocytes and synoviocytes by products based on hyaluronic acid.

Hyaluronic acid is a polysaccharide of the group of glycosaminoglycans, which is a polymer with very high molecular weight (million Dalton), formed by repeating units of N-acetylglucosamine and glucuronic acid linked together by glycosidic bonds.

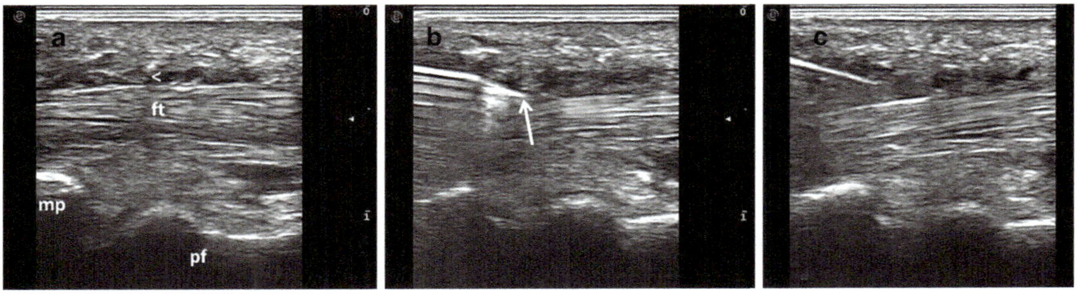

Fig. 28.4 Psoriatic arthritis. Third finger dactylitis. Volar longitudinal view showing finger flexor tendon tenosynovitis. (**a**) Identification of the target area: the synovial tendon sheath. (**b**) Placement of the tip of the needle (*arrow*) at the target area. (**c**) Injection of the steroid, appearing as an echoic material spreading into the synovial tendon sheath. *Arrowhead* synovial hypertrophy, *ft.* finger flexor tendons, *mp* middle phalanx, *pp.* proximal phalanx

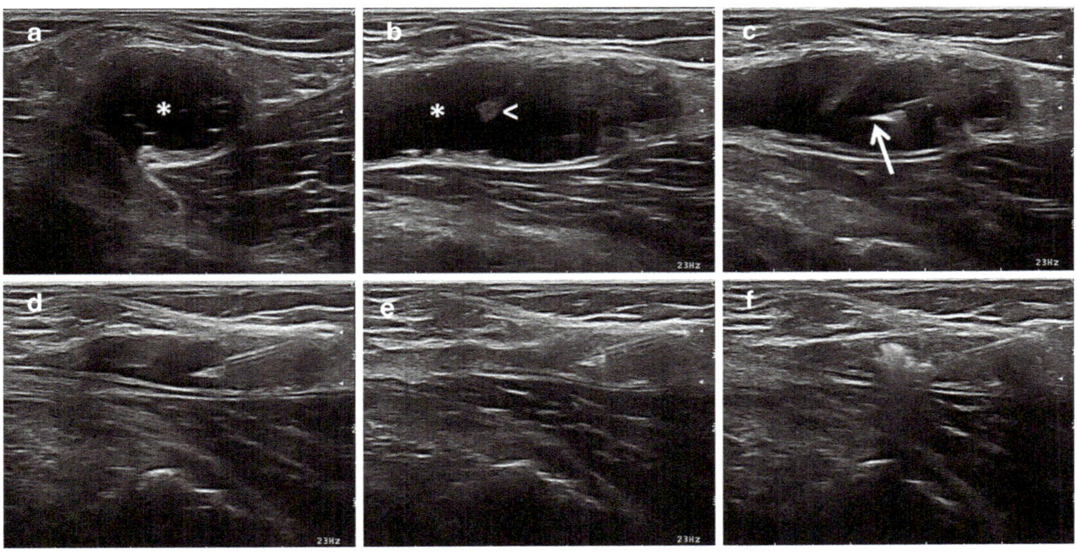

Fig. 28.5 Knee osteoarthritis. Popliteal cyst depicted on transverse (**a**) and longitudinal (**b**) views showing synovial fluid (*) and small areas of synovial hypertrophy (*arrowhead*). Aspiration of synovial fluid (**c–e**) and steroid injection (**f**) were guided using the longitudinal view. (**c**) Placement of the tip of the needle (*arrow*) at the target area. (**d, e**) Aspiration of the synovial fluid. (**f**) Injection of the steroid

It is present in the superficial layer of the hyaline cartilage, the intracellular matrix of the joint capsule, the synovial tissue and the synovial fluid. It is highly absorbent with viscoelastic properties: viscosity (lubrication) in case of static compressive strength and elastic (shock-absorbing) in case of dynamic shear and compressive forces.

You can divide HA in terms of molecular weight:

- Low molecular weight (from 500 to 1000 kDA).
- Average molecular weight (from 1000 to 4000 kDA).
- High molecular weight (>di 4000 kDA).

Molecular weight is related with different effects; low-molecular-weight HA has a greater penetration in the tissues, allowing a greater concentration of the product around the cell surface and producing an increased pharmacological response of chondrocytes, being able to slow down Fas gene-induced apoptosis.

The stabilization of aggregates at high density and high molecular weight (>2000 kDa) results in reduced motility of single molecules of HA and thus they will not be able to be rapidly degraded by the synovial cells that are able to swallow only free molecules of HA. The preparation thus prolonged half-life within the joint (approximately 4 weeks), allowing you to get a single-injection result in long-term treatment of OA.

Ultrasound is an ideal technique for guiding the needle during the joint infiltration procedure and avoiding the extra-articular injection of hyaluronic acid in particular for deep and challenging locations such as the hip.

Intra-articular injection at the level of the hip is generally more complex when compared to other joints (e.g., shoulder, knee) for its deep location and the relative contiguity of the femoral neurovascular bundle.

We hereby describe the standardized ultrasound-guided hip injection technique.

Lateral (in-plane) approach allows a direct and continuous visualization of the needle along the whole path in soft tissues, while out-plane approach may be preferred for being shorter and less painful, but needle visibility is remarkably decreased.

The patient lies in supine position. Slight internal rotation of the leg (about 15°–20°) may help to decrease joint capsule tension and improve tolerability of the procedure. The neurovascular bundle can be visualized with an axial scan at the level of the groin to detect possible vascular or neural anatomic variations and avoid accidental punctures. Then, the probe is rotated about 135° and shifted laterally in order to reach an anterior sagittal-oblique scanning plane over the hip joint. A correct scanning plane should visualize the femoral neck, the femoral head covered by hyaline cartilage, the acetabular labrum, the osseous component of the acetabulum, the joint capsule, and, superficially, the iliopsoas muscle belly. The articular cortex of the femoral head appears as a curve echogenic line and the cortical surface of the anterior acetabular rim as a triangular echogenic structure just distal to this line. The fibrocartilaginous anterior acetabular labrum may be seen as a well-defined, triangular, and uniformly echogenic structure. Of note, in patients with advanced OA, anatomy of this joint can be relatively different, and joint components may not be identified easily.

Using a caudo-cranial approach with the articular joint space centered in the middle of the screen, a 20 G spinal needle is inserted laterally to the distal side of the probe with a caudal-cranial direction. According to the patient's habitus, the depth of the joint may vary, and thus the angle of needle insertion has to be adjusted; generally, the angle of needle insertion ranges from 30° to 60°. This procedure can also be performed with the cranial-caudal approach. Power Doppler module can also be switched on to monitor the flow of the drug within the capsule during injection.

Less experienced operators may take advantage of a metallic needle guide that can be attached to the ultrasound probe. With this approach, the whole path of the needle can be visualized in real time, and slight corrections of the direction can be made. The needle tip can be inserted in within the whole joint capsule. However, inserting the needle exactly in the joint space may result in a very painful injection procedure. The best area to put the needle tip is at the femoral head-neck junction. Once the joint space is reached, the syringe is connected to the needle, and the drug is injected (Fig. 28.6). Of note, in case of high resistance to injection, the needle should be minimally retracted.

In case of arthrosynovitis and/or if iliopsoas bursitis is present, an ultrasound-guided aspiration could be performed during the same procedure just before the intra-articular drug injection (Fig. 28.7).

Using the coaxial approach (Fig. 28.8) the articular joint space is centered on the screen, and a 20 G spinal needle is inserted at the center of the longer side of the probe, with a very slight lateral-to-medial angulation (about 5°) to reach the joint space visualized in the scanning plane. Along its path, the needle tip is visualized indirectly, by means of slight movements

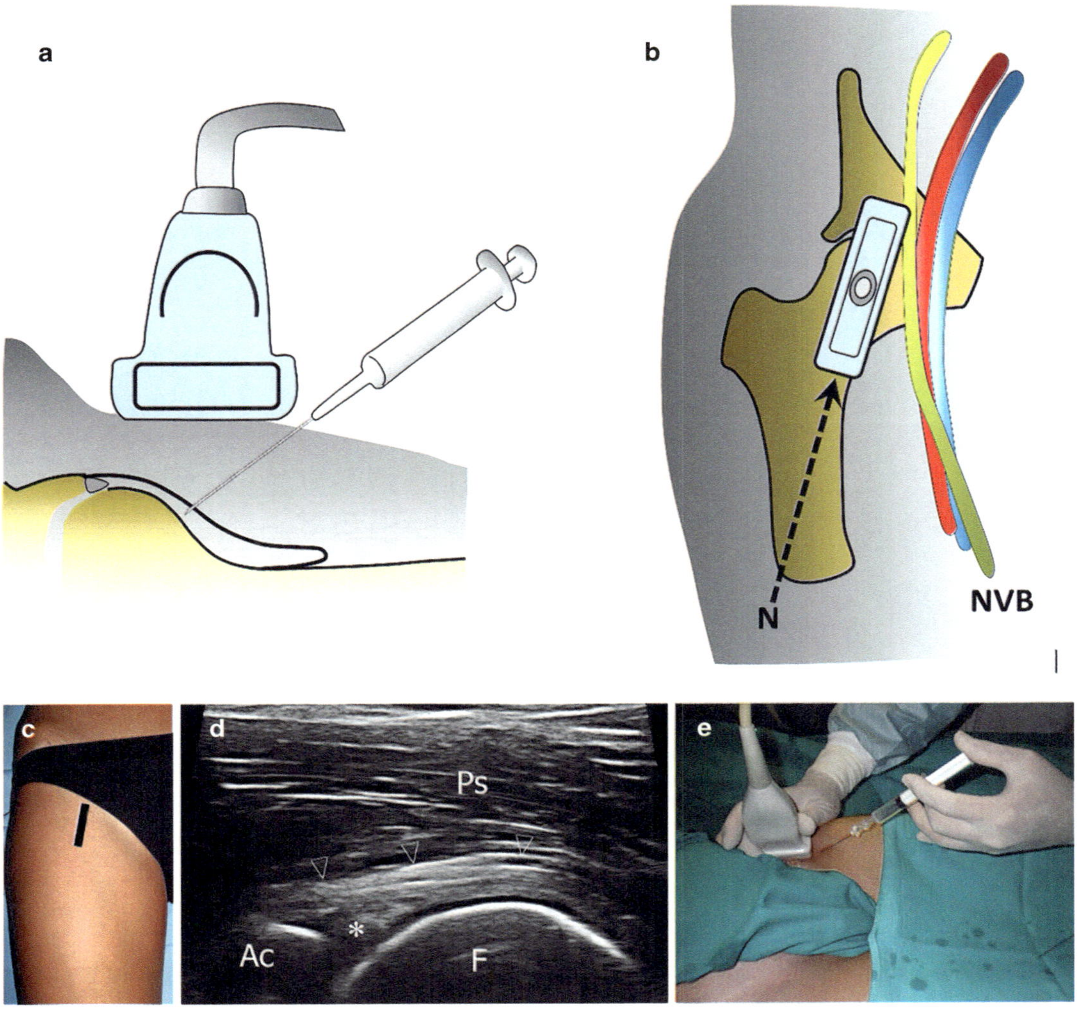

Fig. 28.6 Didactic scheme, probe, and patient position to perform long-axis US-guided intra-articular hip injection (**a**, **b**) with US long-axis view (**d**) and position of the US probe (**c**) and needle (**e**) during acid hyaluronic injection (*PS* iliopsoas muscle, *Ac* acetabulum, *F* femur, *asterisk* labrum, *arrowheads* joint capsule)

of superficial soft tissues; when the joint space is reached, the needle tip should be visible as a hyperechoic dot under the articular capsule. Of note, this procedure is less painful for patients but requires longer experience in US-guided procedures.

After the US-guided hyaluronic acid injection the needle can be removed and a plaster should be applied. Then, patients are usually kept under observation for about 15 min. Pain may occur after treatment and can be managed with a short course of oral NSAIDs.

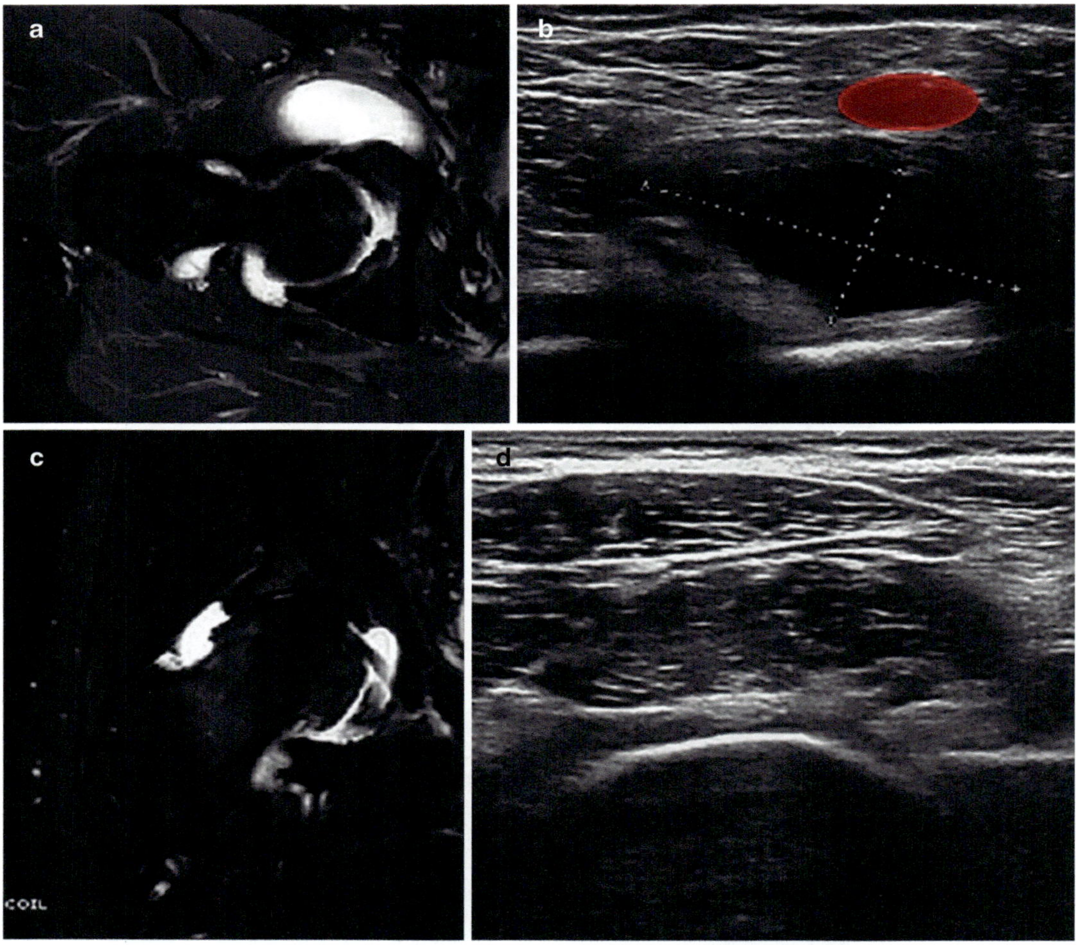

Fig. 28.7 Arthrosynovitis in femur-acetabular conflict with fluid distention of all capsular recesses and the iliopsoas bursa (**a**, **b**). Resolution of exudative distention of the iliopsoas bursitis following arthrocentesis and cycle of US-guided infiltration with PRP and hyaluronic acid (**c**, **d**). Bursa fluid collection evacuation should always be associated with joint US-guided treatment. US-guided bursa evacuation must be obtained with attention in avoiding femoral artery (*red oval*) which runs superficially and anteriorly to the bursa

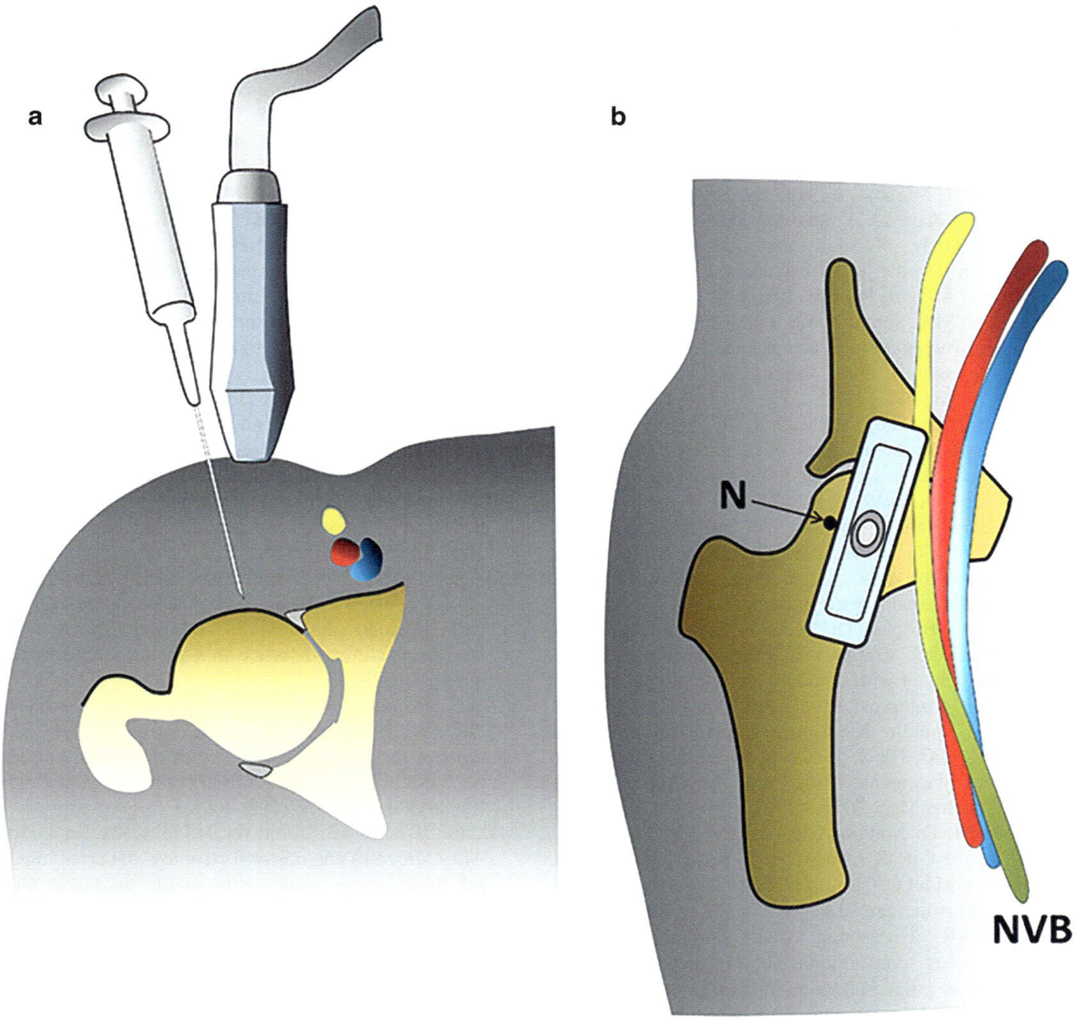

Fig. 28.8 (**a**, **b**). Didactic scheme of ultrasound-guided hip injection performed with coaxial approach. *N* needle, *NVB* neurovascular bundle

Further Readings

Aly AR, Rajasekaran S, Ashworth N. Ultrasound-guided shoulder girdle injections are more accurate and more effective than landmark-guided injections: a systematic review and meta-analysis. Br J Sports Med. 2015;49:1042–9.

Ammitzbøll-Danielsen M, Østergaard M, Fana V, Glinatsi D, Døhn UM, Ørnbjerg LM, et al. Intramuscular versus ultrasound-guided intratenosynovial glucocorticoid injection for tenosynovitis in patients with rheumatoid arthritis: a randomised, double-blind, controlled study. Ann Rheum Dis. 2017;76:666–72.

Bannuru RR, Osani MC, Vaysbrot EE, Arden NK, Bennell K, Bierma-Zeinstra SMA, Kraus VB, Lohmander LS, Abbott JH, Bhandari M, Blanco FJ, Espinosa R, Haugen IK, Lin J, Mandl LA, Moilanen E, Nakamura N, Snyder-Mackler L, Trojian T, Underwood M, McAlindon TE. OARSI guidelines for the non-surgical management of knee, hip, and polyarticular osteoarthritis. Osteoarthr Cartil. 2019;27:1578–89.

Chevalier X. Acide hyaluronique dans la gonarthrose : mécanismes d'action. In: Chevalier X, editor. Injection d'acide hyaluronique et arthrose. Paris: Masson; 2005. p. 9–39.

Cipolletta E, Filippucci E, Incorvaia A, Schettino M, Smerilli G, Di Battista J, Tesei G, Cosatti MA, Di

Donato E, Tardella M, Di Matteo A, Di Carlo M, Grassi W. Ultrasound-guided procedures in rheumatology daily practice: feasibility, accuracy and safety issues. J Clin Rheumatol. 27(6):226–31.

Conrozier T. Is the addition of a polyol to hyaluronic acid a significant advance in the treatment of osteoarthritis? Curr Rheumatol Rev. 2018;14(3):226–30.

Cunnington J, Marshall N, Hide G, Bracewell C, Isaacs J, Platt P, Kane D. A randomized, double-blind, controlled study of ultrasound-guided corticosteroid injection into the joint of patients with inflammatory arthritis. Arthritis Rheum. 2010;62(7):1862–9.

D'Agostino MA, Schmidt WA. Ultrasound-guided injections in rheumatology: actual knowledge on efficacy and procedures. Best Pract Res Clin Rheumatol. 2013;27:283–94.

De Luigi AJ, Saini V, Mathur R, Saini A, Yokel N. Assessing the accuracy of ultrasound-guided needle placement in sacroiliac joint injections. Am J Phys Med Rehabil. 2019;98:666–70.

Di Geso L, Filippucci E, Meenagh G, Gutierrez M, Ciapetti A, Salaffi F, Grassi W. CS injection of tenosynovitis in patients with chronic inflammatory arthritis: the role of US. Rheumatology (Oxford). 2012;51:1299–303.

Eustace JA, Brophy DP, Gibney RP, Bresnihan B, FitzGerald O. Comparison of the accuracy of steroid placement with clinical outcome in patients with shoulder symptoms. Ann Rheum Dis. 1997;56:59–63.

Glattes RC, Spindler KP, Blanchard GM, Rohmiller MT, McCarty EC, Block J. A simple, accurate method to confirm placement of intra-articular knee injection. Am J Sports Med. 2004;32:1029–31.

Gutierrez M, Di Matteo A, Rosemffet M, Cazenave T, Rodriguez-Gil G, Diaz CH, Rios LV, Zamora N, Guzman Mdel C, Carrillo I, Okano T, Salaffi F, Pineda C, Pan-American League against Rheumatisms (PANLAR) Ultrasound Study Group. Short-term efficacy to conventional blind injection versus ultrasound-guided injection of local corticosteroids in tenosynovitis in patients with inflammatory chronic arthritis: a randomized comparative study. Joint Bone Spine. 2016;83:161–6.

Hoeber S, Aly AR, Ashworth N, Rajasekaran S. Ultrasound-guided hip joint injections are more accurate than landmark-guided injections: a systematic review and meta-analysis. Br J Sports Med. 2016;50:392–6.

Johal H, Devji T, Schemitsch EH, Bhandari M. Viscosupplementation in knee osteoarthritis: evidence revisited. JBJS Rev. 2016;4(4):e11–111.

Jones A, Regan M, Ledingham J, Pattrick M, Manhire A, Doherty M. Importance of placement of intra-articular steroid injections. Br Med J. 1993;307:1329–30.

Kane D, Koski J. Musculoskeletal interventional procedures: with or without imaging guidance? Best Pract Res Clin Rheumatol. 2016;30:736–50.

Koski JM, Saarakkala SJ, Heikkinen JO, Hermunen HS. Use of air-steroid-saline mixture as contrast medium in greyscale ultrasound imaging: experimental study and practical applications in rheumatology. Clin Exp Rheumatol. 2005;23:373–8.

Kumar N, Newmon RJ. Complications of intra and peri-articular steroid injections. Br J Gen Pract. 1999;49:465–6.

Kuusalo LA, Puolakka KT, Kautiainen H, Alasaarela EM, Hannonen PJ, Julkunen HA, Kaipiainen-Seppänen OA, Korpela MM, Möttönen TT, Paimela LH, Peltomaa RL, Yli-Kerttula TK, Leirisalo-Repo M, Rantalaiho VM, NEO-RACo Study Group. Intra-articular glucocorticoid injections should not be neglected in the remission targeted treatment of early rheumatoid arthritis: a post hoc analysis from the NEO-RACo trial. Clin Exp Rheumatol. 2016;34:1038–44.

Legre V, Boyer T, Fichez O. Gestes locaux en pathologie sportive: anesthésiques, glucocorticoïdes. Rev Rhum. 2017;74:602–7.

Luc M, Pham T, Chagnaud C, Lafforgue P, Legré V. Placement of intraarticular injection verified by the backflow technique. Osteoarthr Cartil. 2006;14:714–6.

Lussier A, Civino AA, McFarlane CA, Olzinski WP, Potasner WJ, De Medicic R. Viscosupplementation with hylan for the treatment of osteoarthritis: findings from clinical practice in Canada. J Rheumatol. 1996;23:1579–85.

Luz KR, Furtado RN, Nunes CC, Rosenfeld A, Fernandes AR, Natour J. Ultrasound-guided intra-articular injections in the wrist in patients with rheumatoid arthritis: a double-blind, randomised controlled study. Ann Rheum Dis. 2008;67:1198–200.

Makhlouf T, Emil NS, Sibbitt WL Jr, Fields RA, Bankhurst AD. Outcomes and cost-effectiveness of carpal tunnel injections using sonographic needle guidance. Clin Rheumatol. 2014;33:849–58.

Mandl P, Naredo E, Conaghan PG, D'Agostino MA, Wakefield RJ, Bachta A, et al. Practice of ultrasound-guided arthrocentesis and joint injection, including training and implementation, in Europe: results of a survey of experts and scientific societies. Rheumatology. 2012;51:184–90.

Naredo E, Cabero F, Beneyto P, Cruz A, Mondéjar B, Uson J, Palop MJ, Crespo M. A randomized comparative study of short term response to blind injection versus sonographic-guided injection of local corticosteroids in patients with painful shoulder. J Rheumatol. 2004;31:308–14.

Naredo E, Rull M. Aspiration and injection of joints and periarticular tissue and intralesional therapy. Hochberg Rheumat. 6th ed. Section 4, Chapter 69. 2015.

Nordberg LB, Lillegraven S, Aga AB, Sexton J, Lie E, Hammer HB, Olsen IC, Uhlig T, van der Heijde D, Kvien TK, Haavardsholm EA. The impact of ultrasound on the use and efficacy of intraarticular glucocorticoid injections in early rheumatoid arthritis: secondary analyses from a randomized trial examining the benefit of ultrasound in a clinical tight control regimen. Arthritis Rheumatol. 2018;70:1192–9.

Sconfienza LM, Orlandi D, Silvestri E. Ultrasound-guided musculoskeletal procedures: the lower limb. New York: Springer; 2015.

Legré-Boyer V. Viscosupplementation: technique, indications, results. Orthop Traumatol Surg Res. 2015;101:S101–8.

Wang S, Wang X, Liu Y, Sun X, Tang Y. Ultrasound-guided intra-articular triamcinolone acetonide injection for treating refractory small joints arthritis of rheumatoid arthritis patients. Medicine (Baltimore). 2019;98:e16714.

Tendon Infiltrative and Regenerative Treatments

29

Davide Orlandi, Elena Massone, and Enzo Silvestri

Contents

29.1 Introduction

Tendinopathy is generally referred to as a condition causing pain and swelling of a tendon but depending on biomechanical characteristics, the tendons may be affected by various diseases.

Tendons can be distinguished into anchoring tendons which are coated with peritoneum alone (such as the Achilles tendon) and sliding tendons covered with a synovial sheath that facilitates their action (such as flexor or extensor tendons of the wrist and foot).

Inflammatory and degenerative tendinopathy of anchoring tendons is characterized by degenerative-structural changes in collagen fibers associated with fibrotic phenomena and nonconstant presence of inflammatory signs, both intratendinous and of the peritoneum.

This condition may affect the tendon enthesis or the preinsertional tendon portion, resulting in a fusiform thickening of the tendon belly with focal areas of intratendinous degeneration depending on the degree of tendinopathy. When the degenerative disease chronically affects the tendon enthesis it is often associated with the presence of bony spurs and intratendinous enthesopathic lamellar calcifications.

D. Orlandi (✉)
Department of Radiology, Ospedale Evangelico Internazionale, Genova, Italy

E. Massone
Department of Radiology, Ospedale Santa Corona, Pietra Ligure (SV), Italy

E. Silvestri
Radiology, Alliance Medical, Genova, Italy

F. Martino et al. (eds.), *Musculoskeletal Ultrasound in Orthopedic and Rheumatic disease in Adults*,
https://doi.org/10.1007/978-3-030-91202-4_29

Sliding tendons are susceptible to tenosynovitis, with or without inflammatory or degenerative pathology of the underlying tendon. Acute tenosynovitis is characterized by a fluid effusion within the compartment or the tendon sheath, while in chronic tenosynovitis there is synovial thickening or proliferation.

29.2 Tendon Infiltrative Treatments

US guidance is used in the treatment of tendinopathies to guide the injection of steroid anti-inflammatory drugs, low molecular-weight hyaluronic acid, or saline solution into the space between the synovial sheath and the tendon or in the peritenonium.

29.2.1 Tendon Synovial Sheath Injection

US-guided treatment of tenosynovitis is performed injecting steroid anti-inflammatory drugs or low-molecular-weight hyaluronic acid into the space between the synovial sheath and the tendon; it is very important to avoid intratendinous steroid injection as it is associated with an increased risk of tendon rupture.

A special treatment is reserved for stenosing tenosynovitis, where inflammation is partly sustained by the rubbing of the tendon with thickened stabilization structures such as retinaculum or pulleys. In this case, a first intra-sheath steroid injection could be followed by a 1–2-week-delayed forced injection of low-weight hyaluronic acid into the synovial sheath, performing a mechanical stretching and release of the stabilization structures.

Procedure

US-guided synovial sheath injection is generally performed using small-caliber needles (27–29 gauge) in order to minimize the pain perceived by the patient during the procedure (Fig. 29.1).

At the end of the procedure a plaster is applied and the patient is asked to consume NSAIDs for up to 5 days in case of post-procedural pain.

29.2.2 High-Volume Injection

Many studies have focused on non-insertional tendinopathy of the Achilles tendon, a condition that mainly affects runners and in which conservative treatments such as anti-inflammatory drugs and eccentric exercises have limited efficacy.

High-volume injection procedure is based on the peritendinous injection of a large amount (up to 40 ml) of several substances (isolated or in combination) such as saline solution, local anesthetic, corticosteroid, or hyaluronates in cases of inflammatory tendinopathy with high intra-peritendinous vascularity.

In this setting, all the previous substances injected into the peritoneum have been shown to significantly reduce pain and improve tendon functionality in the short and medium terms. The rationale of the procedure would be due to the stretching, rupture, or occlusion of the nerves and vessels responsible for inflammation causing the patient pain.

Procedure

A 21-gauge needle is inserted from the lateral aspect of the tendon under real-time US guidance between the deep aspect of the Achilles tendon and Kager's fat pad. Then, 5 ml of local anesthetic and up to 40 ml of saline solution are injected. Finally 1 ml of long-acting steroid could be injected in the same space. At the end of the procedure a plaster and ice pack are applied.

Patients are allowed to walk on the injected leg immediately, but are advised strictly to refrain from high-impact activity, such as running or jumping, for 72 h.

After 72 h, patients are instructed to restart heavy eccentric loading under the guidance of a chartered physiotherapist.

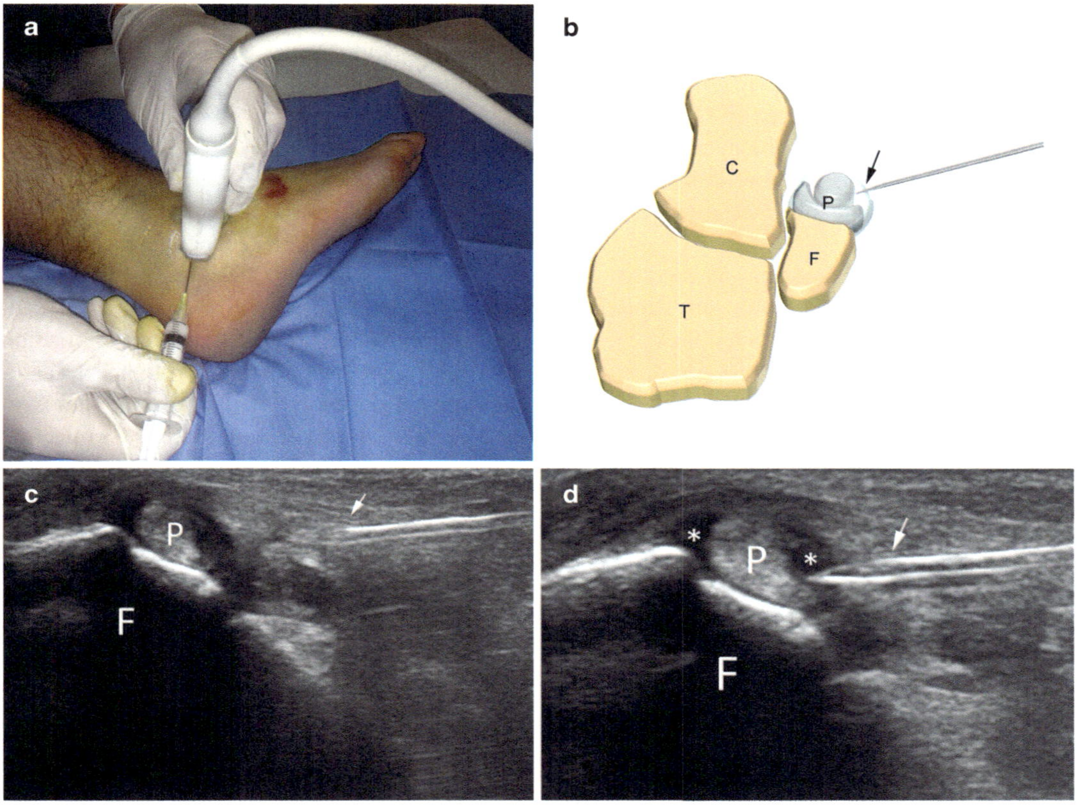

Fig. 29.1 US-guided treatment of peroneal tenosynovitis on a short axis. (**a**) Probe and patient position to perform US-guided treatment of peroneal tenosynovitis. (**b**) Anatomical scheme and (**c**) US image of needle insertion within peroneal tendon sheath, *C* calcaneus, *T* tibia, *F* fibula, *P* peroneal tendons, *arrow* needle tip. (**d**) Steroid injection (asterisks)

29.3 Tendon Regenerative Treatments

The rationale of regenerative treatments of intratendinous tendinopathies is to speed up the physiological tissue regeneration tendon. This could be obtained by a direct bleeding of the tendon induced by scarification (dry needling), by intratendinous injection of platelet-rich plasma (PRP), or by adipose-derived mesenchymal stem cells (ASCs). The latter should participate directly in the process of tendon regeneration, being able to differentiate into different types of cells.

All these treatments have recently been shown to be safe in the orthopedic setting for the regenerative treatment of Achilles tendinopathy and plantar fasciitis.

29.3.1 Tendon Scarification (Dry Needling)

Dry needling is an US-guided procedure for the treatment of anchoring tendons consisting of multiple fenestration of the affected tendon which could be performed alone or combined with simultaneous intratendinous PRP injection.

The purpose of the treatment is to cause local hyperemia and bleeding into the tendon, thus promoting post-procedural platelet-induced recovery phenomena.

Procedure

A 20 G needle is inserted under in-plane ultrasound guidance in the affected portion of the tendon to be treated. Anesthetic (up to 5 ml) is injected along the path of the needle and in the peritendinous soft tissues avoiding intratendinous injection which could slow the regenerative action of the procedure.

The US-guided procedure consists of performing 15–20 small punctures along the entire thickness of the tendon and, when the enthesis is involved, also hitting the periosteum in order to promote a mild bleeding.

At the end of the procedure a plaster and ice pack are applied and the patient is asked to consume paracetamol in case of pain within 48 h and to reduce his/her sports activity for 1–2 weeks.

29.3.2 Platelet-Rich Plasma (PRP)

PRP is a platelet-rich preparation obtained from the centrifugation of peripheral blood. Nowadays PRP is applied in various clinical settings including sports medicine where it has been proposed for the treatment of muscle and tendon injuries, tendinopathies, ligamentous injuries, peripheral neuropathies, and plantar fasciitis. A recent meta-analysis emphasized that PRP was associated with a significant pain reduction at 2 months compared with hyaluronic acid (HA), but no differences were observed at 6- and 12-month follow-up.

The rationale behind PRP use is the ability to stimulate the process of tissue regeneration through angiogenesis, innervation, and release of multiple GFs and cytokines from platelets while the local immune response and fibrinogenesis are modulated.

The most common PRP types are:

1. Pure PRP (P-PRP) with low content of leukocytes
2. Leukocyte- and platelet-rich plasma (L-PRP): preparation with leukocyte and with low-density fibrin network, with greater concentration of platelets than P PRP
3. Pure platelet-rich fibrin (P-PRF): preparation without leukocytes and with a high-density fibrin network

Procedure

The most frequently used PRP preparation in orthopedics and sports medicine is L-PRP with 5–8 more platelets and leukocytes than peripheral blood. The preparation may be obtained by using disposable kit (with predetermined PRP concentration, almost no risk of contamination but higher cost) or obtained from the transfusion medicine service of the hospital. The second method of preparation starts by collecting a whole venous blood sample (40–50 ml) from a patient usually from the cubital vein, and it is mixed with citrate to prevent early clotting. Then, it is centrifuged for about 15 min (depending on the centrifugation method), and a small sample is taken in order to determine the absence of contamination. The centrifugation separates and concentrates platelets and, depending on the type of preparation, leukocytes from other blood components. In the end, usually 4–10 ml of PRP solution is gained. Unactivated PRP must be injected in the site of fiber injury as soon as possible after centrifugation in order to prevent gelification and will be activated by the contact with collagen and other tissue factors.

Sometimes the release of platelet granules is induced by using exogenous substances such as the simultaneous injection of 1–2 ml of calcium gluconate solution by a two-way syringe.

In our experience we recommend the use of inactivated PRP in larger lesions and/or in particular involving the epimysium and/or the fascial planes, where up to 10 ml of PRP may be injected seeking endogenous physiological activation through its contact with collagen and other inflammatory mediators into the site of the injury while exogenously activated 2–6 ml of PRP may be used in particular in small, focal intramuscular strain, where its potential role in the promotion of the fibrin clot may help to speed up the regenerative process (Fig. 29.2). After the procedure a plaster and an ice pack are applied.

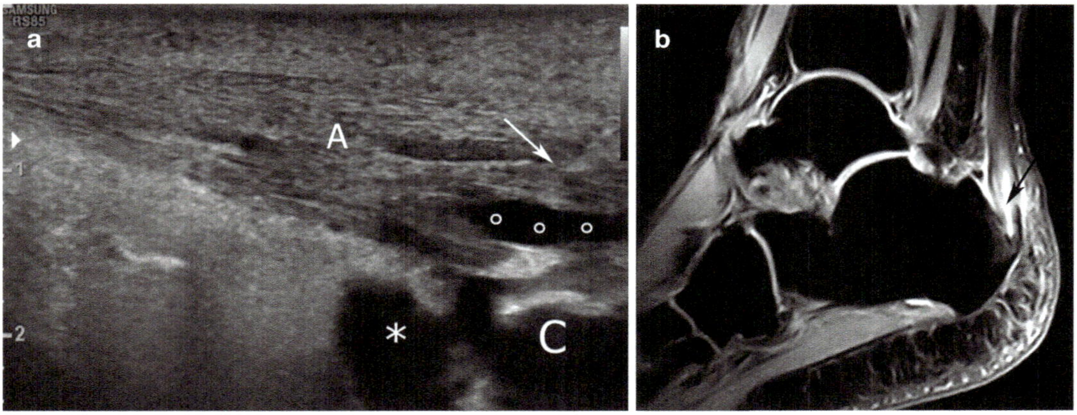

Fig. 29.2 US-guided PRP treatment of Achilles tendinopathy (**a**). *A* Achilles tendon, *C* calcaneus; *asterisk* distended deep retrocalcaneal bursa; *circles* longitudinal tendon tear; *white arrow* needle tip. (**b**) Corresponding sagittal MRI GE-STIR sequence showing Achilles tendinopathy with longitudinal tendon tear (black arrow)

Finally, early rehabilitative mobilization protocol should be considered in order to promote the mechanical stimuli which are essential to the optimal injury recovery (myogenesis stimulation, correct alignment of new fibers, and proper innervation promotion).

29.3.3 Adipose-Derived Mesenchymal Stem Cells (ASCs)

In non-insertional tendinopathy of the Achilles tendon studies agree on the reduction of pain after regenerative treatments, but still have discrepancies on the pathogenic mechanisms; it seems that in the initial stages there is a treatment-induced local inflammation with regional hyperemia and mild thickening of the tendon and then, after a few months, a thickness reduction of the regenerated tendon.

The purpose of ASC tendon treatment is to participate directly in the process of tendon regeneration, being able to differentiate into different types of cells.

ASC preparation and injection procedure:

A small amount of subcutaneous adipose tissue (50 ml) is manually lipoaspirated with a blunt 19 cm, 13 G aspiration cannula.

The adipose tissue is then processed with a dedicated kit, resulting in 10–12 cc of autologous micro-fractured lipoaspirate. The disrupted portion of the tissue, including the SVF, is then centrifuged for 10 min at 400 g. In the last stage of preparation 4 ml of ASCs with SVF is transferred into a syringe ready to be injected.

A 20 G needle is then inserted under in-plane ultrasound guidance in the affected portion of the structure to be treated. Anesthetic (up to 5 ml) is injected along the path of the needle and in the peritendinous soft tissues avoiding intratendinous injection which could slow the regenerative action of the procedure. Care must be taken to inject SVF into the thickest part of the affected structure, covering the entire degenerated area.

After treatment, the patient is advised to walk on crutches for 24 h and to use paracetamol in case of pain within 48 h.

No specific physical therapy is prescribed after the treatment and patients are allowed to progressively resume their normal life and sports activities after 1–2 weeks.

Further Readings

Albano D, Messina C, Usuelli FG, et al. Magnetic resonance and ultrasound in achilles tendinopathy: predictive role and response assessment to platelet-rich plasma and adipose-derived stromal vascular fraction injection. Eur J Radiol. 2017;95:130–5.

Callegari L, Spanò E, Bini A, et al. Ultrasound-guided injection of a corticosteroid and hyaluronic acid: a potential new approach to the treatment of trigger finger. Drugs R D. 2011;11:137–45.

Corazza A, et al. Thigh muscles injuries in professional soccer players: a one year longitudinal study. Muscles, Ligaments Tendons J. 2013;3(4):331–6.

D'Addona A, Maffulli N, Formisano S, Rosa D. Inflammation in tendinopathy. Surgeon. 2017;15(5): 297–302.

Ferrero G, Fabbro E, Orlandi D, et al. Ultrasound-guided injection of platelet rich plasma in chronic Achilles and patellar tendinopathy. J Ultrasound. 2012;15:260–6.

Maffulli N, Sharma P, Luscombe KL. Achilles tendinopathy: aetiology and management. J R Soc Med. 2004;97:472–6.

Maffulli N, Spiezia F, Longo UG, et al. High volume image guided injections for the management of chronic tendinopathy of the main body of the Achilles tendon. Phys Ther Sport. 2013;14:163–7.

Orlandi D, Corazza A, Arcidiacono A, Messina C, Serafini G, Sconfienza LM, et al. Ultrasound-guided procedures to treat sport-related muscle injuries. Br J Radiol. 2016;89:20150484.

Orlandi D, Corazza A, Fabbro E, et al. Ultrasound-guided percutaneous injection to treat de Quervain's disease using three different techniques: a randomized controlled trial. Eur Radiol. 2015;25(5):1512–9.

Orlandi D, Corazza A, Silvestri E, et al. Ultrasound-guided procedures around the wrist and hand: how to do. Eur J Radiol. 2014;83(7):1231–8.

Sconfienza LM, Serafini G, Silvestri E, editors. Ultrasound-guided musculoskeletal procedures. Italia: Springer-Verlag; 2011.

Tagliafico A, Russo G, Boccalini S, et al. Ultrasound-guided interventional procedures around the shoulder. Radiol Med. 2014;119:318–26.

Uygure E, Aktas B, Ozkut A, Erinç S, Yılmazoglu EG. Dry needling in lateral epicondylitis: a prospective controlled study. Int Orthop. 2017;41(11):2321–5.

Shoulder Calcific Tendinitis Treatment

30

Massimo De Filippo, Fabio Martino, and Francesco Pagnini

Contents

30.1 Introduction

The most reasonable diagnostic methods to evaluate shoulder calcifications are X-ray and ultrasonography. X-ray should be considered as the first-line imaging modality, being a panoiramic, fast, and cost-effective imaging modality for the assessment and characterization of the characteristic calcific deposit.

M. De Filippo
Professor of Radiology, Department of Medicine and Surgery, University of Parma, Parma, Italy

Director of Diagnostic an Interventional Unit, Azienda Ospedaliero-Universitaria di Parma, Parma, Italy

F. Martino (✉)
Radiology, Sant'Agata Diagnostic Center, Bari, Italy

F. Pagnini
Radiologist, Diagnostic an Interventional Unit, Azienda Ospedaliero-Universitaria di Parma, Parma, Italy

Ultrasonography is preferable for the correct assessment of the affected tendon, for guiding therapeutic procedures and for the post-procedural evaluation during the follow-up period. Both methods are also effective in evaluating the stage of the calcification process and to establish the timing for its treatment, which is the most important criterion for the therapeutic success.

Multiple classifications have been proposed; among them the most used is the Farin classification, which divides the calcifications into three types on the basis of US appearance (Fig. 30.1):

- Type I: a hyperechoic focus with a well-defined shadow
- Type II: a hyperechoic focus with a faint shadow
- Type III: a hyperechoic focus without an acoustic shadow

F. Martino et al. (eds.), *Musculoskeletal Ultrasound in Orthopedic and Rheumatic disease in Adults*,
https://doi.org/10.1007/978-3-030-91202-4_30

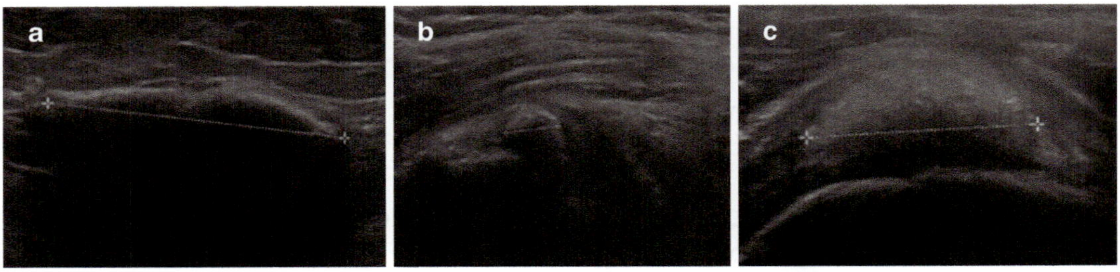

Fig. 30.1 US appearance of shoulder calcifications: (**a**) a hyperechoic focus with a well-defined shadow; (**b**) a hyperechoic focus with a faint shadow; (**c**) a hyperechoic focus without an acoustic shadow

As mentioned in the previous chapters the resorptive phase is usually associated with the development of acute pain that can be very disabling (pseudoparalytic shoulder) and unresponsive to conservative treatments such as nonsteroidal anti-inflammatory drugs (NSAIDs). It happens because of hyperemia detectable with color Doppler ultrasonography, edema, and increased intratendinous pressure with possible extravasation of calcium crystals in the subacromial bursa. This is the moment in which, according to the morphologic type, the treatment can be more effective.

30.2 Therapeutic Options and Clinical Indications

Therapeutic options are subacromial steroid injections, arthroscopy, extracorporeal shock waves, and percutaneous irrigation. Currently ultrasound-guided percutaneous irrigation of calcific tendinopathy (US-PICT), also known as "barbotage" and "lavage," is accepted as the first-line treatment for safety and effectiveness, with significant pain relief and significative improvement in the shoulder function in the short and long terms. It is a procedure that does not require hospitalization, performed under local anesthesia, and that does not need post-procedural immobilization. The patient usually can go home approximately 30 min after the procedure and resume his/her daily activities the day after the treatment without complications.

US-PICT is always indicated in the resorptive phase, in the presence of soft or semifluid calcifications (type II or III). In case of hard calcification (type I) or mildly symptomatic patients, elective treatment should be preferred. With very small calcifications (<5 mm) or migration into the bursal space the procedure is not indicated. Mild or moderate degeneration of the tendon or inflammatory conditions do not represent a contraindication to treatment because the "needling" of the tendon improves the healing process and usually the procedure is combined with a bursal injection of local anesthetics and slow-release steroids in order to relieve inflammation-related symptoms.

30.3 How to Do

30.3.1 Pre-procedural Phase

The patient should lie in semisupine position, with the arm of the affected shoulder completely extended along the body, with an internal/external rotation according to the calcification's location and accessibility. Ordinary antisepsis, with iodopovidone or chlorhexidine, is sufficient to guarantee a safe procedure.

30.3.2 Procedure

The procedure starts with the injection of a small amount of local anesthetic (usually up to 10 ml of lidocaine) along the path of the needles, into the subacromial-subdeltoid bursa and around the calcification.

The size of the needle needed to perform the procedure should be chosen in order to maximize calcium retrieval and to avoid obstruction; in other published studies for RCCT treatment it varies between 16 and 18 G. Every movement is done under continuous US monitoring using a freehand technique which is faster and that allows a more flexible approach, or with needle guidance kit, according to the operator's experience.

The procedure can be done with a double-needle or a single-needle technique: in the double-needle technique (Fig. 30.2) the deeper needle (the furthest from the probe) is first inserted to avoid its own acoustic shadowing, taking care to preserve the integrity of the calcific shell, and then the second needle is inserted superficially.

Both needles should be as perpendicular as possible to the US beam, with an angulation of the needle's tips of approximately 25–30° and with both bevels facing each other. In this way anisotropy artifacts are minimized and needles can be seen entirely. Saline solution is normally injected using a 20/40 ml syringe through one needle; the plunger is pushed repeatedly, and when the calcification starts to dissolve, water and calcium debris are drained from the second needle (Fig. 30.3).

During the irrigation procedure needles can be rotated and displaced to increase calcium disaggregation and fragmentation. The use of warm

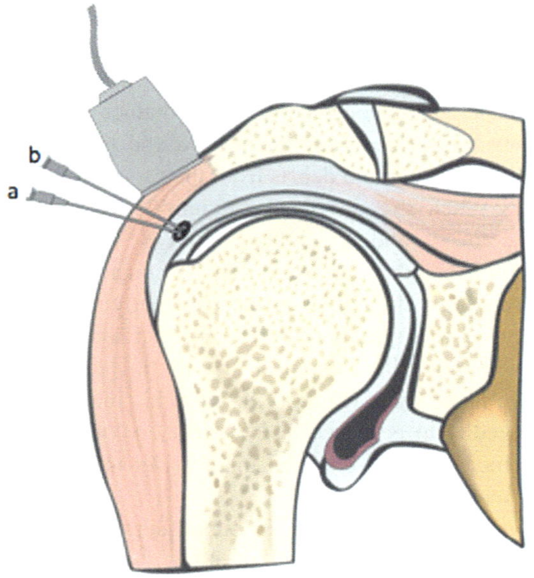

Fig. 30.2 The double-needle technique. The deeper needle (**a**) is positioned, and then the second needle (**b**) is inserted superficially with an angulation of approximately 25–30° to the first one. In order to minimize anisotropy artifacts both needles should be positioned as perpendicular as possible to the US beam

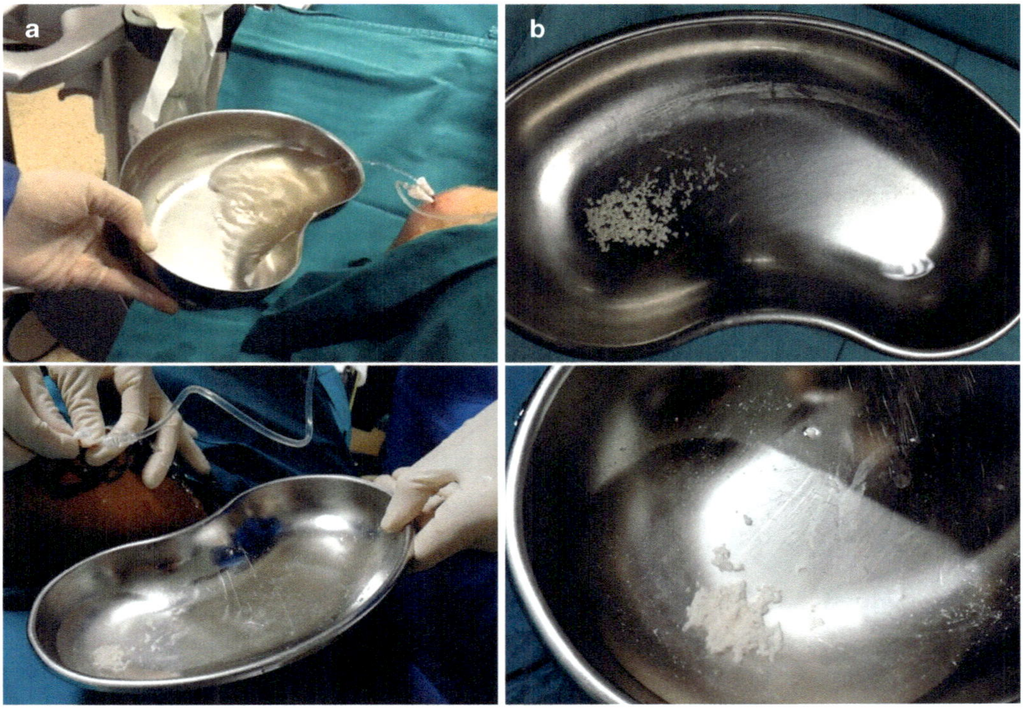

Fig. 30.3 The outflow of saline water and calcium debris, injected from one needle and drained by the other, using warm saline solution with the double-needle technique (**a**). After some minutes of rest the calcific debris tend to form aggregates (**b**)

saline solution may shorten the procedure and improve calcification dissolution.

In the single-needle technique, after the needle placement, calcium retrieval is obtained alternating the saline solution injection and the aspiration of water and debris from the same needle.

When the dissolved calcium is completely removed and calcium debris is no longer retrieved, the procedure can be considered finished. An alternative option, especially useful for type I and type II calcifications, is the approach with a needle composed of a cutting sheet and an inner stylet (Fig. 30.4): with this method the needle tip is placed at the periphery of the calcification, and then the inner stylet is retracted creating vacuum.

The cutting sheet is subsequently inserted applying simultaneous rotations to break the calcification. The needle is completely retracted before getting in touch with the distal side of the calcific shell, in order to retrieve calcium debris and to prevent tendon's injury (Fig. 30.5).

In order to improve the pain relief and to prevent complications the procedure is ended with an US-guided intrabursal injection of local anesthetics and slow-release steroids.

A short course of oral nonsteroidal anti-inflammatory drugs (NSAIDs), a period of relative rest (~15 days), and physiokinetic therapy are suggested to improve the procedure's outcome.

30.4 Clinical Outcome and Complications

In the short-term period the worsening of symptoms is frequent, but normally followed by a quick resolution (~48 h).

Compared to patients who refused the treatment, many authors reported a greater reduction of pain, and a significant improvement of shoulder function in the middle and long-term periods, with reduction of the volume of calcification (Fig. 30.6).

The overall complication rate is about 10%: vasovagal reactions (2%) and seizures (0.2%) are described as immediate reactions, for which it is important to keep an on-site observation period of the patient (~30 min after the procedure) and

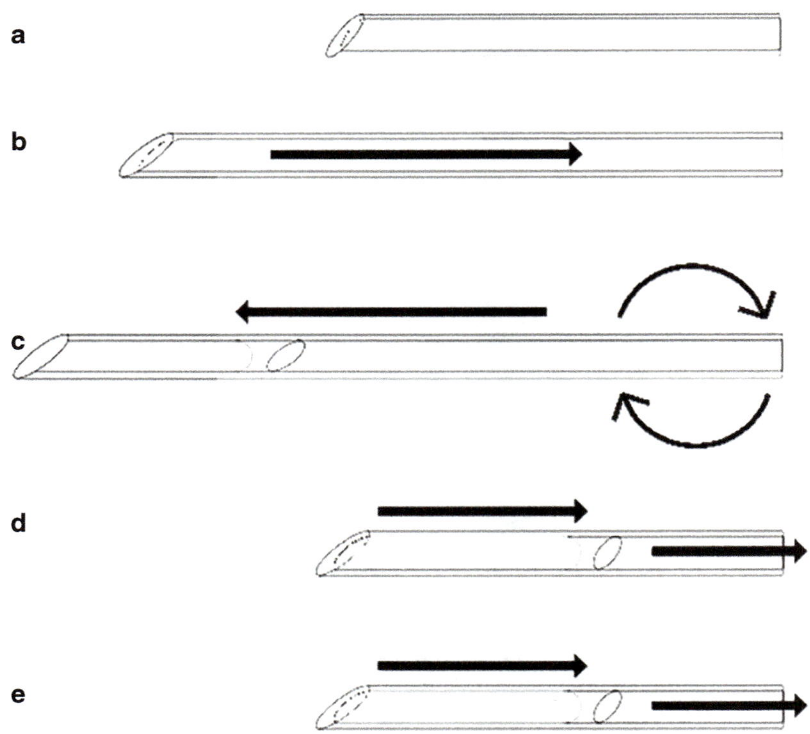

Fig. 30.4 A needle composed of a cutting sheet and an inner stylet (**a**): the needle tip is placed at the periphery of the calcification and the inner stylet is retracted creating vacuum (**b**). The cutting sheet is inserted while rotating to penetrate and break the calcification (**c**). Before getting in touch with the distal side of the calcific shell, the needle is retracted, in order to retrieve calcium debris and to prevent tendon's injury (**d**). Repeating the operation (**a–d**) for multiple times the calcification is completely emptied (**e**)

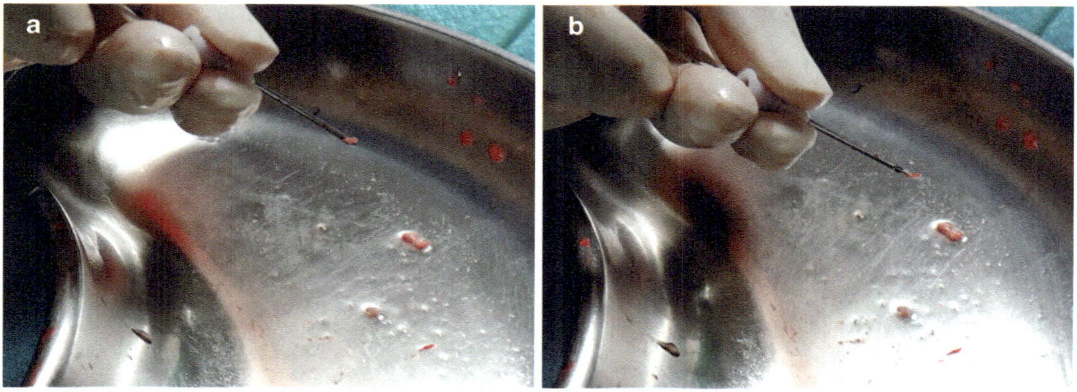

Fig. 30.5 Calcific material retrieved after the procedure (**a**, **b**) in a type I calcification

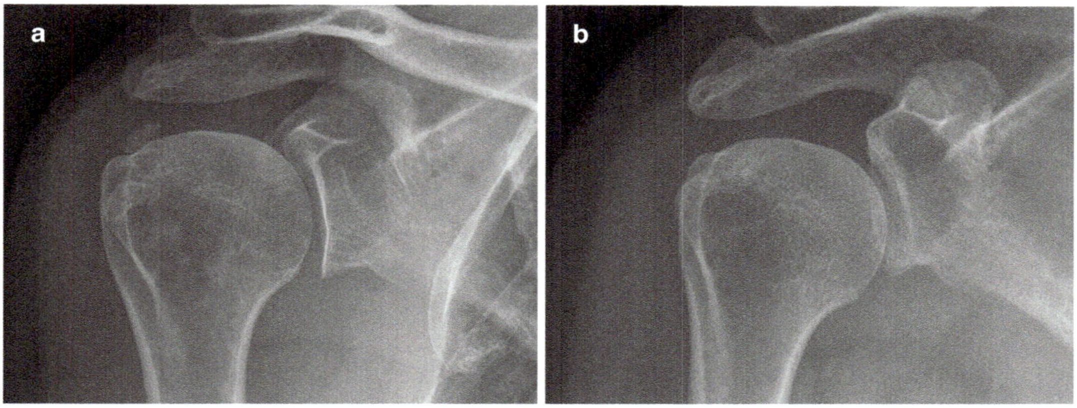

Fig. 30.6 An X-ray of the right shoulder before (**a**) and after (**b**) 3 months of the procedure representing the therapeutic success

to have a prompt pharmacological support for emergencies.

Reported delayed reactions are bursitis (7%), as the most frequent, frozen shoulder (0.2%), and tenosynovitis of the bicipital long head (0.1%).

Further Readings

Barile A, La Marra A, Arrigoni F, et al. Anaesthetics, steroids and platelet-rich plasma (PRP) in ultrasound-guided musculoskeletal procedures. Br J Radiol. 2016; https://doi.org/10.1259/bjr.20150355.

Borchers J, Krey D, McCamey K. Tendon needling for treatment of tendinopathy: a systematic review. Phys Sportsmed. 2015;43(1):80–6.

Di Giacomo V, Trinci M, van der Byl G, Catania VD, Calisti A, Miele V. Ultrasound in newborns and children suffering from non-traumatic acute abdominal pain: imaging with clinical and surgical correlation. J Ultrasound. 2015;18:385–93.

Orlandi D, Mauri G, Lacelli F, Corazza A, Messina C, Silvestri E, Serafini G, Sconfienza LM. Rotator cuff calcific tendinopathy: randomized comparison of US-guided percutaneous treatments by using one or two needles. Radiology. 2017;285(2):518–27.

Oudelaar BW, Schepers-Bok R, Ooms EM, Huis In't Veld R, Vochteloo AJ. Needle aspiration of calcific deposits (NACD) for calcific tendinitis is safe and effective: six months follow-up of clinical results and complications in a series of 431 patients. Eur J Radiol. 2016;85:689–94.

Perrotta FM, Astorri D, Zappia M, Reginelli A, Brunese L, Lubrano E. An ultrasonographic study of enthesis in early psoriatic arthritis patients naive to traditional and biologic DMARDs treatment. Rheumatol Int. 2016;36:1579–83.

Sconfienza LM, Bandirali M, Serafini G, et al. Rotator cuff calcific tendinitis: does warm saline solution improve the short-term outcome of double-needle US-guided treatment? Radiology. 2012;262:560–266.

Sconfienza LM, Serafini G, Sardanelli F. Treatment of calcific tendinitis of the rotator cuff by ultrasound-guided single-needle lavage technique. Am J Roentgenol. 2011;197(2):W366. author reply 367

Serafini G, Sconfienza LM, Lacelli F, Silvestri E, Aliprandi A, Sardanelli F. Rotator cuff calcific tendonitis: short-term and 10-year outcomes after two-needle us-guided percutaneous treatment--nonrandomized controlled trial. Radiology. 2009;252:157–64.

de Witte PB, Selten JW, Navas A, et al. Calcific tendinitis of the rotator cuff: a randomized controlled trial of ultrasound-guided needling and lavage versus subacromial corticosteroids. Am J Sports Med. 2013;41:1665–73.

Zheng F, Wang H, Gong H, Fan H, Zhang K, Du L. Role of ultrasound in the detection of rotator-cuff syndrome: an observational study. Med Sci Monit. 2019;25:5856–63.

Peripheral Nerve Block

31

Giuseppe Sepolvere, Mario Tedesco, and Davide Orlandi

Contents

31.1 Upper Limb Ultrasound-Guided Blocks: How to Do

The ultrasound-guided upper limb nerve blocks allow to anesthetize the peripheral nerve structures of derivation of the brachial plexus (PB) (Fig. 31.1). The latter arises from the ventral branches of the spinal roots from C5 to T1 with variable contributions of C4 and T2 and extends from the neck to the axilla.

The roots merge into three main nerve trunks (interscalene block) moving between the scalene muscles, subsequently above and laterally to the subclavian artery; they are divided into two secondary trunks (supraclavicular block) and from there pass under the clavicle and head towards the armpit group around the axillary artery to form the lateral, medial, and posterior cords (infraclavicular block); joints in the armpit divide into the terminal nerve branches: median nerve; radial; ulnar; and cutaneous and axillary muscle (axillary block).

G. Sepolvere
Department of Anesthesia and Cardiac Surgery Intensive Care Unit, San Michele Hospital, Maddaloni, Italy

M. Tedesco
Department of Anesthesia and Intensive Care Unit and Pain Therapy, Mater Dei Hospital, Bari, Italy

D. Orlandi (✉)
Department of Radiology, Ospedale Evangelico Internazionale, Genova, Italy

F. Martino et al. (eds.), *Musculoskeletal Ultrasound in Orthopedic and Rheumatic disease in Adults*, https://doi.org/10.1007/978-3-030-91202-4_31

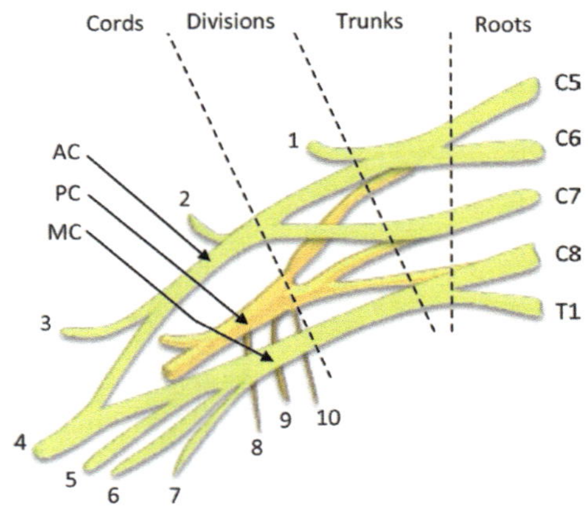

Fig. 31.1 Brachial plexus scheme. *AC* lateral cord (from anterior division), *PC* posterior cord (from posterior division), *MC* medial cord (from posterior division). 1 Suprascapular nerve; 2 lateral pectoral nerve; 3 musculocutaneous nerve; 4 median nerve; 5 ulnar nerve; 6 medial cutaneous nerve of forearm; 7 medial cutaneous nerve of arm; 8 lower subscapular nerve; 9 thoracodorsal nerve; 10 medial pectoral nerve

Materials

- High-frequency linear probe >12 mHz
- 50 mm, 22G atraumatic needle
- Neurostimulator, BSmart® (Injection Pressure Monitor)

31.1.1 Interscalene Block

The interscalene block is used for shoulder surgery, alone or in combination with other approaches (supraclavicular or infraclavicular) when surgery exceeds 1/3 proximal of the humerus.

Patient in supine position with rise under the shoulders and head turned contralaterally (Fig. 31.2a). The main trunks are searched by placing the probe on the supraclavicular sulcus (Fig. 31.2a).

The secondary trunks of the PB are identified laterally to the subclavian artery and, keeping the plexus central to the ultrasound image, the probe is brought up along the sternocleidomastoid muscle with the so-called trace-back technique to observe three vesicles stacked like a traffic light between the scalene muscles (Fig. 31.2a, c). The approach is in lateromedial plane, and the injection of local anesthetic takes place between the upper trunk and the middle trunk with a volume equal to 10–20 ml (Fig. 31.2b).

31.1.2 Supraclavicular Block

Supraclavicular block is used for arm, forearm, and hand surgery, defined as "spinal arm" for its effectiveness. The position of the patient and the probe is the same as that described for the interscalene block, in-plane needle approach (Fig. 31.3a). The plexus is located at the top and side of the subclavian artery, lies on the first rib, and at the top is delimited by the superficial cervical fascia and omohyoid muscle. The injection of about 15–20 ml of local anesthetic takes place between the secondary trunks, which appear as vesicles, and the angle between the subclavian artery and the first "pocket corner" edge (Fig. 31.3b).

31.1.3 Infraclavicular Block

Infraclavicular block has the same indications of the supraclavicular; it is very useful if you decide to place a perineural catheter for elbow surgery rehabilitation. To make the blockage safer, the patient's arm must be abducted (Fig. 31.4); this allows to superficialize the axillary artery and therefore the three ropes, which are all positioned laterally and behind the artery, and move them away from the pleura.

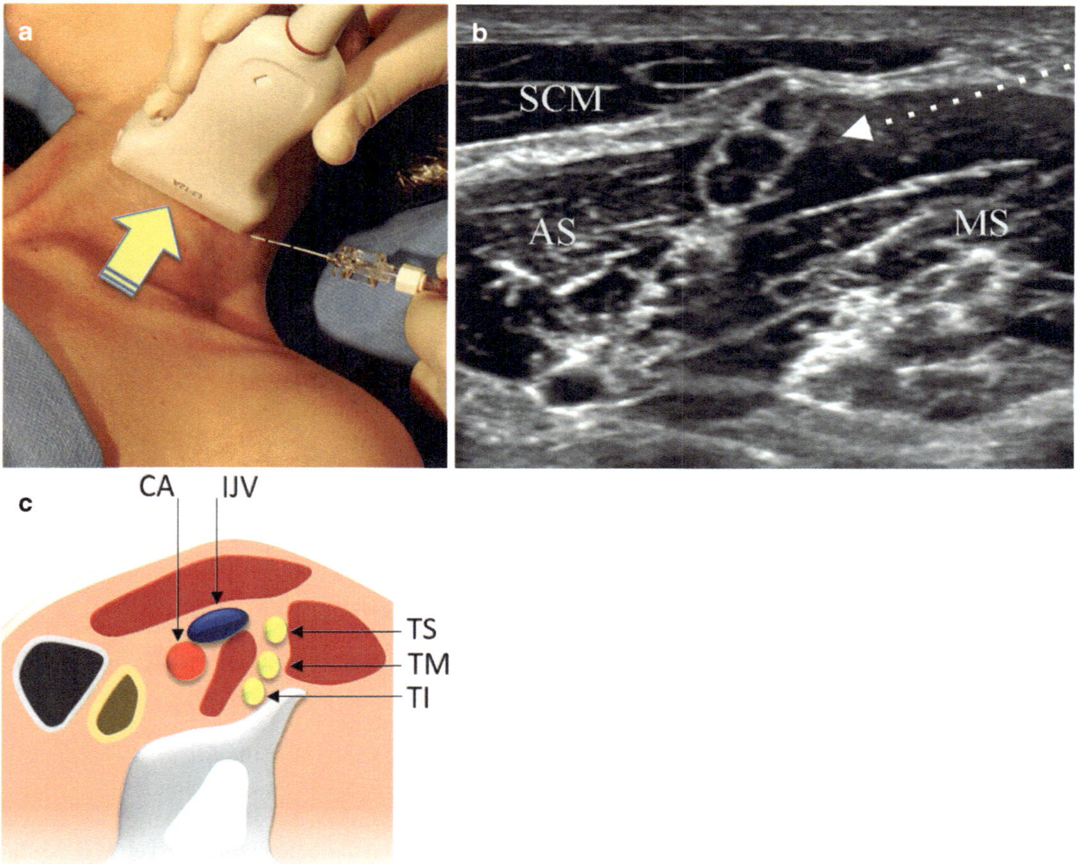

Fig. 31.2 The interscalene groove in a trans-sectional view of the neck. (**a**) Patient position and needle entry point. The *yellow arrow* allows the trajectory of "trace-back method" scanning. (**b**) Sonoanatomy. SCM: sternocleidomastoid muscle; AS: anterior scalene muscle; MS: middle scalene muscle. Long *white arrow*: needle direction and target point. (**c**) Anatomical scheme of the interscalene groove. *TS* superior trunk, *TM* middle trunk, *TI* inferior trunk, *CA* carotid artery, *IJV* internal jugular vein

The probe is positioned in the deltoid-pectoral sulcus (Fig. 31.5a), and the needle enters the plane with direction towards the armpit. The injection of anesthetic about 25–30 ml takes place laterally and posteriorly to the axillary artery (Fig. 31.5b) forming an anechoic bubble (double-bubble sign).

31.1.4 Axillary Block

Axillary block (Fig. 31.6) has similar indications to the supra- and infraclavicular block; it can also be used as a rescue block when the more proximal blocks do not guarantee adequate surgical coverage of some territories.

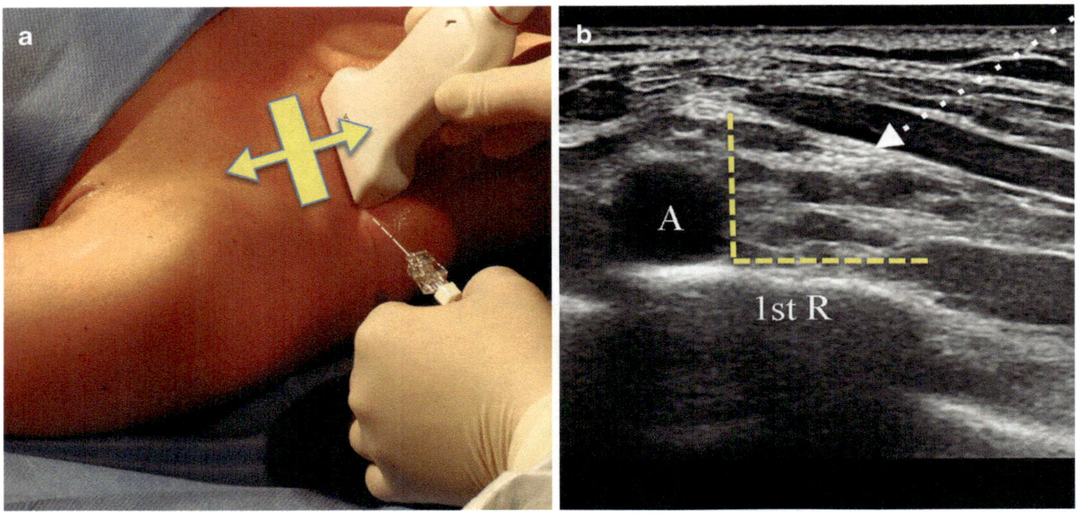

Fig. 31.3 Supraclavicular block. (**a**) Patient position and needle entry point. Probe tilting (*yellow arrows*). (**b**) Sonoanatomy. first R first rib, A subclavian artery. Corner pocket (*yellow dashed lines*). Long *white arrow* needle direction and target point

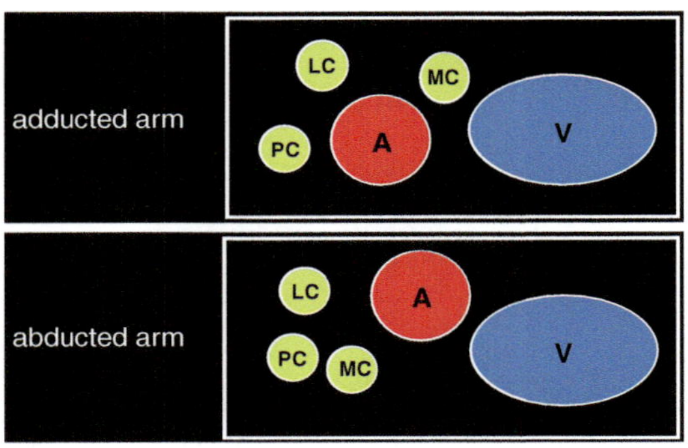

Fig. 31.4 The abduction of the arm shifts the three cords of the brachial plexus laterally and posteriorly to the artery. *MC* medial cord, *LC* lateral cord, *PC* posterior cord, *A* axillary artery, *V* axillary vein

The arm is abducted and the probe is positioned transversely (Fig. 31.7a); an accurate ultrasound scan is performed to identify an image in which all the nerves to be blocked with a single injection are perfectly visible. The needle is introduced into the plane (Fig. 31.7b).

Median, radial, and ulnar nerves are arranged around the axillary artery contained in the nerve vascular fascia (a triangular-shaped space delimited superficially by skin and subcutaneous tissues, deeply by the triceps muscle, and above by the biceps muscle). The musculocutaneous nerve could be located outside the fascia, in the coracobrachialis muscle or between it and the biceps.

Around 5 ml of local anesthetic is injected around the musculocutaneous nerve (Fig. 31.8a, c), then the needle is directed above and below the axillary artery, and up to 20 ml of local anesthetic is injected (perivascular technique).

31.2 Lower Limb Ultrasound-Guided Blocks

The ultrasound-guided blocks of the lower limb ensure anesthetization of the peripheral nervous structures that derive from the lumbar plexus (Fig. 31.9). The lumbar plexus originates from the anterior rami of spinal roots L1–L4 and gives rise to the nervous structures responsible for the sensory and motor innervation of the lower limbs. It is therefore possible to achieve blocks of the femoral, obturator, lateral femoral cutaneous, saphenous, and sciatic nerves.

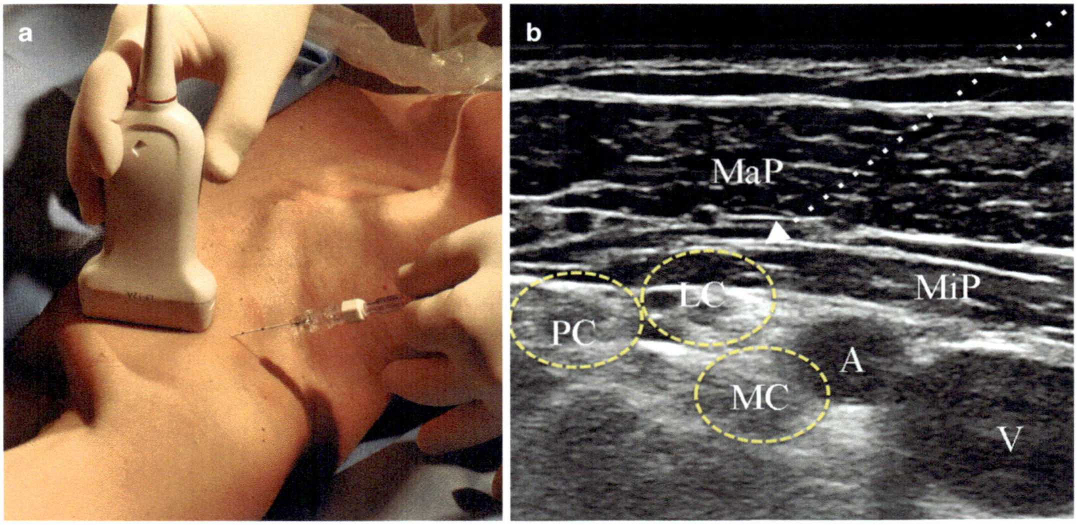

Fig. 31.5 Infraclavicular block (**a**) Patient position and needle entry point, with abducted arm. (**b**) Sonoanatomy. *MaP* major pectoralis muscle, *MiP* minor pectoralis muscle, *A* axillary artery, *V* axillary vein, *MC* medial cord (*yellow outlined*), *LC* lateral cord (*yellow outlined*), *PC* posterior cord (*yellow outlined*). *Long white arrow*: needle direction and target point

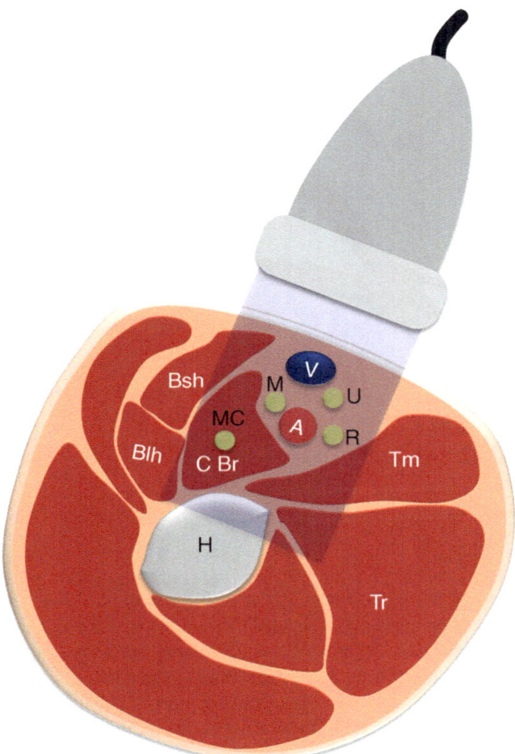

Fig. 31.6 Anatomic slice of axillary area. *Bsh* biceps short head muscle, *Blh* biceps long head muscle, *CBr* coracobrachialis muscle, *H* humerus, *Tm* teres major muscle, *Tr* triceps muscle, *A* axillary artery, *V* axillary vein, *MC* musculocutaneous nerve, *M* median nerve, *U* ulnar nerve, *R* radial nerve

Materials

- High-frequency linear probe >12 mHz for femoral, obturator, and lateral femoral cutaneous nerve blocks
- 6 mHz Convex probe for the sciatic nerve block
- 80–100 mm, 22G atraumatic needle
- Neurostimulator, BSmart® (Injection Pressure Monitor)

31.2.1 Femoral Nerve Block

It is used in anterior thigh surgeries, in combination with obturator, lateral femoral cutaneous, and sciatic nerve blocks. The femoral nerves originate from the posterior divisions of the anterior rami of L2, L3, and L4, and are the most represented branch of the lumbar plexus. Below the inguinal ligament, it divides into an anterior and a posterior division.

The anterior division innervates the anterior and medial cutaneous regions from the inguinal ligament to the knee, and gives off motor branches to the sartorius and pectineus muscles.

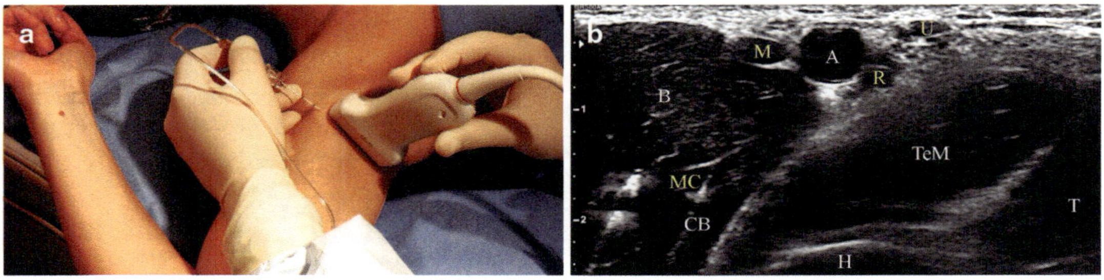

Fig. 31.7 Axillary block (**a**) Patient position and needle entry point, with abducted arm. (**b**) Sonoanatomy of axillary area: *A* axillary artery, *MC* musculocutaneous nerve, *M* median nerve, *U* ulnar nerve, *R* radial nerve, *B* biceps muscle, *CB* coracobrachialis muscle, *TeM* teres major muscle, *T* triceps muscle, *H* humerus

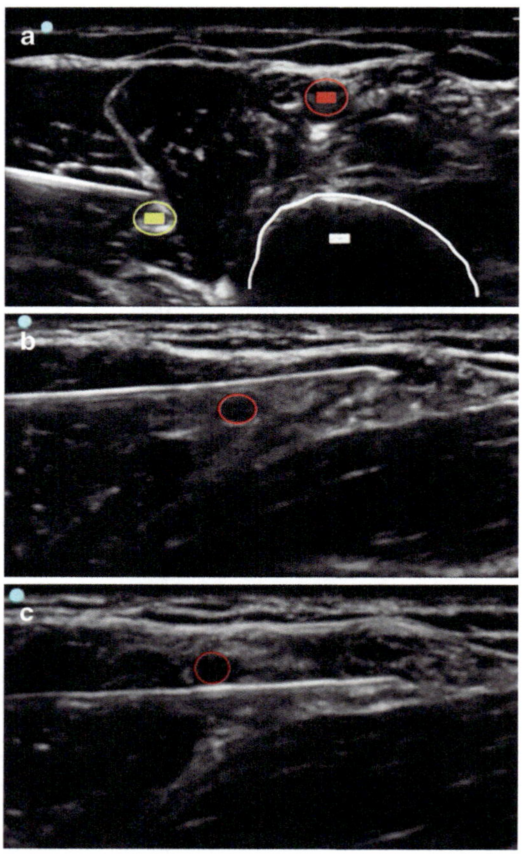

Fig. 31.8 (**a**) Musculocutaneous nerve block. *Yellow* musculocutaneous nerve. *Red circle* axillary artery. (**b**, **c**) "Perivascular technique" of axillary area nerve block. *Red circle*: axillary artery

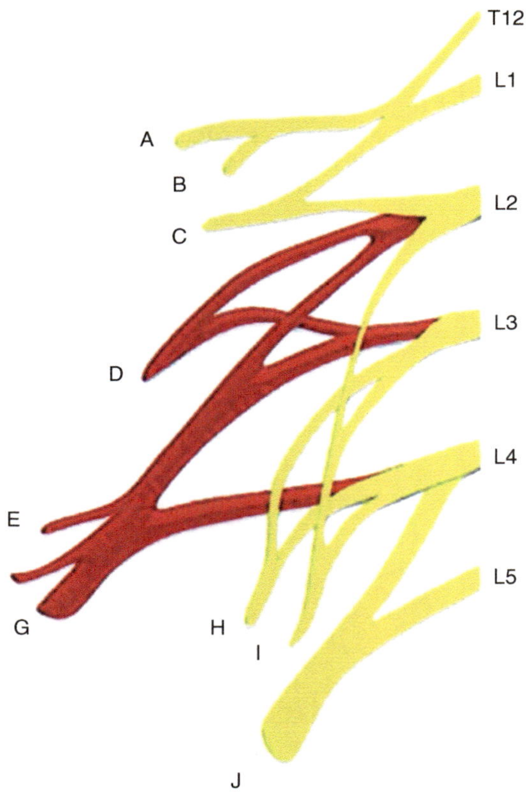

Fig. 31.9 Simplified schema of lumbar plexus anatomy (posterior nerves *red painted*): (**a**) Iliohypogastric nerve, (**b**) ilioinguinal nerve, (**c**) genitofemoral nerve, (**d**) lateral femoral cutaneous nerve, (**e**) and (**f**) branches for psoas and iliacus muscles, (**g**) femoral nerve, (**h**) accessory obturator nerve, (**i**) obturator nerve, (**j**) lumbosacral trunk

The posterior division innervates the medial cutaneous region from the knee to the medial malleolus via the saphenous nerve, and gives off motor branches to the quadriceps muscles. It lies on top the iliopsoas muscles in close anatomical relation to the femoral artery and vein. It runs within the iliac fascia, which is extremely important for the achievement of the nerve block. The iliac fascia envelopes the nerve and then runs medially below the femoral vessels (Fig. 31.10).

The patient is positioned supine and the high-frequency linear probe is placed below the inguinal ligament in order to visualize the femoral nerve and vessels (Fig. 31.11a). Using an in-plane approach, the needle is introduced in a lateromedial direction, past the iliac fascia, to reach the femoral nerve. Then, about 15 ml of local anesthetic is injected circumferentially around the nerve (Fig. 31.11b).

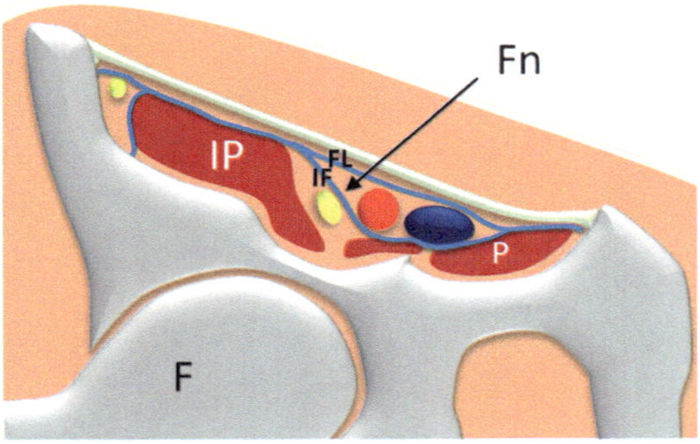

Fig. 31.10 A trans-sectional view of the thigh showing the adductor canal. *IP* iliopsoas muscle, *P* pectineus muscle, *F* femur, *blue line FL* fascia lata, *IF* iliac fascia, *Fn with black arrow* femoral nerve close to femoral artery and vein

31.2.2 Obturator Nerve Block

It is used in surgeries that involve the medial thigh region down to the knee, in association with femoral, lateral femoral cutaneous, and sciatic nerve blocks. The obturator nerve originates from the primary anterior rami of the L2, L3, and L4 roots of the lumbar plexus and descends into the pelvis passing above the psoas at the sacroiliac joint. It exits the pelvis through the obturator foramen and divides into an anterior and a posterior branch (Fig. 31.12a). The anterior branch innervates the skin of the medial and inner thigh and gives off motor branches to the adductor muscles. The posterior branch passes through the adductor muscles and gives rise to a motor branch that innervates most of the adductor magnus, and a sensory branch that innervates the knee joint (joint capsule, synovial membrane, cruciate ligaments). The anterior branch runs in between the adductor longus and adductor brevis muscles, while the posterior branch

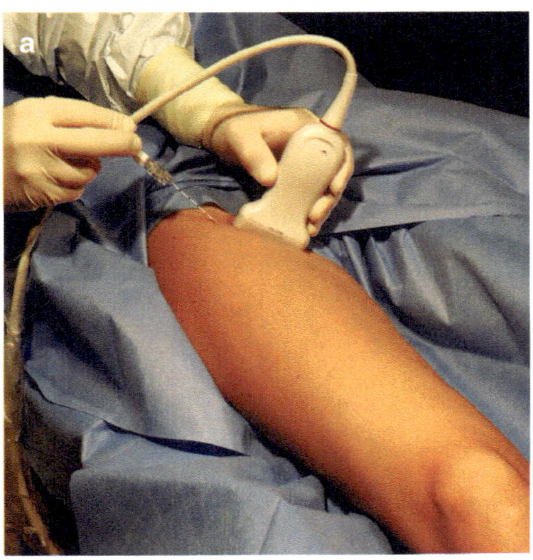

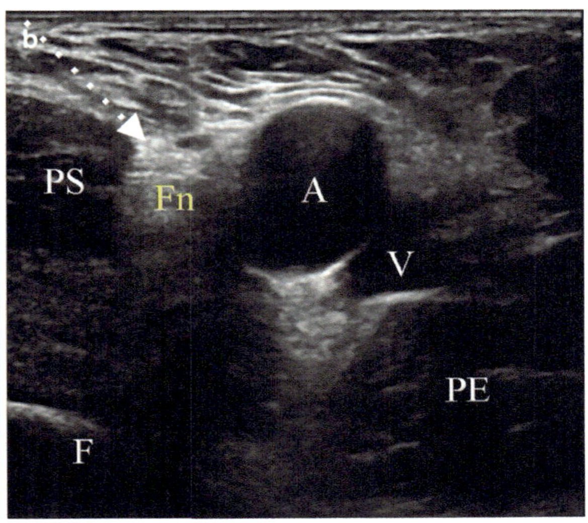

Fig. 31.11 Femoral nerve block. (**a**) Patient position and needle entry point. (**b**) Sonoanatomy of the inguinal area. *Fn* femoral nerve, *PS* iliopsoas muscle, *PE* pectineus muscle, *A* femoral artery, *V* femoral vein, *F* femur. *Long white arrow* needle direction and target point

runs in between the adductor brevis and the adductor magnus (Fig. 31.12b).

At the inguinal level, the medial end of the pectineus muscle comes into strict anatomical relationship with the anterior branch of the nerve. With the patient in supine position, let the high-frequency linear probe slide medially along the inguinal ligament until you find the muscular and nervous structures (Fig. 31.13a). Using an in-plane approach, introduce the needle in a lat-

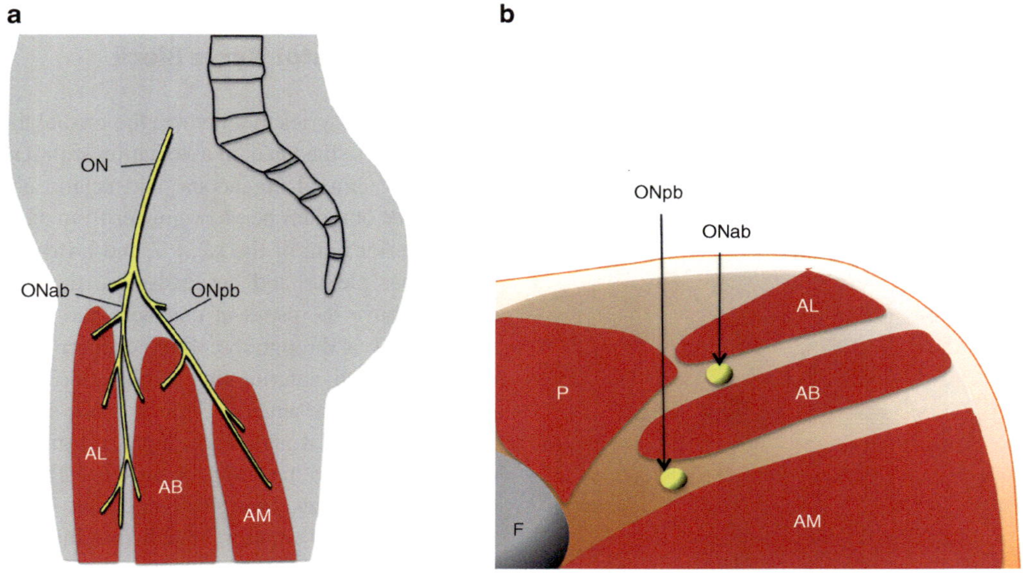

Fig. 31.12 Anatomic scheme in sagittal section (**a**) and in transverse section (**b**) showing the course and distribution in the thigh of obturator nerve. *ON* obturator nerve, *ONab* ON anterior branch, *ONpb* ON posterior branch, *P* pectineus muscle, *AL* adductor longus muscle, *AB* adductor brevis muscle, *AM* adductor magnus muscle, *F* femur

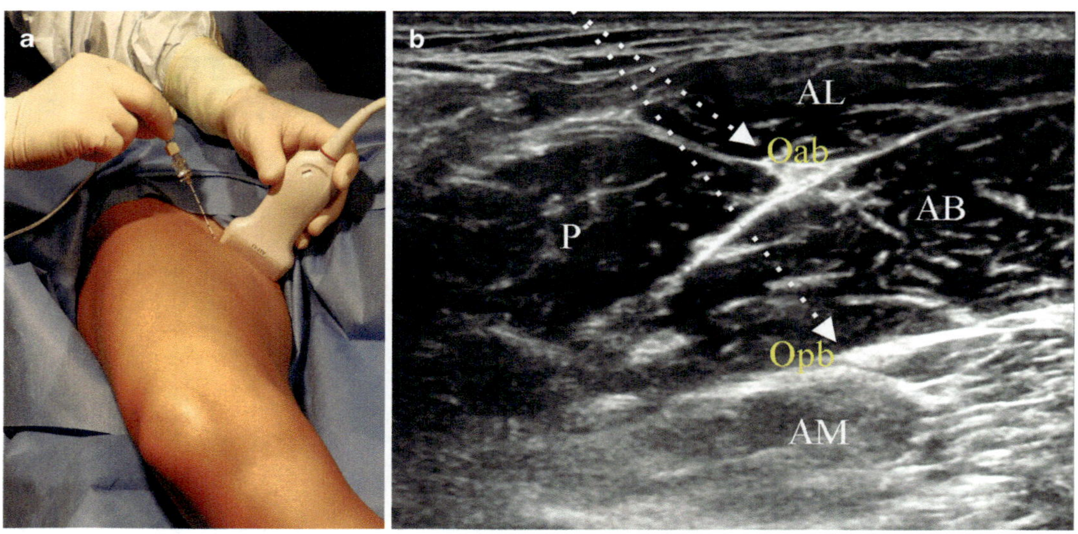

Fig. 31.13 Obturator nerve block. (**a**) Patient position and needle entry point. (**b**) Sonoanatomy medial aspect of upper thigh showing in a transverse view *AL* adductor longus muscle, *AB* adductor brevis muscle, *AM* adductor magnus muscle, *P* pectineus muscle, *Oab* anterior branch and *Opb* posterior branch of obturator nerve. *Double long white arrow* needle direction and target points

eromedial direction until you encounter the anterior and posterior branches of the nerve. Then, inject 8 ml of local anesthetic (Fig. 31.13b).

31.2.3 Lateral Femoral Cutaneous Nerve Block

It is used in association with the femoral, obturator, and sciatic nerve blocks. The lateral femoral cutaneous nerve is exclusively sensory and originates directly from the L2 and L3 roots of the lumbar plexus. It supplies sensory innervation to the anterolateral area of the thigh and knee. It runs underneath the anterior superior iliac spine in between the sartorius and the tensor fasciae latae. It then divides into an anterior and a posterior branch (Fig. 31.14).

With the patient in supine position, slide the high-frequency linear probe laterally along the inguinal ligament (Fig. 31.15a). Using an in-plane approach, introduce the needle in a lateromedial direction until you reach the target nerve, and then inject 5 ml of local anesthetic (Fig. 31.15b).

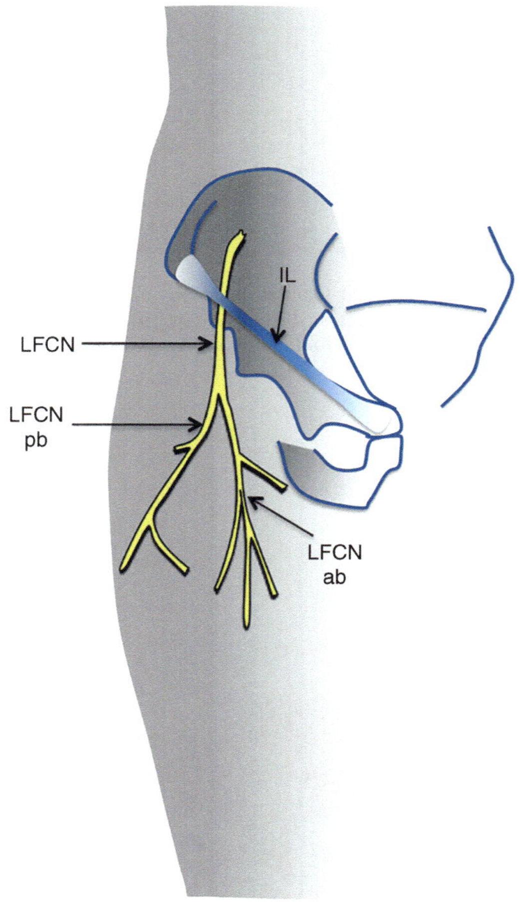

Fig. 31.14 Anatomic scheme of the lateral femoral cutaneous nerve. *IL* inguinal ligament, *LFCN* lateral femoral cutaneous nerve, *LFCNpb* posterior branch, *LFCNab* anterior branch

31.2.4 Saphenous Nerve Block

It is used in association with obturator, lateral femoral cutaneous, and sciatic nerve blocks, or in the management of postoperative pain in prosthetic knee replacement. The saphenous nerve is exclusively sensory and originates from the posterior branch of the femoral nerve in the femoral triangle. It innervates the medial aspect of the leg from the knee to the medial malleolus. It runs lateral to the femoral vessels inside the adductor canal (Hunter's canal). After exiting the subsartorial canal, it divides into two branches: an infrapatellar branch, which supplies sensory innervation to the anteromedial aspect of the knee, and a descending branch, which supplies the anteromedial aspect of the leg and ankle. Below the knee, it follows the same route of the saphenous vein. Hunter's canal is delimited superiorly by the sartorius, laterally by the vastus medialis, and medially by the adductor longus (Fig. 31.16).

With the patient in supine position, place the high-frequency linear probe along Hunter's canal (Fig. 31.17a). Using an in-plane approach, introduce the needle in a lateromedial direction to reach the target nerve. Then, inject 10 ml of local anesthetic (Fig. 31.17b).

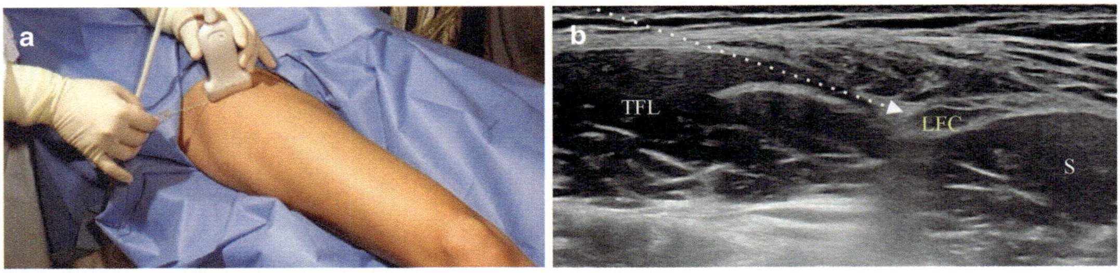

Fig. 31.15 Lateral femoral cutaneous nerve block. (**a**) Patient position and needle entry point. (**b**) Sonoanatomy of the inguinal area. *Fn* femoral nerve, *PS* iliopsoas muscle, *PE* pectineus muscle, *A* femoral artery, *V* femoral vein, *F* femur. *Long white arrow* needle direction and target point

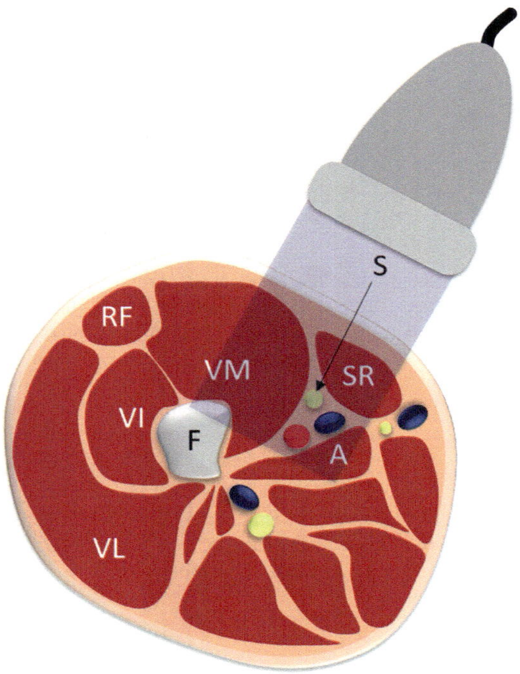

Fig. 31.16 Trans-sectional view of the thigh showing the adductor canal. *RF* rectus femoris muscle, *VL* vastus lateralis muscle, *VI* vastus intermedius muscle, *VM* vastus medialis muscle, *SR* sartorius muscle, *A* adductor longus muscle, *F* femur, *S with black arrow* saphenous nerve

31.2.5 Sciatic Nerve Block

The sciatic nerve is the largest peripheral nerve and the longest nerve in the human body, with a diameter of about 2 cm. It supplies sensorimotor innervation to the posterior aspect of the thigh and to nearly the whole leg, with the exception of the medial aspect of the foot that is innervated by the saphenous nerve. It originates from the spinal roots L4–L5 and S1–S3, then it exits the pelvis, and at the gluteal and subgluteal level it comes in close contact with the gluteus maximus, the piriformis, the quadratus femoris, the greater trochanter laterally, and the ischial tuberosity medially (Fig. 31.18).

With the patient in lateral decubitus, position a convex probe at gluteal level between the greater trochanter and the ischial tuberosity (Fig. 31.19a). Using an in-plane approach, introduce the needle in lateromedial direction to reach the target nerve and inject 15 ml of local anesthetic circumferentially to the nerve (Fig. 31.19b).

Past the gluteal plane, the sciatic nerve descends along the posterior aspect of the thigh to the popliteal fossa, where it divides into a tibial and a common fibular component. The tibial

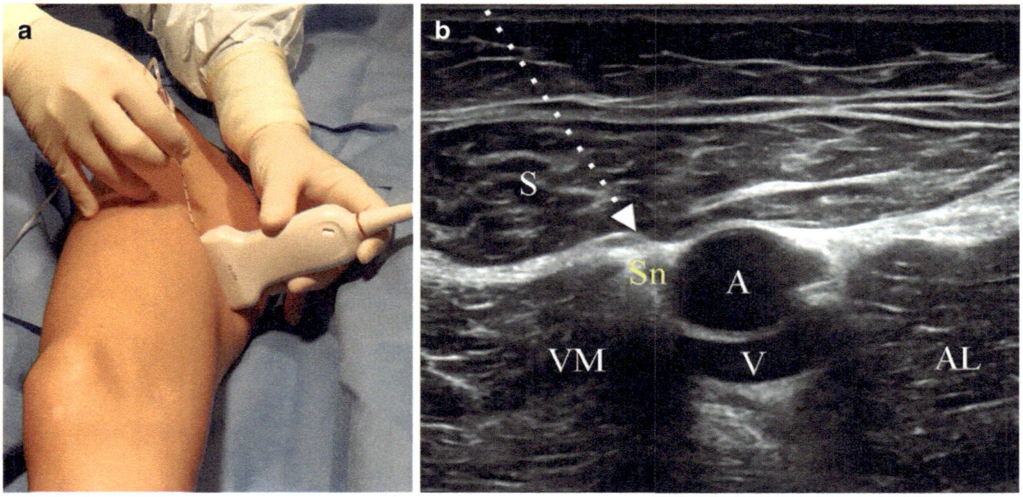

Fig. 31.17 Saphenous Nerve Block (**a**) Patient position and needle entry point. (**b**) Sonoanatomy of the adductor canal. *Sn* saphenous nerve, *S* sartorius muscle, *VM* vastus medialis muscle, *AL* adductor longus muscle, *A* femoral artery, *V* femoral vein. *Long white arrow* needle direction and target point

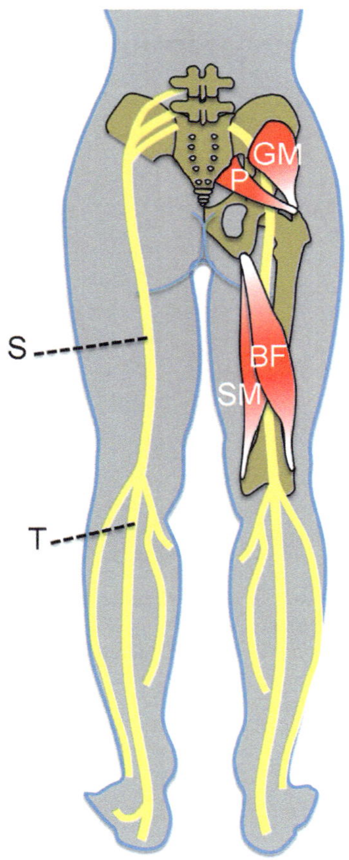

Fig. 31.18 Schema of sciatic nerve anatomy. *S* sciatic nerve, *GM* gluteus maximus muscle, *P* piriform muscle, *BF* biceps femoris muscle, *ST* semitendinosus muscle

component continues to descend along the central aspect of the leg, while the common fibular component moves laterally. Along its posterior route, the sciatic nerve comes in close anatomical contact with the biceps femoris and the vastus lateralis muscles laterally, with the semitendinosus and semimembranosus medially and with the adductor magnus anteriorly (Fig. 31.18). At the level of the popliteal fossa, it is possible to perform a sciatic nerve block by placing the patient in prone position (Fig. 31.20a). With a high-frequency linear probe and in-plane approach, introduce the needle in lateromedial direction until you reach the target nerve. Subsequently, inject 15 ml of local anesthetic in circumferential fashion (Fig. 31.20b).

An alternative approach through the medio-femoral region is described by Sepolvere-Tedesco. The patient is placed supine and a convex probe is placed between the vastus lateralis and the biceps femoris muscles (Fig. 31.21a). The needle is introduced in-plane in lateromedial direction to reach the target nerve, where 15 ml of local anesthetic is injected circumferentially (Fig. 31.21b).

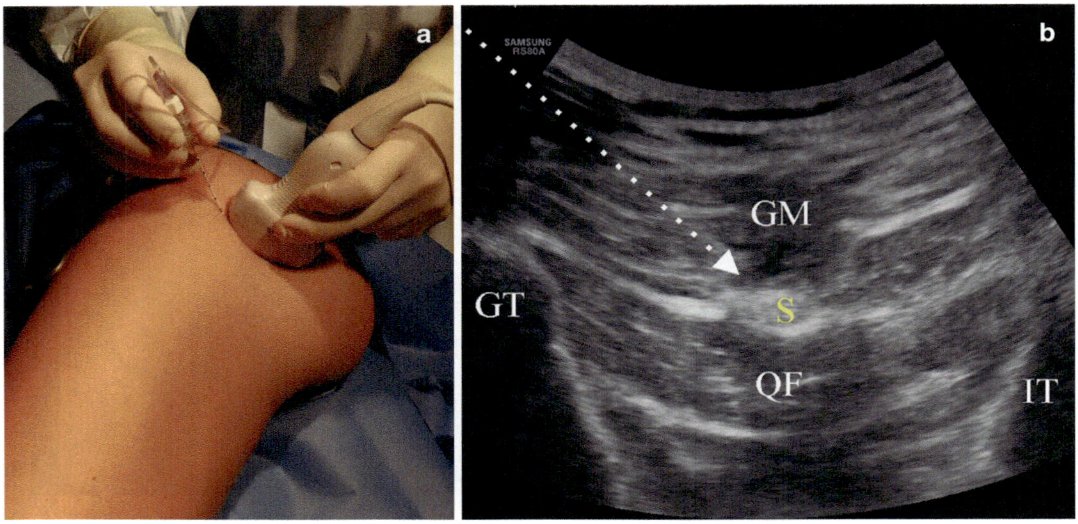

Fig. 31.19 Sciatic nerve block. (**a**) Patient position and needle entry point. (**b**) Sonoanatomy. *S* sciatic nerve, *GT* greater trochanter, *GM* gluteus maximus muscle, *QF* quadratus femoris muscle, *IT* ischial tuberosity. *Long white arrow* needle direction and target point

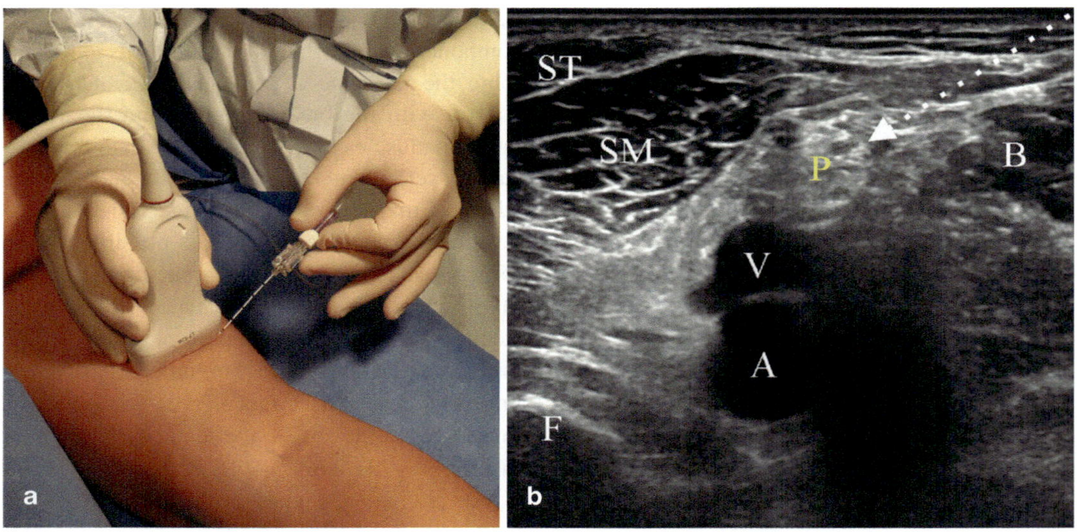

Fig. 31.20 Sciatic nerve block at the popliteal fossa. (**a**) Patient position and needle entry point. (**b**) Sonoanatomy in a transverse section of popliteal region showing popliteal nerve, vein, and artery. *F* femur, *ST* semitendinosus muscle, *SM* semimembranosus muscle, *P* popliteal sciatic nerve. *Long white arrow* needle direction and target point

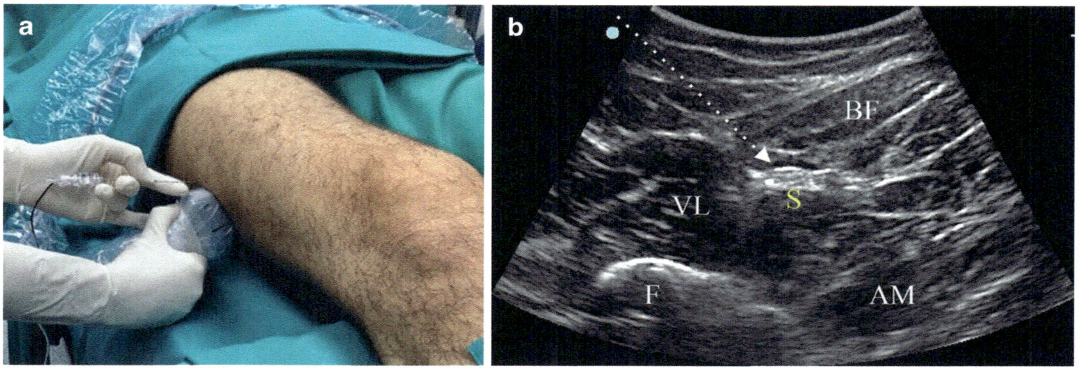

Fig. 31.21 Sciatic nerve block through the medio-femoral region. (**a**) Patient position and needle entry point. (**b**) Sonoanatomy of a lateromedial axial section at mid-shaft of femur. *S* sciatic nerve, *BF* biceps femoris muscle, *VL* vastus lateralis muscle, *AM* adductor magnus, *F* femur. *Long white arrow* needle direction and target point

Further Readings

Bendtsen TF, Moriggl B, Chan V, Børglum J. Basic topography of the saphenous nerve in the femoral triangle and the Adductor Canal. Reg Anesth Pain Med. 2015;40(4):391–2.

Dolan J. Ultrasound-guided anterior sciatic nerve block in the proximal thigh: an in-plane approach improving the needle view and respecting fascial planes. Br J Anaesth. 2013;110:319–20.

Franco CD, Williams JM. Ultrasound-guided Interscalene block: reevaluation of the "stoplight" sign and clinical implications. Reg Anesth Pain Med. 2016;41(4):452–9.

Fredrickson MJ, Wolstencroft P. Evidence-based medicine supports ultrasound-guided infraclavicular block over the corner pocket supraclavicular technique. Reg Anesth Pain Med. 2011;36(5):525–6.

Galluccio F, Arnay EG, Salazar C, Altinpulluk EY, Capassoni M, Garcia DS, Espinoza K, Olea MS, Perez MF. Ultrasound-guided block of the axillary nerve: a prospective, randomized, single-blind study comparing Interfascial and perivascular injections. Pain Physician. 2020;23(1):E61–70.

Goffin P, Lecoq JP, Ninane V, Brichant JF, Sala-Blanch X, Gautier PE, et al. Interfascial spread of Injectate after Adductor Canal injection in fresh human cadavers. Anesth Analg. 2016;123(2):501–3.

Kirkpatrick JD, Sites BD, Antonakakis JG. Preliminary experience with a new approach to performing an ultrasound-guided saphenous nerve block in the mid- to proximal femur. Reg Anesth Pain Med. 2010;35:222–3.

Sahin L, Sahin M, Isikay N. A different approach to an ultrasound-guided saphenous nerve block. Acta Anaesthesiol Scand. 2011;55:1030–1.

Silvestri E, Martino F, Puntillo F. Ultrasound-guided peripheral nerve blocks. Milan, Berlin, Heidelberg, New York: Springer; 2018.

Snaith R, Dolan J. Ultrasound-guided interfascial injection for peripheral obturator nerve block in the thigh. Reg Anesth Pain Med. 2010;35:314–5.

Taha AM. Brief reports: ultrasound-guided obturator nerve block: a proximal interfascial technique. Anesth Analg. 2012;114:236–9.

Tedesco M, Sepolvere G, Cibelli M. Ultrasound-guided lateral, mid-shaft approach for proximal sciatic nerve block. Reg Anesth Pain Med. 2019;7:100657. https://doi.org/10.1136/rapm-2019-100657.

Tran DQ, Charghi R, Finlayson RJ. The "double bubble" sign for successful infraclavicular brachial plexus blockade. Anesth Analg. 2006;103(4):1048–9.

Wong WY, Bjørn S, Strid JMC, Børglum J, Bendtsen TF. Defining the location of the Adductor Canal using ultrasound. Reg Anesth Pain Med. 2017;42(2):241–5.

Fluid Collection Evacuation

32

Ernesto La Paglia, Enzo Silvestri,
and Davide Orlandi

Contents

32.1 Introduction

One of the most important prognostic factors in patients with musculoskeletal fluid collection is the delay in establishing therapy, both in order to get a diagnosis of septic process which requires analysis of fluid and in order to avoid compartment syndrome. Ultrasonography is a rapid, portable, sensitive technique for fluid collection management. The study can be easily repeated for follow-up of lesions.

Fluid collection must be completely aspirated and the cavity is irrigated with a volume of saline that is half of the aspirated fluid volume and the irrigation is continued until the aspirated fluid is clear. Typically needle drainage is chosen for smaller abscesses and catheter drainage is preferred for the drainage of multiloculated abscesses and for larger ones. This technique avoids unnecessary catheter insertions into sterile fluid collection such as lymphoceles and hematomas.

32.2 Abscess

US allows real-time guidance of fluid aspiration and can reduce the risk of contaminating other anatomic compartments, especially in the hands, wrists, and feet. Radiography provides complementary information and should be performed in conjunction with US. US is the imaging modality of choice for diagnosis of superficial abscesses. Dynamic compression with the US probe and color Doppler imaging can facilitate the detection of superficial abscesses. US may help in the early diagnosis of osteomyelitis by demonstrating subperiosteal or juxtacortical fluid collections and by providing guidance for aspiration of these collections.

E. La Paglia
Department of Radiology, Humanitas Cellini, Torino, Italy

E. Silvestri
Radiology, Alliance Medical, Genova, Italy

D. Orlandi (✉)
Department of Radiology, Ospedale Evangelico Internazionale, Genova, Italy

F. Martino et al. (eds.), *Musculoskeletal Ultrasound in Orthopedic and Rheumatic disease in Adults*,
https://doi.org/10.1007/978-3-030-91202-4_32

Abscesses may have different features at US. The lesion may appear as an anechoic or diffusely hypoechoic mass which increases through transmission or may be hyperechoic or isoechoic relative to surrounding tissues and lack mass effect. The margins may be well circumscribed or blend in with the surrounding tissues. Sometimes, an echogenic rim is seen. Septa may be present, as well as internal echoes, which represent debris or gas. Power or color Doppler imaging may be used to demonstrate hyperemia at the periphery of the mass and absence of flow in the center (Fig. 32.1).

Dynamic evaluation of the soft-tissue area by palpation or gentle compression with the US probe is useful to reveal the motion of the liquefied purulent material in cases of isoechoic or hyperechoic abscesses. US plays a major role in the detection and management of superficial abscesses, being deeper fluid collections, particularly in the lumbar and pelvic regions, more easily managed by the guidance of magnetic resonance imaging or computed tomography (diagnosis, determination of location and extent, and percutaneous management). MR imaging and CT also provide detailed information regarding osseous involvement, which would not be available with US (Fig. 32.2).

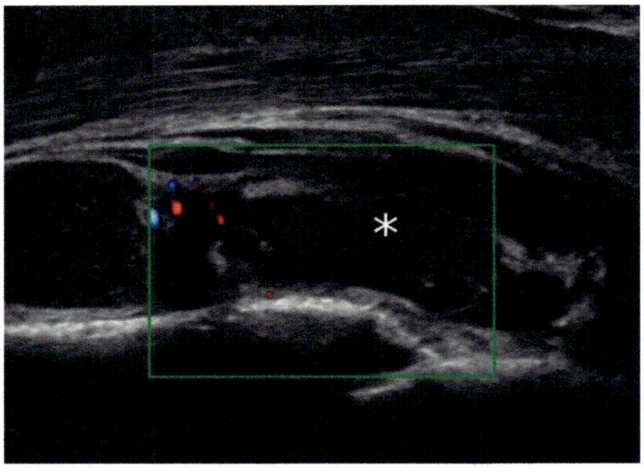

Fig. 32.1 Longitudinal US scan of an anechoic collection with multiple internal echoes (*asterisk*). The margins are well circumscribed and septa are present with color Doppler imaging demonstrating hyperemia at the level of the septum and absence of flow in the center. The abscess is lying on the cortical bony surface of the tibia

Ultrasound-guided drainage of soft tissues' abscesses is a safe and effective treatment approach. Needle drainage is the most common first-line treatment approach because of the simplicity of the procedure, improved patient comfort, and reduced costs. Catheter drainage will be reserved for large multiloculated abscesses. Follow-up US may show that a repeat puncture and drainage are necessary. Most drainage procedures are performed without any anesthesia and apart from minor discomfort during the drainage procedure and the subsequent indwelling catheter period, there were no serious complications related to the drainage procedures. All procedures must be performed under aseptic conditions, which include sterile draping of the transducer. Patient must be prepared for the drainage procedure, which includes being informed about the nature of the procedure and the possible related discomfort in compliance with medicolegal legislation. A diagnostic puncture must be performed in all patients introducing a spinal needle (16–18 G) into the fluid collection under continuous US guidance and fluid from the cavity is aspirated with a syringe. When pus is aspirated, either the needle drainage or the catheter drainage protocol may be implemented, with the latter being an extension of the diagnostic puncture introducing a guidewire and a self-retaining pigtail catheter over the guidewire into the cavity.

32.3 Hematoma

Ultrasound-guided hematoma evacuation is a well-tolerated procedure. However, the proportion of unsuccessful evacuations and hematoma recurrence is substantial (13%). Such a rate of unsuccessful evacuation is because of excessive density and/or viscosity of the content. Ideally, hematoma evacuation must be performed before 3–5 days since the beginning of the muscular

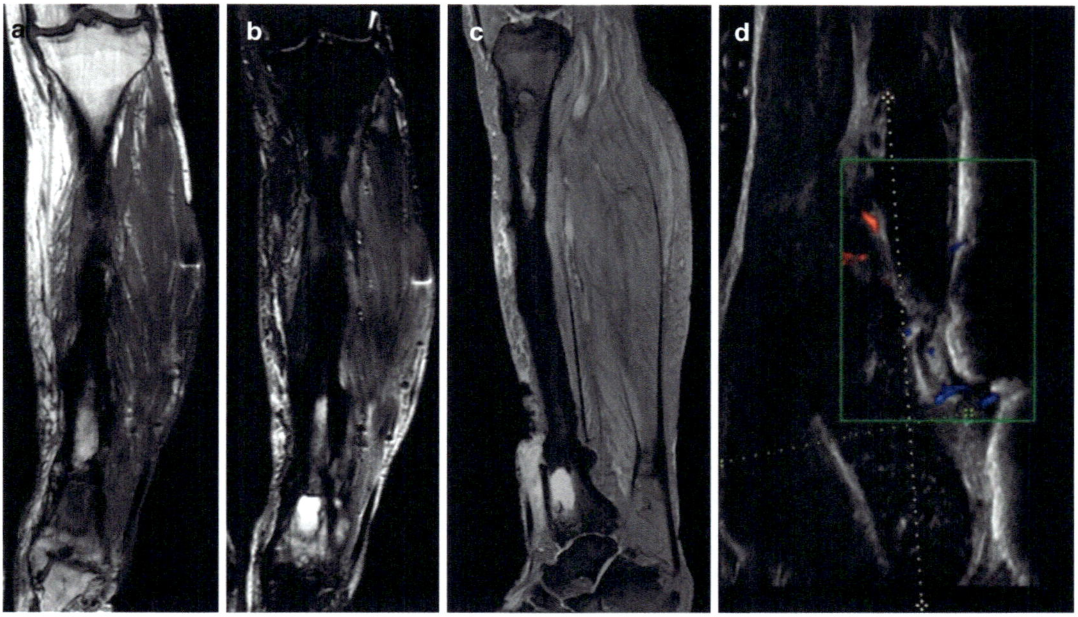

Fig. 32.2 Reactivated chronic osteomyelitis. (**a–c**) MRI T1w and STIR coronal sequences and GRE T2*w sagittal sequence of left tibia show signs of chronic osteomyelitis with widening of the diaphysis, cortical thickening, and irregular periosteal reaction. Multiple central medullary lesions consistent with sequestrum are also visible. (**c**, **d**) GRE T2*w sagittal sequence and longitudinal sonogram of the distal thigh demonstrate a large hypoechoic heterogeneous abscess that communicates with the bone marrow cavity through a cortical break. During US study, compression with the transducer demonstrated in-and-out motion of debris from the bone through the opening in the cortex

bleed, especially in the case of large hematomas in the liquid phase.

Between 10% and 23% of bleeding episodes in the musculoskeletal system of hemophilia patients occur in the muscles. When a muscle bleed is suspected, confirmation must be achieved by means of imaging tests (ultrasound, MRI, CT). Then, immediate (early) enhanced on-demand hematological treatment must be started until the full disappearance of the hematoma. If untreated, muscle bleeds can cause complications such as nerve injury, compartment syndrome, myositis ossificans, pseudotumor, and even infection (abscess). Currently, the literature for muscle hematomas in the nonhemophilic population suggests that ultrasound-guided percutaneous drainage, or surgical drainage performed as open surgery if percutaneous drainage fails, could be beneficial in terms of achieving better and faster symptom relief.

Further Readings

Baoge L, et al. Treatment of skeletal injury: a review. ISRN Orthopaed. 2012;2102:7.

Cardinal E, et al. Role of ultrasound in musculoskeletal infections. Imag Musculosk Spinal Infect. 2001;39(2):191–201.

De la Corte-Rodriguez H, et al. Treatment of muscle haematomas in haemophiliacs with special emphasis on percutaneous drainage. Blood Coagul Fibrinolysis. 2014;25(8):787–94.

Lorentzen T, et al. Ultrasound-guided drainage of deep pelvic abscesses: experience with 33 cases. Ultrasound Med Biol. 2011;37(5):723–8.

Querol F, Rodriguez-Merchan EC. The role of ultrasonography in the diagnosis of the musculo-skeletal problems of haemophilia. Haemophilia. 2012;18:e215–26.

Stainsby BE, et al. Management approaches to acute muscular strain and hematoma in national level soccer players: a report of two cases. J Can Chiropr Assoc. 2012;56:262–8.

Index

F. Martino et al. (eds.), *Musculoskeletal Ultrasound in Orthopedic and Rheumatic disease in Adults*,
https://doi.org/10.1007/978-3-030-91202-4

GPSR Compliance

The European Union's (EU) General Product Safety Regulation (GPSR) is a set of rules that requires consumer products to be safe and our obligations to ensure this.

If you have any concerns about our products, you can contact us on ProductSafety@springernature.com

In case Publisher is established outside the EU, the EU authorized representative is:

Springer Nature Customer Service Center GmbH
Europaplatz 3
69115 Heidelberg, Germany

Batch number: 10732801

Printed by Printforce, the Netherlands